INTERNATIONAL ENCYCLOPEDIA OF PHARMACOLOGY AND THERAPEUTICS

Sponsored by the International Union of Pharmacology (IUPHAR)
(Chairman: B. UVNÄS, Stockholm)

Executive Editor: G. PETERS, Lausanne

Section 79

SULFUR-CONTAINING RADIOPROTECTIVE AGENTS

Section Editor

Z. M. BACQ

Liège

INTERNATIONAL ENCYCLOPEDIA OF
PHARMACOLOGY AND THERAPEUTICS

SULFUR-CONTAINING RADIOPROTECTIVE AGENTS

CONTRIBUTORS

Z. M. Bacq   J. Lecomte
M. L. Beaumariage   P. Lelièvre
R. Goutier   C. Liébecq
J. S. Hugon   J. R. Maisin

P. Van Caneghem

PERGAMON PRESS

OXFORD · NEW YORK · TORONTO
SYDNEY · BRAUNSCHWEIG

Pergamon Press Ltd., Headington Hill Hall, Oxford

Pergamon Press Inc., Maxwell House, Fairview Park, Elmsford,
New York 10523

Pergamon of Canada Ltd., 207 Queen's Quay West, Toronto 1

Pergamon Press (Aust.) Pty. Ltd., 19a Boundary Street,
Rushcutters Bay, N.S.W. 2011, Australia

Pergamon Press GmbH, Burgplatz 1, Braunschweig 3300, West Germany

First edition 1975

Library of Congress Cataloging in Publication Data

Main entry under title:

Sulfur-containing radioprotective agents.
(International encyclopedia of pharmacology and
therapeutics. Section 79)
1. Radiation-protective agents. 2. Sulphur compounds.
I. Bacq, Zénon M. II. Series.
[DNLM: 1. Radiation—Protective agents. 2. Radio-
chemistry. 3. Sulfur. QV4 158 section 79]
RA1231.R2S786 1975   614.8′39   74–10909
ISBN 0-08-016298-3

*Printed and bound in Great Britain by
Hazell Watson & Viney Ltd, Aylesbury, Bucks*

CONTENTS

LIST OF CONTRIBUTORS   vii

CHAPTER 1.   INTRODUCTION   1
Z. M. Bacq, Liège, Belgium

CHAPTER 2.   TOXICITY   15
J. R. Maisin, Mol, Belgium and Z. M. Bacq,
Liège, Belgium

CHAPTER 3.   GENERAL PHARMACOLOGY   39
Introduction
J. Lecomte, Liège, Belgium

   3.1. CARDIOVASCULAR EFFECTS   41
J. Lecomte, Liège, Belgium

   3.2. VASCULAR PERMEABILITY AND
INFLAMMATORY PHENOMENA   59
M. L. Beaumariage, Liège, Belgium

   3.3. SHOCK AND BLOOD COMPOSITION   77
P. Van Caneghem, Liège, Belgium

   3.4. ENDOCRINE GLANDS   91
M. L. Beaumariage, Liège, Belgium

   3.5. NERVOUS SYSTEM AND RECEPTORS   105
M. L. Beaumariage, Liège, Belgium

   3.6. SMOOTH MUSCLES *IN VIVO* AND
IN VITRO   129
J. Lecomte, Liège, Belgium

   3.7. EFFECTS OF CYSTAMINE AND
CYSTEAMINE ON THE SKIN   137
P. Van Caneghem, Liège, Belgium

CHAPTER 4.   CELLULAR EFFECTS AS SEEN WITH
THE ELECTRON MICROSCOPE   143
J. S. Hugon, Sherbrooke, Quebec, Canada

CHAPTER 5.   DISTRIBUTION, METABOLISM AND
EXCRETION   161
P. Lelièvre, Liège, Belgium, J. R. Maisin,
Mol, Belgium, and Z. M. Bacq,
Liège, Belgium

v

CHAPTER 6.   METABOLIC EFFECTS OF SULFUR-
             CONTAINING RADIOPROTECTIVE
             AGENTS   205
             P. Lelièvre and C. Liébecq, Liège, Belgium
CHAPTER 7.   EFFECTS ON CELL GROWTH
             PROCESSES (MITOSIS, SYNTHESIS OF
             NUCLEIC ACIDS AND OF PROTEINS)   283
             R. Goutier, Liège, Belgium
CHAPTER 8.   PROTECTION BY THIOLS AGAINST
             POISONING BY RADIOMIMETIC
             AGENTS   303
             Z. M. Bacq, Liège, Belgium
CHAPTER 9.   IMPORTANCE OF PHARMACOLOGICAL
             EFFECTS FOR RADIOPROTECTIVE
             ACTION   319
             Z. M. Bacq, Liège, Belgium
AUTHOR INDEX   325
SUBJECT INDEX   337

LIST OF CONTRIBUTORS

BACQ, Z. M., Laboratoire de Physiopathologie, 32 bd de la Constitution, 4000 Liège, Belgium.

BEAUMARIAGE, M. L., Laboratoire de Physiopathologie, 32 bd. de la Constitution, 4000 Liège, Belgium.

GOUTIER, R., Laboratoire de Physiopathologie, 32 bd de la Constitution, 4000 Liège, Belgium.

HUGON, J. S., Faculté de Médecine, Université de Sherbrooke, Sherbrooke, Quebec, Canada.

LECOMTE, J., Institut de Physiologie, 17 place Delcour, 4000 Liège, Belgium.

LELIÈVRE, P., Laboratoire d'Anatomie Pathologique, 1 rue des Bonnes Villes, 4000 Liège, Belgium.

LIÉBECQ, C., Laboratoire de Biochimie, 1 rue des Bonnes Villes, 4000 Liège, Belgium.

MAISIN, J. R., Laboratoire de Radiobiologie, Centre de l'Energie Nucléaire, 2400 Mol, Belgium.

VAN CANEGHEM, P., Laboratoire de Physiopathologie, 32 bd de la Constitution, 4000 Liége, Belgium,

CHAPTER 1

INTRODUCTION

Z. M. Bacq

Liège, Belgium

1.1. DEFINITION, NOMENCLATURE AND ABBREVIATIONS

Chemical protective agents or radioprotective agents are substances which, administered to an animal or added to a culture medium shortly before exposure to ionizing radiation, significantly decrease the effects of this radiation; administration after irradiation does not have this favorable effect.

Some substances are known to be slightly effective when given both before and after irradiation; these cannot be considered to be true protective agents. Such terms as "post-irradiation protection" or "preprotection" should be excluded from the literature because they are misleading; we have often stressed the necessity of a logical and clear terminology.

Books, reviews and general discussions are numerous; the following list is certainly not exhaustive. Alexander (1960, 1963); Alexander *et al.* (1955); Bacq (1951, 1954, 1959, 1961, 1966); Bacq and Alexander (1955, 1961, 1964a, b); Bacq and Herve (1952, 1954); van Bekkum and Zaalberg (1959); Brues and Patt (1953); Doherty (1960); Eldjarn and Pihl (1960); Eldjarn (1962); Hollaender and Stapleton (1953); Hollaender *et al.* (1958); Kalkwarf (1960); Koch and Melching (1959); Koch *et al.* (1961); Langendorff (1957); Maisin (1961); Melching (1960, 1963); Moreau (1954); Patt (1953, 1954, 1960); Pihl and Eldjarn (1958); Scott (1963); Stapleton (1960); Straube and Patt (1963). The most recent monograph written essentially for radiobiologists is that of Bacq (1965).*

---

* Several catalogs of radioprotective substances have been published or are available to interested scientists. Unfortunately, it is not very easy to obtain copies of them. The following are in the hands of Z. M. Bacq (see page 2).

According to a decision taken by Bacq *et al.* in 1954, β-mercapto-ethylamine (MEA) has received the common name of cysteamine (and not cysteinamine); its disulfide is called cystamine. Modern purists of the Office of Biochemical Nomenclature insist on the fact that 2-amino-ethylthiol is the only correct name for this substance.

The abbreviations or patented names currently used in radiobiology are as follows:

$MEA = \beta$-mercaptoethylamine, cysteamine $= HS-CH_2-CH_2-NH_2$

Becaptan disulfure® (Labaz) $=$ cystamine $= \begin{cases} \overset{.}{S}-CH_2-CH_2-NH_2 \\ S-CH_2-CH_2-NH_2 \end{cases}$

Becaptan® (Labaz, Brussels) $= MEA$

Mercaptamine $= MEA$

Merkamin $= MEA$

Lambratene® (Bracco, Milano) $= MEA$

MPA $=$ mercaptopropylamine

AET $=$ S-2, aminoethylisothiourea (Br. HBr)

APT $=$ S-2, aminopropylisothiourea (Br. HBr)

MEG $=$ mercaptoethylguanidine (rearrangement in water of AET, see p. 11)

GED $=$ guanidoethyl disulfide, S—S form of MEG

1. Doull, J., Plzak, V. and Brois, S. J. (1962) *A Survey of Compounds for Radiation Protection,* document 62–29–USAF Aerospace Medical Division, Brooks Air Force Base, Texas, U.S.A., 124 pages.

2. Two catalogs edited in Russian by the Institute of Cytology of the Acad. Sc. U.S.S.R.: (a) Tiunov, L. A., Vasilyev, G. A. and Paribok, V. P. (1961), 172 pages; (b) Tiunov, L. A., Vasilyev, G. A. and Valdsteyn, E. A. (1964). V. P. Paribok (Ed.), 318 pages.

3. An English translation of this 1964 Russian catalog prepared by the Translation division, Foreign Technology division, Wright–Patterson Air Force Base, Ohio, U.S.A. Unclassified no. AD/633268, February 1966, 581 pages.

4. A catalog in four volumes published in German by the Akademie-Verlag, Berlin (East): Huber, R. and Spode, E. (1961, 1963) *Biologisch-Chemischer Strahlenschutz.*

5. A French catalog in five volumes (1965–8) and an index (1969) established by Robbe, Y., Sablayrolles, C., Randon, M., Valentin, M., Chevron, F. and Fernandez, J. P., under the direction of Granger, R. (Faculty of Pharmacy, Montpellier, France) with the help of the Ministère des Armées. This catalog exists only in stenciled copies.

6. A typewritten catalog of the work of fourteen Japanese scientists, prepared in 1965 by Fukuda, M., Onoyama, Y. and Abe, M. of the Department of Radiology, Faculty of Medicine, Kyoto University.

MPG   = mercaptopropylguanidine
ABMT   = 2-aminobutylisothiuronium bromide hydrobromide
AEMT   = 2-aminoethyl-N'-methylisothiuronium bromide hydro-
            bromide
AEMMT   = 2-aminoethyl-N',N''-methylisothiuronium bromide
            hydrobromide
AEdiMT = 2-aminoethyl-N'-dimethylisothiuronium bromide
            hydrobromide
EbAET   = 2,2'-bis(2-aminoethyl)-1,1'-ethylenebisisothiuronium
            bromide dihydrobromide
APMMT   = 3-aminopropyl-N,N'-dimethylisothiuronium bromide
            hydrobromide
APdiMT = 3-aminopropyl-N'-dimethylisothiuronium bromide
            hydrobromide
APMHET = 3-aminopropyl-N'-methyl-N''-(2-hydroxyethyl)
            isothiuronium bromide hydrobromide
EbAPT   = 2,2'-bis(3-aminopropyl)-1,1'-ethylenebisisothiuronium
            bromide hydrobromide
GSH   = reduced glutathione
GSSG   = oxidized glutathione
PAPP   = para-aminopropiophenone
DEDTC   = diethyldithiocarbamate
5-HT   = 5-hydroxytryptamine = serotonine
DRF   = dose reduction factor

1.2. HISTORICAL INTRODUCTION

Four main steps must be earmarked in the development of our knowledge of chemical protection against ionizing radiations.

In 1942, W. M. Dale, of Manchester University, showed that addition
of certain substances (colloidal sulfur, thiourea, formate, etc.) to an
aqueous solution of carboxypeptidase and D-aminoacid-oxidase decreases
the inactivation of these enzymes by X-rays (see Dale *et al.,* 1949).

In 1948, Latarjet and Ephrati tested certain substances on a bacteriophage which, logically, on the basis of the theory of indirect action,
might act as chemical protective agents. They obtained positive results
with thioglycollic acid, tryptophane, glutathione, cystine, and cysteine,
even in the absence of oxygen. They also pointed out the importance of

certain active groups (SH and NH$_2$). This fact was emphasized a few years later by Bacq and Herve (1952) when discussing their results in mice.

The author was impressed by the fact that irradiated frog muscles when stimulated repeatedly show contracture and inexcitability (known as the Lundsgaard effect) which can be produced not only by iodoacetate, but also by oxidizing agents like H$_2$O$_2$ (Bacq *et al.*, 1949). Since peroxides were known to be produced by ionizing radiation in water and aqueous solutions and since the peroxides have some radiomimetic properties, he tried to modify the effects of X-irradiation of mice by using cyanide to inhibit the catalases and peroxidases present in nearly all living systems; these enzymes rapidly eliminate the peroxides normally formed by various metabolic processes. This experiment yielded an unexpected result: some effect was expected when cyanide was injected after irradiation; in fact cyanide decreased mortality only if injected before irradiation (Herve and Bacq, 1949).

The second note published later in 1949 came from the Argonne Laboratory in Chicago, where H. M. Patt and his associates put to clear-cut experimental test a general hypothesis built by G. Barrón during the last war. Barrón and his associates have shown that pure crystallized thiol enzymes are much more sensitive to ionizing radiation in aqueous solution than non-SH enzymes; moreover, he succeeded in reactivating radiation-altered SH enzymes by adding an excess of cysteine or reduced glutathione (GSH). For Barrón, the main mechanism of action of ionizing radiation is the oxidation of —SH functions to form S—S bridges with inactivation of enzyme or coenzyme activity depending on these functions. This theory has not been substantiated and has now

TABLE 1. EFFECT OF TIME OF INJECTION OF CYSTEINE (875 mg/kg, i.v.) ON SURVIVAL OF RATS AFTER X-IRRADIATION WITH 800 R. CONTROLS RECEIVED EQUAL VOLUME OF 5% NaCl I.V. (Patt *et al.*, 1949)

Treatment group	Time of injection relative to X-irradiation	Number of rats	% survival after irradiation			
			1st week	2nd week	3rd week	4th week
Control	5 min before	15	73	20	13	13
Cysteine	5 min before	15	87	87	87	87
Control	1 hr before	15	80	20	20	20
Cysteine	1 hr before	15	100	87	80	80
Control	5 min after	16	88	19	13	6
Cysteine	5 min after	15	60	20	13	13

been abandoned. It suggested the possibility of repairing the elementary chemical lesions produced during irradiation by injecting mice or rats with large quantities of a physiological —SH compound, the amino acid cysteine, just as Sir Rudolph Peters had succeeded in inhibiting the development of lewisite-induced lesions with 2,3-dithiopropanol (BAL). The result of an experiment by Patt *et al.* (1949) was as clear as that of the author's: pure protection (Table 1), no difference between controls and injected rats even as early as 5 min after irradiation. Mole *et al.* (1950) showed that thiourea, which protects enzymes in solution, reduces radiation mortality in mice if injected before irradiation.

The work of Patt *et al.* was centered around the role of the —SH function. Bacq was also interested in the NH_2 group, not only because he is a pharmacologist and amines were a favorite subject of W. B. Cannon and Sir Henry Dale with whom he had worked in 1929 and 1936, but also because amines are known to inhibit the action of mustards, the radiomimetic properties of which had just been discovered in England by Auerbach and Robson (1944) and which are used in human cases of Hodgkin's disease and tumors of lymphoid tissue. The simplest amine,

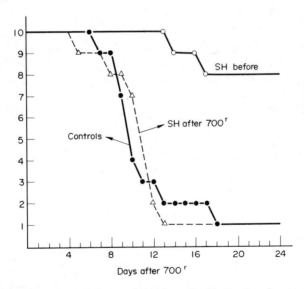

FIG. 1. Survival curves of three groups of ten C_{57} black mice after exposure to 700 r of 200 kV X-rays. Protection by mercaptoethylamine 150 mg/kg; no effect if MEA is injected after irradiation. This is the less favorable series in the observations of Bacq *et al.* (1951).

methylamine, has a slight but undeniable radioprotective activity (Bacq and Herve, 1951). The author tried to increase the effectiveness of cysteine by applying a well-known rule in pharmacology, of "liberating" the NH_2 function of this amino acid by removal of the carboxyl group; MEA was synthesized and immediately proved to be much more active than cysteine (Fig. 1). Cystamine (the S—S derivative) was found to be as active as MEA, a surprising fact at that time since it was known that cystine, the S—S form of cysteine, is totally inactive (Patt *et al.*, 1949). In 1952, it was already known that not all —SH substances are radioprotective and that many amines (including histamine, tryptamine, 5-hydroxytryptamine (5-HT), norepinephrine, tyramine) were also good protective agents (Bacq and Herve, 1952; Bacq, 1954).

Since 1952 research has taken many directions:

(a) During the 1951/2 outburst, the author was convinced that in a few years, compounds much more powerful than MEA would be synthesized; with the exception of aminoethylisothiourea (AET) developed at Oak Ridge, this line of research has so far been of little use. Probably more than three thousand compounds were tested and found to be too toxic, inactive, or at least less active than MEA. There has been a tendency in the last years to forget about new possible protective chemicals and to concentrate on studying the most active of those already known.

(b) The metabolism of the radioprotective agents, their distribution in the body, and their pharmacological and biochemical effects have been actively investigated.

(c) The detailed knowledge of what happens in the cells and tissues of an animal or a cell irradiated under chemical protection has attracted and retained the attention of many radiobiologists.

(d) Finally, much progress has been made in investigating the fascinating problem of the mechanisms of action of the various important protective compounds: agreement has been reached on many aspects of this question.

1.3. PROTECTIVE COMPOUNDS

The interested reader will find in Bacq's monograph (1965) a long list of protective chemicals. Several series of compounds are active, probably by different mechanisms. The ideas prevalent in 1969 may be summarized as follows (see also Bacq, 1966; Bacq and Goutier, 1967).

1. Cyanide, nitriles, and azide act either because they produce a

transitory true anoxia (i.e. a decrease of O_2 partial pressure in the tissues) or because they induce in mammals some metabolic disturbance which renders their cells more resistant to ionizing radiation.

2. A rule of radiobiology (and even of radiochemistry) states that with few exceptions the presence of O_2 in a system during exposure enhances the effects of X- or γ-radiation.

3. The so-called biological amines (acetylcholine, histamine, and the catecholamines) decrease the O_2 partial pressure in mammalian tissues and the dose reduction factor (DRF), i.e. the factor by which resistance to irradiation is increased, is proportional to the degree of anoxia. Pharmacological antagonists inhibit the radioprotective effect of the amines. On isolated cells or non-living systems, these amines are totally incapable of decreasing radiation damage.*

4. The case of 5-HT is much more complex (see Bacq, 1965). There are some arguments in favor of anoxia as the main mechanism of the radioprotective action by 5-HT, but certain bacterial strains and mucopolysaccharides in aqueous solution are also well protected against X-irradiation by 5-HT. Furthermore, 5-HT considerably lessens the lethal effects following head irradiation much more than after exposure of the rest of the body.

5. The sulfur-containing radioprotective agents have been extensively studied since 1949 and are still the subject of many publications. There are many reasons for this persistent interest:

(a) Cysteine, glutathione, MEA (as a fragment of CoA), which are normal cell constituents, are among the best-known protective agents.

(b) The SH or S—S protective agents when present in high enough concentrations in any kind of system and almost under any conditions decrease radiation damage by mechanisms in which free radicals are clearly involved. These systems range from dry films of synthetic polymers exposed to millions of rads in an atomic pile to mammals. Bacteria, viruses, DNA, proteins or enzyme solutions, spores, spermatozoa in liquid nitrogen, yeast cells, seeds, isolated mammalian cells in culture and invertebrates are all protected more or less effectively against ionizing radiation. For bacteria, the DRF may reach the value of 6, i.e. six times more energy in the form of ionizing radiation must be given in the presence of MEA in order to obtain the same mortality as in the non-protected controls. In mammals, a DRF of 2 is considered as high; the reason

---

* The radioprotective effect of histamine has been reviewed by Bacq in Section 74 on *Histamines and Antihistamines* of the *Encyclopedia of Pharmacology and Therapeutics* (Section Ed. M. Schachter), Pergamon Press, 1973.

for this discrepancy is that the *toxicity* of the sulfur-containing radio-protective agents is much higher for mammals than for bacteria.

(c) A careful study of the literature shows that in order to get protection in non-living systems or in bacteria or yeast cells, one must reach concentrations which are never obtained in whole mammals. Thus the mechanism of free radical scavenging (involving a competition with molecular oxygen) which is well established for non-living and certain cellular systems cannot explain the protection of mammals (see Bacq and Alexander, 1964b; Bacq, 1965). The anoxia mechanism may also be ruled out (Bacq and Alexander, 1964a; Bacq, 1965, 1966); MEA remains active as a protective agent in rats irradiated under a pressure of 5 atm pure O_2. There remains the possibility that after injection of large amounts of protective disulfides (cystamine for instance) the O_2 partial pressure in the tissue is significantly lowered and therefore part of the radioprotective action results from hypoxia; but the main mechanism of protection must be sought elsewhere.

(d) Accordingly, a "biochemical shock" hypothesis was proposed in 1964 by Bacq and Alexander; interest was again stimulated in pharmacological and biochemical research with these thiols and disulfides.

How far can the observations centered around this hypothesis explain the phenomenon of radioprotection in mammals?

This point will be discussed in the final chapter of this monograph.

1.4. THE MOST ACTIVE SH S—S COMPOUNDS

Table 2 gives a list of sulfur-containing protective chemicals (and related substances) based on observations in mammals. Aminothiols are by far the most interesting compounds, and practically all the research work in radiobiology, as well as in pharmacology or toxicology, is concerned with only a few substances. These are MEA and its disulfide cystamine, cysteine (and occasionally glutathione) and AET which in phosphate buffer isomerizes quantitatively in a few minutes at room temperature to MEG (mercaptoethylguanidine), by intramolecular transguanylation (Fig. 2). This last point is very important; the authors always mention AET, but in every case it is MEG which is present in solution. As in the case of MEA, MEG in the presence of oxygen is oxidized to guanidoethyl disulfide (GED); this reaction, like all thiol dimerizations, is greatly accelerated at alkaline pH.

Table 2 shows that in this series of compounds the structure of the most active protective agents is a two or three carbon chain with a strong basic

TABLE 2. RADIOPROTECTIVE CHEMICALS IN MAMMALS. CYSTEINE, CYSTEAMINE,
RELATED THIOLS AND DISULFIDES (adapted from Bacq, 1965)

Compound	Animal	Dose (mg/kg)[a]	Protective effect[b]
N-Alkyl and *N*-aryl Derivatives of Cysteine and Cysteamine			
Cysteine	Mice, rats	950–1200 i.p.	3
Cysteine	Rats	1900 or.	2
Cysteamine	Mice, rats	75–250 i.p.	3
Cystine	Mice, rats	240–280 i.p.	0
Cystamine	Mice	150–300 i.p.	3
Cystamine	Mice, rats	400–600 or.	3
N-Monomethylcysteamine	Mice	60–120 i.p.	2
N-Dimethylcysteamine	Mice, rats	40–70 i.p.	1
N,N'-Tetramethylcystamine	Rats	60 i.p.	2
N-Diethylcysteamine	Mice	50–60 i.p.	2
N-Piperidylcysteamine	Mice	25 i.p.	0
N-Methylphenylcysteamine	Mice	250 i.p.	0
N-Phenylcysteamine	Rats	150 i.p.	0
Cysteamine-*N*-acetic acid	Mice	220–1500 i.p.	2–3
S-2, Aminoethylisothiourea Br. HBr (AET)	Mice	240–480 i.p.	3
		1500 or.	3
S-2, Aminoethylisothiourea Br. HBr	Dogs	100 i.p.	0
		150 i.v.	2
S-2, Aminoethylisothiourea Br. HBr	*Macaca mulat-ta* (monkey)	200–250 i.p.	3
S-2, Aminoethyl-*N*-methylisothiourea Cl. HCl	Mice	150 i.p.	2
S-2, Aminoethylthiosulfuric acid	Mice	450 i.p.	2
Guanylthiourea	Mice	1000 i.p.	2
N-Acyl Derivatives of Cysteine and Cysteamine			
Glutathione	Mice, rats	800–1000 i.p.	2
Glutathione	Rats	2000 or.	0
N-Acetylcysteamine	Mice, rats	120–250 i.p.	2
N-Acetoacetylcysteamine	Mice	240 i.p.	0
Aletheine	Mice	250–300 i.p.	1
Pantetheine	Mice	350–550 i.p.	0
N-Acetylmethylcysteamine	Mice	150 i.p.	0
Compounds with Covered Sulfur Function			
Homocysteine thiolactone	Mice	700 i.p.	2
		1000 or.	2
N,S-Diacetylcysteamine	Mice	280–320 i.p.	0–1
S-Methylcysteamine	Mice	850 i.p.	0
S-Benzylcysteamine	Mice	160 i.p.	0
Methionine	Mice	500–1500 i.p.	0
S-2, Dimethylaminoethylisothiourea Cl. HCl	Mice	350 i.p.	0
S-2 (1-Morpholyl), ethylisothiourea Br. HBr	Mice	150 i.p.	0
Di(ethylaminoethyl) sulfide	Mice	140 i.p.	0

(*For key to notes*[a,b] *see* p. 10.)

TABLE 2 (*cont.*)

Compound	Animal	Dose (mg/kg)[a]	Protective effect[b]
Compounds with Branched or Prolonged Carbon Chain			
3-Mercaptopropylamine	Mice	90 i.p.	3
3-Mercaptopropylguanidine	Mice	125–250 i.p.	3
Homocysteine	Mice	450 i.p.	2
1-Mercapto-5-diethylaminopentane	Mice	35 i.p.	0
1-Mercapto-7-aminoheptane	Mice	40 i.p.	0
α-Methylcysteine	Rats	100 i.p.	0
Thiols with Alcoholic or Carboxylic Acid Groups			
Thioglycolic acid	Mice	180 i.p.	0
Mercaptosuccinic acid	Mice	350 i.p.	0
2,3-Dithiopropanol (BAL)	Mice, rats	150–200 i.p. and s.c.	0 1
Dithiopentaerythrit	Mice	75 i.p.	0
Cyclic Compounds			
2-Mercaptothiazoline	Mice	100 i.p.	0
1(–)-2-Thiolhistidine	Mice	420 i.p.	0
Ergothioneine	Mice	500 i.p.	0
4,6-Dimethyl-2-mercaptopyrimidine	Mice	270 i.p.	0
o-Aminothiophenol	Mice	50 i.p.	0
Miscellaneous Sulfur-containing Substances			
Ammonium dithiocarbamate	Mice	500 i.p.	3
Diethyldithiocarbamate	Mice	600 i.p.	3
Thiourea	Mice	2500 i.p.	2
Thiocyanate	Mice	200 i.p.	0
Thioacetamide	Mice	150 i.p.	0
Sodium tetrathionate	Mice	150 i.p.	0
Sodium sulfide	Rats	5 i.v.	0

[a] i.p. = intraperitoneally; i.v. = intravenously; i.m. = intramuscularly; s.c. = subcutaneously; or. = orally.

[b] *Protective effect.* The grading of the optimal protective effect has been carried out according to the following arbitrary scale: 0 = No protective effect; 1 = slight or dubious protective effect; 2 = moderate protective effect; 3 = strong protective effect (e.g. MEA, AET).

group (amino or guanidino) at one end and a thiol at the other. They have chelating properties.

In certain systems (isolated mammalian cells), the disulfide cystamine does not cross the cell membrane and is not effective. Some authors maintain that only the reduced thiol form is active, and that cystamine is a good protective agent in whole mammals because it is rapidly reduced to the thiol form by an intracellular enzymatic system. On the other

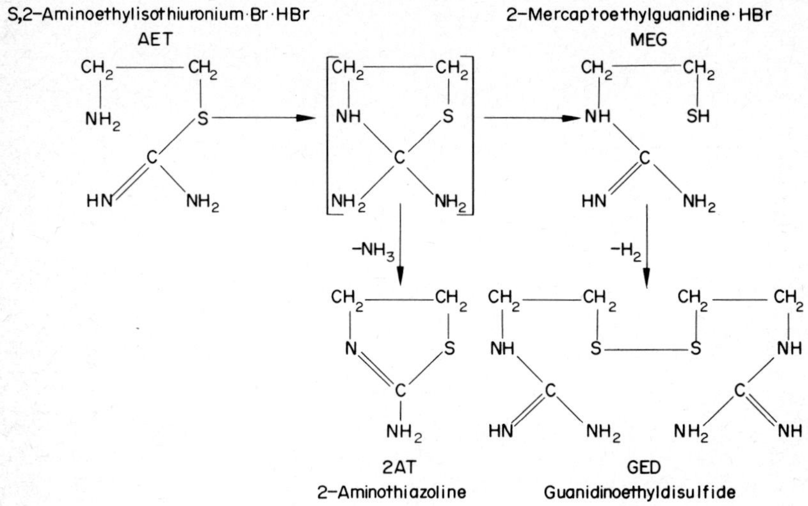

FIG. 2. Transguanylation of AET and oxidation of MEG to GED.

hand it is quite clear (see Bacq, 1965) that cystamine *in vitro* in non-living systems, or in systems where it is certainly not reduced, may act as a powerful protector against ionizing radiation.

The fate of these molecules in mammals is rather complicated and is of great importance in understanding their mode of action. Recent observations have revealed peculiar, rapid transient toxic effects (at the dose required for radioprotective action) which have never been observed with other drugs or toxic substances. These two facts (radioprotective action and a peculiar type of toxicity) are important enough criteria for considering the sulfur-containing radioprotective substances as a particular class of drugs.

Section 79 of the *Encyclopedia* is devoted to the study of the various pharmacological and biochemical actions of these compounds.

REFERENCES

ALEXANDER, P. (1960) Protection of macromolecules *in vitro* against damage by ionizing radiations. In: *Radiation Protection and Recovery*, A. HOLLAENDER (Ed.), Pergamon Press, Oxford, pp. 3–44.

ALEXANDER, P. (1963) Chemical protection in chemical systems. In: *Radiation Effects in Physics, Chemistry and Biology.* Proc. 2nd Intern. Congress Radiation Research, Harrogate, 1962. North-Holland Publ. Co., Amsterdam, pp. 254–74.

ALEXANDER, P., BACQ, Z. M., COUSENS, S., FOX, M., HERVE, A. and LAZAR, J. (1955) Mode of action of some substances which protect against the lethal effects of X-rays. *Radiation Res.* **2**: 392–415.

AUERBACH, C. and ROBSON, J. (1944) Production of mutations by allyl isothiocyanate. *Nature* **154**: 81.

BACQ, Z. M. (1951) L'action indirecte du rayonnement X et ultraviolet. *Experientia* **7**: 11–19.

BACQ, Z. M. (1954) The amines and particularly cysteamine as protectors against roentgen rays. *Acta radiol.* **41**: 47–55.

BACQ, Z. M. (1959) Chemical protection against ionizing radiation in vertebrates. XXIst Intern. Congress Physiol. Sci., Buenos Aires, Symposia and Conferences.

BACQ, Z. M. (1961) Chemical protection against ionizing radiation. *Triangle* **5**: 2–11.

BACQ, Z. M. (1965) *Chemical Protection against Ionizing Radiation.* Ch. C. Thomas, Springfield, Ill., U.S.A., 344 pages.

BACQ, Z. M. (1966) La protection chimique contre les radiations ionisantes chez les mammifères. *Bull. Acad. Roy. Méd. Belg.*, VIIth series **6**: 115–41.

BACQ, Z. M. and ALEXANDER, P. (1955) *Fundamentals of Radiobiology.* 1st ed., Butterworths, London, 1955, 389 pages. 2nd ed., Pergamon Press, Oxford, 1961, 562 pages.

BACQ, Z. M. and ALEXANDER, P. (1961) Mechanism of chemical radiation protection. In: *The Initial Effects of Ionizing Radiation on Cells.* A Symposium, Moscow, Oct. 1960. Academic Press, London, pp. 301–14.

BACQ, Z. M. and ALEXANDER, P. (1964a) The rôle of oxygen in the phenomenon of chemical protection against ionizing radiation. A symposium on *Oxygen in the Animal Organism,* London, 1963. Pergamon Press, Oxford, pp. 509–36.

BACQ, Z. M. and ALEXANDER, P. (1964b) Importance for radioprotection of the reaction of cells to sulphydryl and disulphide compounds. *Nature* **203**: 162–4.

BACQ, Z. M. and GOUTIER, R. (1967) Mechanisms of action of sulfur-containing radioprotectors. In: *Recovery and Repair Mechanisms in Radiobiology,* Brookhaven Symposia in Biology, No. 20, pp. 241–62.

BACQ, Z. M. and HERVE, A. (1951) Protective action of methylamine against X-irradiation. *Nature* **168**:1126.

BACQ, Z. M. and HERVE, A. (1952) Protection chimique contre le rayonnement X. *Bull. Acad. Roy. Méd. Belg.*, VIth series **17**: 13–58.

BACQ, Z. M. and HERVE, A. (1954) Ein chemischer Schutz gegen Roentgenstrahlungen. *Strahlentherapie* **95**:215–37.

BACQ, Z. M., LECOMTE, J. and HERVE, A. (1949) Action des radiations ionisantes sur le muscle strié de grenouille. *Arch. internat. Physiol.* **67**: 142–53.

BACQ, Z. M., HERVE, A., LECOMTE, J., FISCHER, P., BLAVIER, J., DECHAMPS, G., LE BIHAN, H. and RAYET, P. (1951) Protection contre le rayonnement X par la β-mercaptoéthylamine. *Arch. internat. Physiol.* **59**: 442–7.

BACQ, Z. M., BADDILEY, J., ELDJARN, L., LIPMANN, F. and LYNEN, F. (1954) Nomenclature of the amines derived by decarboxylation of cysteine and cystine. *Science* **119**: 163–4.

BEKKUM, D. VAN and ZAALBERG, O. (1959) Mechanisms of chemical protection against ionizing radiation in living organisms. *Intern. J. Rad. Biol.* **1**: 155–60.

BRUES, A. and PATT, H. (1953) Mechanisms of protection against mammalian radiation injury. *Physiol. Rev.* **33**: 85–9.

DALE, W. M., GRAY, L. H. and MEREDITH, W. J. (1949) The inactivation of an enzyme (carboxypeptidase) by X- and γ-radiation. *Phil. Trans. Roy. Soc.* **242A**: 33–52.

DOHERTY, D. (1960) Chemical protection to mammals against ionizing radiation. In: *Radiation Protection and Recovery.* HOLLAENDER (Ed.), Pergamon Press, Oxford, pp. 45–86.

ELDJARN, L. (1962) Chemical protection against ionizing radiation. Radiochemistry or cellular physiology? In: *Strahlenwirkung und Milieu,* FRITZ-NIGGLI (Ed.), Urban u. Schwatzenberg, München, pp. 232–44.

ELDJARN, L. and PIHL, A. (1960) Mechanisms of protective and sensitizing action. In: *Mechanisms in Radiobiology*, ERRERA, M. and FORSSBERG, A. (Eds.), Academic Press, New York, vol. II, pp. 231–96.

HERVE, A. and BACQ, Z. M. (1949) Cyanure et dose léthale de rayons X. *C.R. Soc. Biol.* **143**: 881–3.

HOLLAENDER, A. and STAPLETON, G. (1953) Fundamental aspects of radiation protection from a microbiological point of view. *Physiol. Rev.* **33**: 77–84.

HOLLAENDER, A., CONGDON, C., DOHERTY, D., MAKINODAN, T. and UPTON, A. (1958) New developments in radiation protection and recovery. *Proc. 2nd Int. U.N. Conf. on Peaceful Uses of Atomic Energy, Geneva* **23**: 3–22.

KALKWARF, D. (1960) Chemical protection from radiation effects. *Nucleonics* **185**: 76–130.

KOCH, R. and MELCHING, H. (1959) Der gegenwärtige Stand der chemischen Strahlenschutzforschung. *Medizinische Klinik* **54**: 1635–9.

KOCH, R., LANGENDORFF, H. and MELCHING, H. (1961) Der chemische Strahlenschutz. *Chemoterapia* **3**: 153–65.

LANGENDORFF, H. (1957) Zur Chemie des biologischen Strahlenschutzes. *Atomwirtschaft* **2**: 132–50.

LATARJET, R. and EPHRATI, E. (1948) Influence protectrice de certaines substances contre l'inactivation d'un bactériophage par les rayons X. *C.R. Soc. Biol.* **142**: 497–9.

MAISIN, J. R. (1961) Protection chimique des Mammifères contre les radiations. *Rev. Franç. Et. Clin. Biol.* **6**: 378–93.

MELCHING, H. (1960) Untersuchungen über den chemischen Strahlenschutz. *Dtsch. med. Wochenschr.* **86**: 2284–6.

MELCHING, H. (1963) Zur Frage einer Beeinflussung der Strahlenempfindlichkeit beim Saügetier. *Strahlentherapie* **120**: 34–73.

MOLE, R., PHILPOT, J. and HODGES, C. (1950) Reduction in lethal effect of X-irradiation by pretreatment with thiourea or sodium ethane-dithiophosphonate. *Nature* **166**: 515.

MOREAU, R. (1954) Les radioprotecteurs chimiques. *Revue Générale des Sciences* **61**: 197–220.

PATT, H. (1953) Protective mechanisms in ionizing radiation injury. *Physiol. Rev.* **33**: 35–76.

PATT, H. (1954) Radiation effects on mammalian systems. *Ann. Rev. Physiol.* **16**: 51–80.

PATT, H. (1960) Chemical approaches to radiation protection in mammals. *Fed. Proc.* **19**: 549–53.

PATT, H., TYREE, E., STRAUBE, R. and SMITH, D. (1949) Cysteine protection against X-irradiation. *Science* **110**: 213–14.

PIHL, A. and ELDJARN, L. (1958) Pharmacological aspects of ionizing radiation and of chemical protection in mammals. *Pharmacol. Rev.* **10**: 437–74.

SCOTT, O. (1963) The modification of tissue response to injury. *Ann. Rev. Medic.* **14**: 371–80.

STAPLETON, G. (1960) Protection and recovery in bacteria and fungi. In: *Radiation and Recovery*, HOLLAENDER (Ed.), Pergamon Press, Oxford, pp. 87–116.

STRAUBE, R. L. and PATT, H. M. (1963) Chemical protection against ionizing radiation. *Ann. Rev. Pharmacol.* **3**: 293–306.

CHAPTER 2

TOXICITY

J. R. Maisin (*Mol*) and Z. M. Bacq (*Liège*)

Belgium

2.1. INTRODUCTION

The problem of the safety of an antiradiation compound for eventual use in man is the same as that presented by any new drug proposed for the treatment of a disease. Complete pharmacological testing and determination of acute, subacute and chronic effects in many mammalian species are required. Particular care must be given to the study of teratogenecity, premature ageing, and carcinogenesis. The findings must permit an accurate estimation of the safety factor (Griffith and Dyer, 1966). The degree of protection and the toxicity of a given compound appear to be correlated (DiStefano, 1964). Protective compounds show deleterious effects at the cellular, tissue, and general levels. As recent results indicate, toxicity at the cellular level, at least in mammals, is probably the factor on which protective efficiency depends; some of the general toxic effects following administration of a sulfhydryl protective agent are probably side effects not related to the protective potency of the drug (Bacq, 1965; Bacq and Goutier, 1967; Maisin, 1968). The acute general symptoms in mice after the administration of a toxic dose of aminoethyl-isothiourea (AET) or cysteamine (MEA), the most powerful protective agents known today, differ greatly (Hulse, 1963).

So far no agent has been found sufficiently protective and safe to justify the expense and labor required in complete long-term toxicological testing. As it has now become possible, with mixtures of chemical compounds, to obtain a dose reduction factor of about 3 in mice (Maisin *et al.*, 1968), a detailed study of the toxicity of different protective agents appears warranted.

Experience shows that the results of toxicological studies vary from one

15

laboratory to another. This is due mainly to the degree of purity of the compounds tested, and to the use of different strains of animals. We have tested preparations from many sources. Some commercial batches of MEA or cystamine are very impure (up to 20% impurities), unduly toxic, and devoid of radioprotective activity, causing necrosis of the skin after subcutaneous injections of only moderately concentrated solutions.

Some ampoules of MEA neutral solution sealed under nitrogen become toxic in a few years. Cysteamine ($-SH$) in contact with air is oxidized to cystamine ($S-S$) either in solution or in the solid state. One way to avoid the formation of cystamine during handling of MEA solutions is to take advantage of the reducing properties of thiolated Sephadex. Cystamine is more stable; some authors therefore prepare their solutions of MEA when required by electrolytic reduction of cystamine. Some batches of MEA (and less frequently of cystamine) kept either as base or as a salt, without special precautions, may become yellow. Logically MEA should be kept in hydrogen.

The various stocks of AET used by radiobiologists or pharmacologists are not only unstable and change with time despite all protective measures (vacuum, cold, darkness) but also are of variable quality from the start. We have known the presence in a laboratory of two samples of AET, the first well tolerated but devoid of radioprotective action, the second active as a protective agent but more toxic than reported in the literature.

Many experiments lose a good deal of their value because the purity of the thiol under study has not been ascertained. It is neither difficult nor time-consuming to check the purity by paper chromatography and recrystallization of the material.

Since the sulfhydryl and disulfide protective agents are basic substances, they are administered in neutralized solution or used as salts. The nature of the acid is of little importance; the hydrochloride of MEA or cystamine is generally used, but Soviet scientists prefer the nicotinate (Arbusow *et al.*, 1959).

As far as AET is concerned, the most frequently used salt is the bromide, hydrobromide as defined by Doherty and Burnett (1955); the chloride, hydrochloride has been used with equal success. In certain experiments, for example with bacteria, in which fairly concentrated solutions are used, the bromide ion may have some action of its own in increasing the lethal action of X-rays (Hollaender and Doudney, 1955); otherwise the toxicity is all due to the sulfur base (Melville and Leffingwell, 1962).

2.2. TOXICITY OF SULFHYDRYL COMPOUNDS GIVEN SEPARATELY

2.2.1. ACUTE AND SUBACUTE TOXICITY

Details of the toxicity of sulfhydryl compounds are found in the following books, reviews, or articles : Doherty and Burnett, 1955; Doherty *et al.,* 1957; Koch and Schwarze, 1957; Koch *et al.,* 1960; Bacq, 1965; and in the catalogs of Huber and Spode, 1961, 1963.

The clinical symptoms vary greatly from one compound to another and, for a given compound, with the dose administered. For instance in dogs, MEA causes salivation, vomiting, diarrhea, agitation, ataxia, tonic and clonic convulsions, and an increase in depth and rate of respiration. Low doses of AET cause a fall in blood pressure and apnea mediated by a vagal reflex. Larger doses elevate blood pressure, and still larger ones lower the blood pressure by ganglionic blocking. Oral administration of 500 mg of AET in man produces nausea and vomiting; 750–1000 mg causes dizziness, drowsiness, sweating, dyspnea, and diarrhea. These effects on the blood pressure, circulation, and nervous system are discussed in following chapters. In contrast to the general symptoms, the cellular effect appears similar for all sulfhydryl compounds. A few minutes after administration of AET or any other sulfhydryl compound, the ultrastructure of the cell changes, in a manner similar to that found after X-ray irradiation, although the former are reversible whereas the latter are not (see Chapter 4). In parallel to the structural alteration, the cellular metabolism, nucleic acid synthesis and mitotic activity are affected by administration of sulfur protective agents (see Chapters 6 and 7). The degree of these changes seems to be related to the protective action of sulfhydryl compounds (see Chapter 9). Studies *in vitro* also show the great cellular toxicity of chemical protective drugs (Therkelsen, 1958b).

Some biochemical signs of cellular toxicity have been correlated with the ability of thiols to protect against ionizing radiation. The injection of MEA in radioprotective amounts in rats induces a rapid but temporary increase in the blood concentration of several enzymes, normally located in the cytoplasm, mitochondria, or lysosomes; we interpret this phenomenon as a sign of shock (see Chapter 3.3). Mercaptoethanol, a non-protective thiol in equal amounts, does not produce shock, or enzyme liberation, and has no radioprotective activity. Two isomers are of particular interest: 5-mercaptopyridoxine protects against irradiation: 4-mercaptopyridoxine does not. The 5-isomer produces ultrastructural lesions of mitochondria and enzyme liberation; the 4-isomer, administered in similar doses, has strictly none of these effects, although it is not devoid of toxicity (Plomteux *et al.,* 1967, 1968). Proliferation of HeLa S$_3$ cells *in vitro* was markedly inhibited by mercaptoethylguanidine (MEG) when the compound was present in the medium for a long period even in a concentration as low as 0.1 mM (Takagi *et al.,* 1970).

2.2.2.   LD$_{50}$ AND TOLERATED DOSES

Table 1 gives the available data about acute LD$_{50}$ values.

Table 2 summarizes data concerning the quantities of compounds frequently used in adult animals of different species in studies of radioprotective activity. The reader should understand that these doses are generally the maximum tolerated amounts. This is because investigators are interested in injecting the largest possible doses in order to obtain the highest possible dose reduction factors against ionizing radiations or radiomimetic alkylating agents (see Chapter 8). The two most active compounds, MEA or MEG (AET), are equally toxic on a per mol basis (Koch and Schwarze, 1957).

As far as AET is concerned, the rapidity of the intravenous (i.v.) injection is very important. When the compound is injected slowly, doses six times higher than after rapid injection are tolerated. This is due to a vagal reflex (see Chapter 3), the intensity of which depends on the concentration of the drug in the blood. There is one more reason for discrepancy in LD$_{50}$ values. Lethal doses in mammals range from 350 to 650 mg/kg with i.p. injection and from 50 to 450 mg/kg with i.v. injection. Aminoethylisothiourea is less toxic when injected at an acid pH, rather than at pH 7 or 8.

In general, the toxicity of compounds related to AET increases with the number of carbon atoms in the alkyl chain (Doherty *et al.,* 1957). In order to obtain less toxic and longer-acting derivatives of MEA, Foye and Zaim (1964) prepared thio-esters of different α-amino acids. Esters of MEA would slowly liberate MEA *in vivo* and might thus provide more active radioprotective agents than MEA itself.

Åkerfeldt *et al.* (1968) have described the radioprotective effect of diammonium-amidophosphorothioate (AO 331). The dose reduction factors of this compound in mice appears to be at least as high as that of MEA, but only one-fifteenth of AO 331 (on a per mol basis) needs to be administered compared with other protective thiols. The therapeutic index found reaches 2.9 whereas it is only 1.3 for MEA.

The oral administration is less toxic than other routes of administration, although starvation may increase the toxicity (Hanna and Colclough,

TABLE 1. LD$_{50}$ OF CLASSICAL SH OR S—S PROTECTIVE AGENTS AGAINST IONIZING RADIATION

Substance	Animal species	Route of administration[a]	LD$_{50}$ (mg/kg)	Reference
MEA	Mouse	i.p.	350 (base)	Bacq et al., 1951
		i.p.	425	Doull et al., 1958[b]
		i.p.	260	Therkelsen, 1958a
		i.p.	270	Doherty et al., 1957[c]
	Rat	i.p.	143 ±9	Maisin et al., 1964[d]
		or.	359 ±20	Maisin et al., 1964[d]
	Rabbit	i.v.	150	Beccari et al., 1955
Cystamine	Mouse	i.p.	215	Koch and Schwarze, 1957
	Rat	i.p.	126 ±4	Maisin et al., 1964[d]
		or.	1035	Maisin et al., 1964[d]
MPA[e]	Mouse	i.p.	125	Doherty et al., 1957
AET Br, HBr[f]	Rat	i.p.	410	Benson et al., 1961
		i.p.	288	Hanna and Colclough, 1963
		i.p.	375 ±23	Melville and Leffingwell, 1962
	Mouse	i.p.	600	Shapira et al., 1957
	Mouse	i.p.	400—500	Doull et al., 1958[b]
	Mouse	i.p.	690	Doherty and Burnett, 1955
	Adult	i.p.	475	Rousanov and Novoselova, 1962
	2–3 weeks	i.p.	335	Rousanov and Novoselova, 1962
	Newborn	i.p.	520	Rousanov and Novoselova, 1962
	Rabbit	i.v.	236	Hanna and Colclough, 1963
	Dog	i.v.	113	Hanna and Colclough, 1963

(For key to notes[a-f] see p. 20.)

(continued overleaf)

TABLE 1 (*cont.*)

Substance	Animal species	Route of administration[a]	LD_{50} (mg/kg)	Reference
APT Br, HBr	Mice	i.p.	340–400	Shapira *et al.*, 1957
Cysteine	Rat	i.p.	7000	

[a] i.p. = intraperitoneal injection; i.v. = intravenous injection; or. = oral administration.
[b] The toxicity of other salts of 2-aminoethylisothiourea is given in Doull *et al.*, 1962. The dichloride and diiodide derivatives are less toxic and protect against radiation at suitable dose. The acetate is very well tolerated (LD_{50} exceeds 2 g/kg) but does not protect even at high dose (1.5 g/kg).
[c] The toxicity for mice of twelve compounds related to MEA is given by Doherty *et al.*, 1957.
[d] The toxicity of MEA and cystamine is significantly greater in irradiated rats (i.e. when administered after exposure to 600 r of X-ray irradiation).
[e] MPA = mercaptopropylamine; APT = aminopropylthiourea.
[f] The toxicity of seventy-four mercaptoalkylguanidines (protective or non-protective) and related isothiouronium compounds is given by Shapira *et al.*, 1957).

TABLE 2. PROTECTIVE DOSES[a] OF THE MOST EXTENSIVELY STUDIED COMPOUNDS FOR ADULT ANIMALS OF DIFFERENT SPECIES

(See also Pihl and Eldjarn, 1958 for other derivatives of these series)

Compound	Species	Dose (mg/kg)	Route of administration[b]	Reference
Cysteine	Mouse	950–1200	i.p.	Bacq and Herve, 1952
	Mouse	500	i.v.	Caffarati, 1951a, b
	Rat	1900	or.	Patt et al., 1950
	Rat	950–1200	i.p.	Patt et al., 1950
	Dog	550	or.	Jakovlev and Ivanov, 1958
	Dog	250	i.p.	Jakovlev and Ivanov, 1958
	Dog	500	i.v.	Jakovlev and Ivanov, 1958
	Man	300–900	i.m.	Kolář, 1958
	Man	100	i.v.	Theismann, 1955
MEA	Mouse	75–250	i.p.	Bacq et al., 1951
	Rat	75–250	i.p.	Bacq et al., 1951
	Dog	75–110	i.v.	Razorenova and Sherbova, 1961
	Man	200	i.v.	Bacq et al., 1953; Bacq and Herve, 1955; Herve and Bacq, 1952; Van de Berg and Van de Berg, 1954
	Man	150–400	i.v.	Albano and Oliva, 1955
	Man	200–300	i.v.	Juliani and Orso, 1956
Cystamine	Mouse	400–600	or.	Bacq, 1953
	Mouse	150–300	i.p.	Bacq et al., 1951
	Rat	400–600	or.	Bacq, 1953

(For key to notes[a,b] see p. 22.)

(continued overleaf)

TABLE 2 (cont.)

Compound	Species	Dose (mg/kg)	Route of administration[b]	Reference
AET	Mouse	1500	or.	Dacquisto and Blackburn, 1961
	Mouse	240–480	i.p.	Doherty and Burnett, 1955
	Rat	300	i.p.	Hanna and Colclough, 1963
	Dog	100	i.p.	Benson et al., 1961
	Dog	150	i.v.	Newsome et al., 1962
	Macaca mulatta	200–250	i.p.	Crough and Overman, 1957
Glutathione	Mouse	800–1000	i.p.	Chapman and Cronkite, 1950
	Rat	2000	or.	Patt et al., 1950
	Rat	800–1000	i.p.	Chapman and Cronkite, 1950
Diammonium–amidophosphorothioate	Mouse	20	i.p.	Åkerfeldt et al., 1968

[a] Generally equal to maximal tolerated doses.
[b] i.p. = intraperitoneal injection; i.v. = intravenous injection; i.m. = intramuscular injection; or. = oral administration.

1963; Maisin *et al.*, 1964). The protective activity of the compounds administered orally is lower but more prolonged (Bacq, 1956; Maisin *et al.*, 1964). Guanidoethyl disulfide is less toxic (and equally less protective) than MEG by oral route because it is not so well absorbed, a fact which suggests failure of reduction by the intestinal flora (Kollmann *et al.*, 1963). Rousanov and Novoselova (1962) claim that the toxicity of AET in the mouse varies with age; the most resistant are newborn mice.

Rats are more sensitive to radioprotective agents after partial hepatectomy, since sulfhydryl compounds are mostly metabolized in the liver (Maisin *et al.*, 1965). Aminoethylisothiourea administered intraperitoneally (i.p.) can cause local pathological changes such as necrosis (Hanna and Colclough, 1963).

In general, protective compounds are more toxic when exposure to X-ray irradiation follows the administration. Only if the X-ray dose is small and follows within 2–15 min does toxicity decrease (Hulse, 1963). Intraperitoneal administration of AET is also better tolerated by rats after repeated oral doses of AET or repeated increasing i.p. doses over fourteen days (Hanna and Colclough, 1963). Dogs (but not rabbits) may develop tolerance to AET.

Introduction of a methyl group into N and N' nitrogen of the guanido group of MEG significantly increased acute toxicity in mice of the mother compound. When compared on an equimolar basis in some narrow ranges, N-methyl, N'-methyl and N',N''-dimethyl derivatives showed the same magnitude of prophylactic action against X-ray irradiation in mice as MEG. However, the radioprophylactic range of these compounds was obviously narrower than that of MEG (Takagi *et al.*, 1970).

A multiple emulsion of an 8% solution of MEA (an equal volume of light liquid paraffin containing 10% of the detergent "Arlacel 83" and a 2% aqueous solution of "Tween 80") considerably prolonged protection against the lethal effects of X-ray exposure (Gresham *et al.*, 1971).

Landahl and Hasegawa (1970) have injected as much as 600 mg/kg (i.v.) and 900 mg/kg (i.p.) of MEA into mice with very high mortality. The toxicity was greater in mice kept at 30°C than in those kept at 22°C. Pentobarbital counteracts the toxity of high doses of MEA.

2.2.3. LONG-TERM AND EMBRYONIC TOXICITY

Long-term toxicity of single doses of sulfhydryl protective agents has not been adequately investigated. Figures 1a, 1b show the long-term

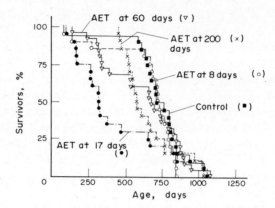

FIG. 1a. Male rats cumulative percent survival as a function of time after treatment at 8, 17, 60, or 200 days of age.

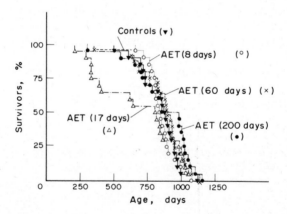

FIG. 1b. Female rats cumulative percent survival as a function of time after treatment at 8, 17, 60, or 200 days of age.

survival of male and female Wistar rats treated at 8, 17, 60, and 200 days of age with a single dose of 200 mg/kg of AET (Br-HBr). Rats treated at 17 days of age are more sensitive than those treated at 8, 60, or 200 days. At an age of 17 days, male rats appear more susceptible than female ones (Léonard *et al.,* 1969a), and similar results are obtained when the dose of AET is increased (Fig. 2). The kidneys of rats treated at 17 days of age frequently show a marked intercapillary glomerulosclerosis. Such changes are, however, not seen in all strains of rats. When the

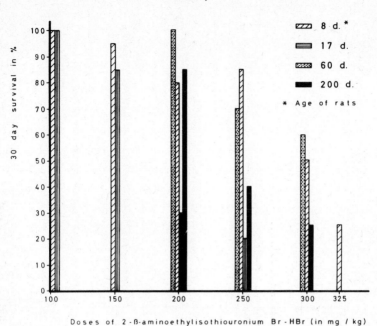

Fig. 2a. Thirty days survival of normal male rats treated at 8, 17, 60, or 200 days
of age with increasing doses of AET.

administration of AET is followed by an X-ray dose of 300 r, the lesions
in the kidney are more pronounced and appear sooner. The mechanism
of production of these lesions is unknown, but it appears to be related to
the excretion of the protective drug and its metabolites by the kidney.
Glomeruli of 8-day-old rats may still be capable of partially repairing
the damage induced by AET, whereas those of 17-day-old rats may have
reached a state of differentiation which makes this impossible. The
ingestion of AET also causes tubular damage after a few days, but this
seems to be reversible.

No satisfactory study has been published so far on the effects of
radioprotective agents on mammalian embryos. Good embryonic
protection against acute X-ray irradiation by MEA or cystamine has
been repeatedly observed (see Bacq, 1965 for references). Onkelinx (1961)
found that MEA is quite toxic to the chicken embryo. If a drop of MEA
solution is deposited on the beating heart of a seven-day-old chicken
embryo, 10–20% of embryos do not survive and reduction of the caudal

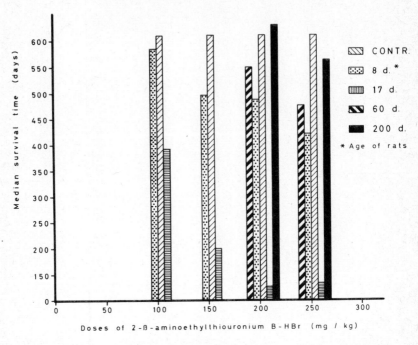

FIG. 2b. Median survival of rats treated at 8, 17, 60, or 200 days with increasing doses of AET.

burgeon is seen (Reyss-Brion, 1962; for figures, see Bacq, 1965). A disc of paraffin which prevents the amine spreading too rapidly and ensures slow absorption and distribution by the circulation to all tissues is used in these experiments. This effect again may be classified as radiomimetic.

A single dose of AET does not have any influence on the long-term survival of male and female Balb/c mice (Léonard and Mattelin, 1970). During the course of assaying tolerance of chick embryos (ages ranging from 4 to 8 days) to radioprotective substances it was observed that chicks from embryos treated at 7 days of age with AET were disoriented and unable to maintain an upright posture (Morgan *et al.*, 1969).

2.2.4. REPEATED INJECTIONS

The cumulative toxicity of repeated i.p. administration of AET or MEA (or mixtures of protective agents) introduces some difficulty in studying protection against repeated X-ray doses (Maisin, 1969). As early as 1958 DuBois and Raymund observed that pyruvic dehydrogenase in rat kidney is depressed when AET (300 mg/kg) is administered at 2-day, but not at 3-day, intervals.

Repeated injections of large doses of MEA or cystamine are generally well tolerated by mice provided that an interval of 4–6 hr is maintained between the injections, i.e. when all the signs of shock have disappeared, in particular the increased blood levels of intracellular enzymes (see Chapter 3.3). During the shock induced by a first injection of a maximal tolerated dose, the animal is extremely sensitive and dies rapidly if a second injection of a small dose is given.

Good tolerance to MEA has been observed by Therkelsen (1958a) in AKA mice ($\pm$24 g); no deaths occurred after i.p. injection of 3 mg each day for 14 consecutive days, but a weight loss of 3 g was observed. Seven out of eight mice survived two daily injections of 3 mg at 4–6 hr intervals with a similar weight loss. No shrinkage of the spleen was seen at the end of the series of injections (at variance with Peczenik's observation, 1953), but there was a very significant decrease in the weight of the thymus, which may be related to increased glucocorticoid secretion (see Chapter 3.4).

Mice treated daily during 24 days with an i.p. dose of 3 mg of MEA generally survived; i.p. injection of MEA once a week for 40 weeks also caused few fatalities (Nelson *et al.*, 1967).

2.2.5. CONTINUOUS FEEDING

Mitchell (1935), Jackson and Bloch (1936), and Wellers (1954) have given cystamine mixed in the food (up to 0.5%) for periods of 20–27 days and failed, like Bacq (1956), to observe any toxic reaction. The experience of Sebrell and Daft (1939) is completely different; all young rats fed a normal diet in which 0.5% cystamine had been mixed died in 12–19 days; their bones were unusually brittle, and the epiphyses were easily detachable. This fact has been confirmed by Dasler (1955) using MEA; he considered the lesions to be identical with those of lathyrism due to aminopropionitrile (the active principle of the sweet pea). Dasler accordingly suggested that the presence of a nitrile may not be required for lathyric action. Our experience (Bacq and Ponlot, 1955; Bacq, 1956) is that young rats tolerated 1% cystamine (2HCl = 0.67% base) in food during 45 days, but growth was markedly retarded; when killed, these rats showed intense pulmonary vasodilatation and serosity in the alveoli. The concentration of 0.5% cystamine (2HCl) in food, for 2 months, slightly slowed down the increase in weight. No bone lesions have been seen. No reasonable explanation can be suggested for the toxicity of the stock of MEA used by Dasler.

A decrease in weight was also observed in mice when cystamine was mixed in the food at a concentration of 1 or 0.5% (Bacq and Van Caneghem, 1966; Van Caneghem, 1969). Decreased food consumption is the simple reason; appetite did not seem to be specifically inhibited but food was rendered rather unpalatable. This phenomenon may be of some importance for the interpretation of Harman's (1962, 1969) results. Apparently the introduction of cysteine (1%), MEA (1%), or cystamine (0.5%) in food throughout life (beginning shortly after weaning) resulted in an *increased* life span in certain strains of mice. Harman claims this fact as argument in favor of his hypothesis that ageing is due to damage by constantly occurring free radicals which would be "scavenged" by the protective agents.

Apart from the fact that we know very little about the frequency, quality, life span, etc. of the free radicals which occur naturally within mammalian tissues, there are three important objections to this interpretation:

1. The concentration of free MEA reached in the tissues, even at the optimum time after injection of a single maximal tolerated dose, is not sufficient to affect the fate of free radicals produced by exposure to ionizing radiation (MEA must be free in order to react with free radicals) (see Bacq, 1965 for this discussion). The tissue concentration of free MEA when the amine is constantly absorbed by the gastrointestinal tract has not been determined but must be very small owing to rapid liver detoxication.

2. Bacq and Van Caneghem (1966) failed to find the slightest protection against continuous exposure to low levels of X-rays by continuous feeding with cystamine.

3. The life span of control pair-fed mice (i.e. of mice which would, by food restriction, show similar weight reduction) is not given by Harman (1962, 1969); one cannot exclude that underfeeding is the cause of the increased life span.

It is not surprising that sulfhydryl amines are toxic when administered regularly in sufficient amounts over a long period of time. Rats treated for 4 weeks with an excess of certain amino acids such as phenylalanine showed an inhibition of growth, marked damage to the pancreas, slight damage to the liver, hyperkeratosis of the skin and an inhibition of spermatogenesis by failure of spermatids to mature (Klavins, 1967).

Benson *et al.* (1961) found no effect on growth in rats fed 0.1, 0.3, and 0.5% AET for a period of one month. One per cent AET in the diet produced a moderate depression of growth, whereas an increase in white blood cells was observed at all dietary levels of AET. Histological lesions attributable to the ingestion of AET were not detected. Preston *et al.* (1959) described a retardation of growth when 0.5% AET was fed to rats; 1% did not afford protection.

2.3. TOXICITY OF MIXTURES OF CHEMICAL RADIOPROTECTIVE AGENTS

All recent attempts to discover chemical protective agents more active than MEA, AET, or 5-HT against acute radiation death in mammals have failed. For 10 years, mixtures of chemical protective agents have

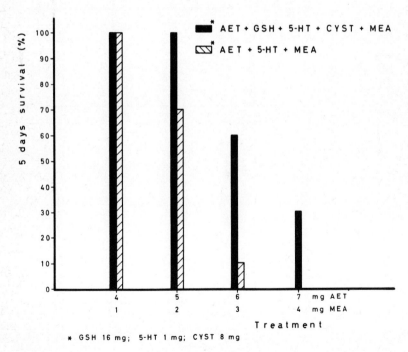

FIG. 3. Five days survival of normal mice treated with different doses of a mixture of AET + MEA + 5-HT or AET + MEA + 5-HT + cysteine + GSH.

been used by several investigators to increase protection against radiation damage (see Maisin *et al.*, 1968, 1970).

Some of these mixtures of radioprotective compounds are of value since the protection obtained by separate administration of each compound is potentiated, and their general toxicity decreased (Fig. 3). These mixtures have, however, no favorable effect on cellular toxicity, which may even increase. Thus, the toxicity of i.p. administration of AET to mice is lessened by ingestion of glutathione 15 min before the administration of the

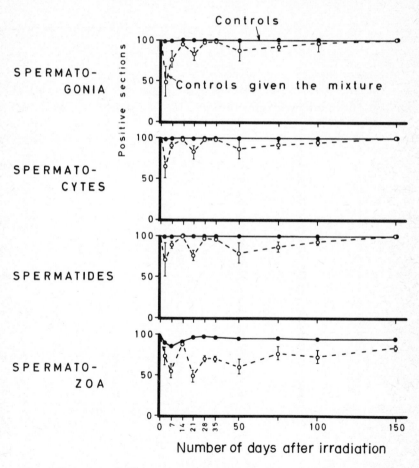

Fig. 4. Percentage of different types of germ-cells in tubule sections of testis of mice treated with a mixture of AET + MEA + 5-HT + cysteine + GSH.

AET, or by i.p. administration of cysteine simultaneously with the AET. Such lowering of toxicity is possible also for repeated doses of AET. Diethyldithiocarbamate, AET, and MEA diminish the glutathione content of liver and kidney; treatment with glutathione may, therefore, compensate for certain effects of these substances (Zins *et al.*, 1959). Similar observations on mice have been reported by Gantz and Wang (1964) and by Therkelsen (1958b) in tissue culture.

Mixtures of certain chemical protective drugs are, however, not less toxic than the single compounds (Maisin and Doherty, 1963; Plzak *et al.*, 1958; Zherebchenko *et al.*, 1962). Simultaneous administration of AET (100 mg/kg) and dimethylammonium-dimethyldithiocarbamate (300 mg/kg) damaged kidneys and liver more severely than each compound given separately at the same dose level (DuBois *et al.*, 1958).

Potent mixtures of protective drugs may have side effects not seen with single substances. For example, a mixture of MEA, AET, 5-HT, cysteine, and reduced glutathione (Maisin *et al.*, 1968) provided good radioprotection to spermatogenic cells, but also significantly decreased the number of cells in the various stages of germination from treatment. A difference between non-treated and treated animals persisted for 100 days after treatment with respect to the number of spermatogonia, spermatocytes, and spermatids; normal sperm counts in testis and epididymis were not seen even 150 days after the treatment (Fig. 4) (Léonard *et al.*, 1969b).

Pretreatment with chlorpromazine reduced the magnitude of the rise in hematocrit which followed the administration of a mixture of (5-HT) + AET + MEA and prevented death from chemical toxicity during multiple radiation exposures. Chlorpromazine also slightly reduced the radioprotective efficacy of the chemical mixture (Hasegawa and Wang, 1971).

2.4. VARIOUS OBSERVATIONS

Attempts have been made to diminish the toxicity of protective compounds by giving substances counteracting their general deleterious effects. Administration of chlorpromazine (12 mg/kg), ether, magnesium sulfate, and phenobarbital have indeed successfully decreased the toxicity of MEA in mice. Pyridoxine, reserpine, diphenylhydantoin, and antihistaminics are not effective (Yam and DuBois, 1965; Yam *et al.*, 1964). Anesthesia in dogs reduces the emetic and convulsive reactions to 100 mg of MEA, but does not affect the cardiovascular changes (Mundy and Heiffer, 1960).

The toxicity of *N,N*-diethylcysteamine (but not of MEA) in mice is markedly potentiated by copper sulfate injected 15 min before, together with, or 15 min after the thiol. The tremor caused by *N,N*-diethylcysteamine is increased by copper sulfate (Curzon and Schnieden, 1965).

2.5. CONCLUSIONS

The most active sulfur-containing radioprotective chemicals are toxic to all living systems and particularly to mammals; the range between the active and the toxic dose is narrow. Deleterious effects of protective compounds occur at the cellular, tissue, and general levels. Some of the general toxic effects following the administration of a sulfur-containing radioprotective agent are secondary in nature, and not related to the protective capacity of the drug. Cellular toxicity appears to be the responsible factor for the protective power, at least in mammals (see Chapter 9). Certain mixtures of radioprotective agents are of value since they provide greater protection than each compound given separately and simultaneously decrease some of the general toxic effects.

Further investigations are necessary before single substances or mixtures of substances may be tried in man as protective agents against the effects of exposure to ionizing radiation .

REFERENCES

ÅKERFELDT, S., RÖNNBACK, C., HELLSTRÖM, M. and NELSON, A. (1968) Radioprotective agents: Further results with amidophosphorotioate and· related compounds. *Radiat. Res.* **35**: 61–7.

ALBANO, V. and OLIVA, L. (1955) Profilassi e terapia del male da raggi mediante bete-mercaptoetilamina. *Radiologia* (*Roma*) **11**: 37–61.

ARBUSOW, S. J., BASANOW, V. A., NEKATSCHALOWA, I. J., PATALOWA, W. N., PETELINA, W. W. and SCHAMOWA, E. K. (1959) Über die Verteilung des ^{35}S-β-Merkaptoethyla-mins in den Organen und Geweben bestrahlter und nicht bestrahlter Ratten. *Acta Biol. Med. Germ.* **3**: 417–32.

BACQ, Z. M. (1953) La cystamine, protecteur par voie orale contre le rayonnement X. *Bull. Acad. Roy. Méd. Belg.,* VIth series **18**: 426–35.

BACQ, Z. M. (1956) Efficacité et absence de toxicité de la cystamine en ingestion chez le rat. *Bull. Acad. Roy. Méd. Belg.,* VIth series **21**: 121–9.

BACQ, Z. M. (1965) *Chemical Protection against Ionizing Radiation.* Charles Thomas Publ., Springfield, Illinois, U.S.A., 344 p.

BACQ, Z. M. and GOUTIER, R. (1967) Mechanisms of action of sulfur-containing radio-protectors. In: *Recovery and Repair Mechanisms in Radiobiology,* Brookhaven Symposium No. 20, pp. 241–62.

BACQ, Z. M. and HERVE, A. (1952) Protection chimique contre le rayonnement X. *Bull. Acad. Roy. Méd. Belg.*, VIth series **17**: 13–58.

BACQ, Z. M. and HERVE, A. (1955) Nouvelles obsèrvations sur l'action radioprotectrice de la cystamine administrée en ingestion. *C.R. Soc. Biol.* **149**: 1509–12.

BACQ, Z. M. and PONLOT, R. (1955) Toxicité chronique de la cystamine. *C.R. Soc. Biol.* **149**: 2012–14.

BACQ, Z. M. and VAN CANEGHEM, P. (1966) The influence of cystamine administered by mouth to mice irradiated with gamma-rays at a low dose-rate. *Int. J. Rad. Biol.* **10**: 595–9.

BACQ, Z. M., HERVE, A., LECOMTE, J., FISCHER, P., BLAVIER, J., DECHAMPS, G., LE BIHAN, H. and RAYET, P. (1951) Protection contre le rayonnement X par la mercaptoéthylamine. *Arch. internat. Physiol.* **59**: 442–7.

BACQ, Z. M., DECHAMPS, G., FISCHER, P., HERVE, A., LE BIHAN, H., LECOMTE, J., PIROTTE, M. and RAYET, P. (1953) Protection against X-rays and therapy of radiation sickness with β-mercaptoethylamine. *Science* **117**: 633–6.

BACQ, Z. M., BEAUMARIAGE, M. L., GOUTIER, R. and VAN CANEGHEM, P. (1968) The state of shock induced by cystamine and cysteamine. *Brit. J. Pharmacol.* **34**: 202 p.

BECCARI, E., BIANCHI, C. and FELDER, E. (1955) Chemisch-physikalische, pharmakologische und klinische Untersuchungen über β-mercaptoaethylamin, besonders im Hinblick auf die Bleivergiftung. *Arzneim. Forsch.* **5**: 421–8.

BEAUMARIAGE, M. L., VAN CANEGHEM, P., PLOMTEUX, G., BACQ, Z. M. and HEUSGHEM, C. (1970) Accroissement du taux sangium de différents enzymes cellulaires après radioprotecteurs soufrés. IVe Congrès International de Physiopathologie et de Physicochimie des Rayonnements, 29 June–4 July, Evian.

BENSON, R. E., MICHAELSON, S. M., DOWNS, W. L., MAYNARD, E. A., SCOTT, J. K., HODGE, H. C. and HOWLAND, J. W. (1961) Toxicological and radioprotection studies on S, β-aminoethylisothiouronium bromide (AET). *Radiat. Res.* **15**: 561–72.

CAFFARATI, E. (1951a) Alcune sostanze ad azione riducente (cisteina, acido tioglicolico acido ascorbico, associazione cisteina ed acido ascorbico) come agenti protettivi nelle lesioni biochimiche da raggi X. Nota I. *Radioter. Radiobiol.* **4**: 378–94.

CAFFARATI, E. (1951b) Alcune sostanze ad azione riducente come agenti protettivi nelle lesioni biochimiche da raggi X. Nota II. *Radioter. Radiobiol.* **4**: 395–410.

CHAPMAN, W. H. and CRONKITE, E. P. (1950) Further studies of the beneficial effect of glutathione on X-irradiated mice. *Proc. Soc. Exptl. Biol. Med.* **75**: 318–22.

CROUGH, B. G. and OVERMAN, R. R. (1957) Chemical protection against X-irradiation death primates: A preliminary report. *Science* **125**: 1092.

CURZON, G. and SCHNIEDEN, H. (1965) The effect of copper sulphate on the LD_{50} of cysteamine and *N,N*-diethyl-cysteamine and on tremor induced by these compounds. *Biochem. Pharmacol.* **14**: 289–94.

DACQUISTO, M. P. and BLACKBURN, E. W. (1961) Protective effect of orally administered S,β-aminoethylisothiouronium-Br-HBr against X-radiation death in mice. *Nature* **190**: 270.

DASLER, W. (1955) Production of experimental lathyrism in the rat by two different beta-substituted ethylamines. *Proc. Soc. Exptl. Biol. Med.* **88**: 196–9.

DISTEFANO, V. (1964) Some remarks on the pharmacology of radioprotectant agents. *Ann. N.Y. Acad. Sci.* **114**: 588–96.

DOHERTY, D. G. and BURNETT, W. T., JR. (1955) Protective effect of S,β-aminoethylisothiouronium-Br-HBr and related compounds against X-radiation death in mice. *Proc. Soc. Exptl. Biol. Med.* **89**: 312–14.

DOHERTY, D. G., BURNETT, W. T., JR. and SHAPIRA, R. (1957) Chemical protection against ionizing radiation. II. Mercaptoalkylamines and related compounds with protective activity. *Radiat. Res.* **7**: 13–21.

DOULL, J., PLZAK, V., BROIS, S. J. and NOBLE, J. F. (1958) The influence of various chemical compounds on radiation lethality in mice. *USAFRL Quart. Report,* No. **29**: 46.

DOULL, J., PLZAK, V. and BROIS, S. J. (1962) A survey of compounds for radiation protection. Document 62–29–USAF Aerospace Medical Division. Brooks Air Force Base, Texas, U.S.A. 124 p.

DUBOIS, K. P., RAYMUND, A. B. and HIETBRINK, B. E. (1958) The effect of ionizing radiations on the biochemistry of mammalian tissues. I. Enzymatic measurements of cumulative toxic effect of repeated doses of sulfur-containing radioprotective agents. *Chicago Univ. Air Force Radiation Lab.* NP-11359, pp. 1–15.

FOYE, W. D. and ZAIM, R. H. (1964) Antiradiation compounds. V. α-Amino acid esters of 2-mercaptoethylamine. *J. Pharm. Sci.* **53**: 906–8.

GANTZ, J. A. and WANG, R. I. H. (1964) Reduction in radiation lethality by chemical mixture and bone-marrow in mice. *J. Nucl. Med.* **5**: 606–12.

GRESHAM, P. A., BARNETT, M., VAUGHAN SMITH, S. and SCHNEIDER, R. (1971) Use of sustained-release multiple emulsion to extend the period of radioprotection conferred by cystamine. *Nature* **234**: 149–50.

GRIFFITH, W. H. and DYER, H. M. (1966) *A Study of Research Methodology for Use in the Development of Antiradiation Agents.* Life Sciences Research Office, Washington, D.C., p. 45.

HANNA, C. and COLCLOUGH, N. V. (1963) Toxicity and tolerance studies on AET. *Arch. int. Pharmacodyn.* **142**: 510–15.

HARMAN, D. (1962) Role of free radicals in mutation, cancer, ageing and the maintenance of life. *Radiat. Res.* **16**: 753–63.

HARMAN, D. (1969) Chemical protection against ageing. *Agents and Actions.* **1**: 3–8.

HASEGAWA, A. T. and WANG, R. I. H. (1971) Attenuation of increased vascular permeability of a radioprotective chemical mixture by chlorpromazine in mice. *Radiation Res.* **45**: 364–72.

HASEGAWA, A. T. and LANDAHL, H. D. (1970) Dose reduction factor for radiation lethality in mice as a function of the dose of mercaptoethylamine. *Radiation Res.* **44**: 738–47.

HERVE, A. and BACQ, Z. M. (1952) Protection chimique contre le rayonnement X. Essais thérapeutiques. *J. Radiol. Electrol.* **33**: 651–5.

HOLLAENDER, A. and DOUDNEY, C. O. (1955) Studies on the mechanism of radiation protection and recovery with cysteamine and β-mercaptoethanol. *Radiobiology Symposium, Liège* 1955, Butterworth, London, 112–15.

HUBER, R. and SPODE, E. (1961, 1963) *Biologisch-Chemischer Strahlenschutz,* II and IV, Akademie-Verlag, Berlin.

HULSE, E. V. (1963) The acute toxic effects of cysteamine and their modification by X-irradiation. *Intern. J. Radiat. Biol.* **6**: 323–9.

JACKSON, R. W. and BLOCH, R. J. (1936) Does bis (2-aminoethyl) disulfide (cystamine) promote growth in the rat limited to an inadequate intake of cystine and methionine? *J. Biol. Chem.* **113**: 135–9.

JAKOVLEV, V. G. and IVANOV, I. I. (1958) Chemical protection of animals from the effect of X-rays. *Med. Radiol. (Mosk.)* **3**: 14.

JULIANI, G. and ORSO, G. P. (1956) Observazioni sulla cura del male da raggi con cisteamina per os. *Gaz. Med. ital.* **115/8**: 1.

KLAVINS, J. V. (1967) Pathology of amino acid excess. VII. Phenylalanine and tyrosine. *Arch. Pathol.* **84**: 238–50.

KOCH, R. and SCHWARZE, W. (1957) Toxikologische und chemische Untersuchungen und β-Aminoäthylisothiouronium Verbindungen. *Arzneim. Forsch.* **7**: 476–9.

KOCH, R., KLEMM, D. and SEITER, I. (1960) Zur Toxikologie schwefelhaltiger Pyridoxin-Derivate. *Arzneim. Forsch.* **10**: 683–6.

KOLÀŘ, V. (1958) Léceni irradiacniho syndrom. *Vnitrni Lek.* **4**: 708–15.

KOLLMANN, G., SHAPIRO, B. and SCHWARTZ, E. E. (1963) The mechanism of action of AET. V. The distribution and the chemical forms of 2-mercaptoethylguanidine and bis(2-guanidoethyl)disulfide given orally in protective doses to mice. *Radiat. Res.* **20:** 17–23.

LANDAHL, H. D. and HASEGAWA, A. T. (1970) Pharmacological and toxicological compounds as protective or therapeutic agents against radiation injury in experimental animals. III. Studies on the dose reduction factor for irradiation lethality in mice as a function of the dose mercaptoethylamine. *Chicago Univ. Air Force Radiation Lab.* NP-11966, pp. 123–7.

LÉONARD, A., MAISIN, J. R., and DEKNUDT, GH. (1969a) Effect of age and AET on lifespan of irradiated male and female rats. *Strahlentherapie* **137:** 92–100.

LÉONARD, A., MAISIN, J. R. and MATTELIN, G. (1969b) Effect of mixture of chemical protectors against X-irradiation induced testis injury in mice. *Strahlentherapie* **137:** 92–100.

LÉONARD, A. and MATTELIN, G. (1970) Effets à long terme de la S-(2-aminoéthyl)-iso-thiourée-Br HBr administrée aux souris. *Compt. Rend. Soc. Biol.* **164:** 907–9.

MAISIN, J. (1966) Au sujet de la lecture de M. Z. M. Bacq intitulée "La protection chimique contre les radiations ionisantes chez les mammifères. *Bul. Acad. Roy. Méd. Belg.,* VIIth series **6:** 293–300.

MAISIN, J. R. (1968) Effet protecteur toxicité et mécanisme d'action des associations de substances radioprotectrices. *Bul. Acad. Roy. Méd. Belg.,* VIIth series **8:** 149–82.

MAISIN, J. R. (1969) Reduction of long-term radiation lethality by mixtures of chemical protectors. *Atomkernenergie* **14:** 226–8.

MAISIN, J. R. and DOHERTY, D. G. (1963) Comparative chemical protection to the intestinal hematopoietic systems of whole-body X-irradiated mice. *Radiat. Res.* **19:** 474–84.

MAISIN, J. R. and LAMBIET, M. (1967) Influence of a mixture of chemical radioprotectors on the cellular renewal in the duodenum of mice. *Nature* **214:** 412–13.

MAISIN, J., DUNJIC, A. and COUVREUR, P. (1964) Protective effects of cysteamine and cystamine on the irradiated rats. *J. Belg. Radiol.* **47:** 755–71.

MAISIN, J. R., LÉONARD, A. and HUGON, J. (1965) Tissue and cellular distribution of tritium labeled AET in mice. *J. Nat. Cancer Inst.* **35:** 103–12.

MAISIN, J. R., MATTELIN, G., FRIDMAN-MANDUZIO, A. and VAN DER PARREN, J. (1968) Reduction of short- and long-term radiation lethality by mixture of chemical protectors. *Radiat. Res.* **35:** 26–44.

MAISIN, J. R., MATTELIN, G. and LAMBIET-COLLIER, M. (1970) Reduction of short- and long-term radiation effects by mixtures of chemical protectors. *Intern. J. Rad. Biol.* **19:** 355–61.

MELVILLE, G. S., JR. and LEFFINGWELL, T. P. (1962) Toxic and protective effects of AET upon normal and irradiated female rats. *Brit. J. Radiol.* **35:** 563–71.

MITCHELL, H. H. (1935) The substitution of dithio-ethylamine (cystine amine) for cystine in the diet of the white rat. *J. Biol. Chem.* **111:** 699–705.

MORGAN, W., MAISIN, J. R., CALLEBAUT, M. and MATTELIN, G. (1969) Disorientation response of chicks which survived 2-β-aminoethylisothiouronium-Br-HBr (AET) administration during early embryogenesis. *Intern. J. Rad. Biol.,* Intern. Symp. on Radiosensitizing and Radioprotective Drugs, Rome, 6–8 May.

MUNDY, R. L. and HEIFFER, M. H. (1960) The pharmacology of radioprotectant chemicals. General pharmacology of β-mercaptoethylamine. *Radiat. Res.* **13:** 381–94.

NELSON, A., HERTZBERG, O. and RÖNNBÁCK, C. (1967) Protective effect of cysteamine at fractionated irradiation. II. Shortening of life span. *Acta Radiol. Therapy Physics Biol.* **6:** 449–63.

NEWSOME, J. R., KNOTT, D. H. and OVERMAN, R. R. (1962) Radioprotective effects of β-aminoethylisothiouronium-Br-HBr in the dog. *Radiat. Res.* **17:** 847–54.

ONKELINX, C. (1961) Absence de radioprotection chimique chez l'embryon de poulet irradié "in toto". *C.R. Soc. Biol.* **155:** 1604–7.

PATT, H. M., SMITH, D. E., TYREE, E. B. and STRAUBE, R. L. (1950) Further studies on modification of sensitivity to X-rays by cysteine. *Proc. Soc. Exptl. Biol. Med.* **73**: 18–21.

PECZENIK, O. (1953) Influence of cysteinamine, methylamine and cortisone on the toxicity and activity of nitrogen mustard. *Nature* **172**: 454–6.

PIHL, A. and ELDJARN, L. (1958) Pharmacological aspects of ionizing radiation and of chemical protection in mammals. *Pharmacol. Rev.* **10**: 437–75.

PLOMTEUX, G., BEAUMARIAGE, M. L., BACQ, Z. M. and HEUSGHEM, C. (1967) Variations enzymatiques dans le plasma du rat après injection d'une dose radioprotectrice de cystéamine. *Biochem. Pharmacol.* **16**: 1601–7.

PLOMTEUX, G., BEAUMARIAGE, M. L., BACQ, Z. M. and HEUSGHEM, C. (1968) Influence du β-mercaptoethanol sur certains enzymes plasmatiques du rat. *Biochem. Pharmacol.* **17**: 1998–2002.

PLZAK, V., DOULL, J. and ROOT, M. (1958) Pharmacological and toxicological compounds as protective or therapeutic agents against radiation injury in experimental animals. I. Dose–mortality relationship for the toxic and radioprotective effects of various chemical agents. *Chicago Univ. Air Force Radiat. Lab.* NP-11660, pp. 1–15.

PRESTON, R. L., WELLS, A. and ERSHOFF, B. H. (1959) Comparative effects of intraperitoneal and oral administration of AET on survival of X-irradiated rats. *Radiat. Res.* **11**: 255–9.

RAZORENOVA, V. A. and SHERBOVA, E. N. (1961) The use of cysteamine and cystamine for preventive purpose in acute radiation sickness. *Med. Radiol. (Mosk.)* **6/3**: 11.

REYSS-BRION, M. (1962) Protection par la cystéamine de jeunes embryons de poulet soumis ultérieurement à une irradiation aux rayons X. *Arch. Anat. Histol. Embryol. Norm. et Exper.* Suppl. to Vol. **44**: 197–216.

ROUSANOV, A. M. and NOVOSELOVA, G. S. (1962) The protective effects of aminoethylisothiourea against ionizing radiations and its toxic effects according to the age of the white mice. *Ann. Radiol.* **5**: 225–41.

SEBRELL, W. H. and DAFT, F. S. (1939) The effect of cystamine on the albino rat. *J. Biol. Chem.* **128**: 89p.

SHAPIRA, R., DOHERTY, D. G. and BURNETT, W. T., JR. (1957) Chemical protection against ionizing radiation. III. Mercaptoalkylguanidines and related isothiouronium compounds with protective activity. *Radiat. Res.* **7**: 22–34.

TAKAGI, Y., SATO, F., SHIKITA, M., SHINODA, M., TERASIMA, T. and AKABOSHI, S. (1970) Toxicity and radioprophylactic action of 2-mercaptoethylguanidine and its derivatives in mice and Hela S$_3$ cells. *Radiation Res.* **42**: 79–89.

THEISMANN, H. (1955) Érythemhemmung durch Aminosäuren. *Strahlentherapie* **96**: 107–10.

THERKELSEN, A. J. (1958a) Combined treatment of a transplantable mouse tumour with cysteamine (β-mercaptoethylamine) and nitrogen mustard (HN2). *Biochem. Pharmacol.* **1**: 245–57.

THERKELSEN, A. J. (1958b) Studies on the cytotoxicity of cysteamine and related compounds in tissue culture. *Acta Pathol. Microbiol. Scand.* **42**: 201–15.

VAN CANEGHEM, P. (1969) Essais de protection de la souris contre l'action létale de radiations ionisantes à faible débit. *Int. J. Rad. Biol.* **16**: 51–5.

VAN DE BERG, F. and VAN DE BERG, L. (1954) Protection chimique et mal des rayons. *J. Belge Radiol.* **37**: 562–71.

WELLERS, G. (1954) Recherches sur la sulfoconjugaison de l'indol. III. Rôle des sulfures, du soufre élémentaire et de la cystéamine. Importance de la tautomérie ceto-énolique. *Bull. Soc. Chim. Biol.* **36**: 1655–64.

YAM, KEI-MING and DUBOIS, K. P. (1965) The effects of ionizing radiations on the biochemistry of mammalian tissues. I. Studies on the toxicity and mechanism of action of 2-mercaptoethylamine (MEA). *Chicago Univ. Air Force Radiat. Lab.* NP-15072, pp. 1–6.

YAM, KEI-MING, HEITBRINK, B. E. and DuBois, K. P. (1964) Pharmacological and toxicological compounds as protective or therapeutic agents against radiation injury in experimental animals. III. Studies on the toxicity and mechanism of action of mercaptoethylamine (MEA). *Chicago Univ. Air Force Radiat. Lab.* NP-14448, pp. 98–107.

ZHEREBCHENKO, P. G., KRASNYKH, I. G., KUZNETS, E. I., SUVOROV, N. N., SHASHKOV, V. S. and YARMONENKO, S. P. (1962) The radioprotective effect in combined use of preparations. *Med. Radiol.* 7: 67–81.

ZINS, G. R., RAYMUND, A. B. and SEIDEL, D. M. (1959) The effect of radioprotective agents on the reduced glutathione levels in the tissues of rats. *USAFRL Quart. Report,* No. 32: 14.

CHAPTER 3

GENERAL PHARMACOLOGY

INTRODUCTION

J. Lecomte

Liège, Belgium

THE cardiovascular effects of radioprotective substances are related to the changes they cause in peripheral distribution of oxygen. As oxygen deficiency of circulatory origin results in tissue anoxia, the role of vasomotor disturbance has often been used in interpreting radioprotective activity itself; hence the importance given here to the cardiovascular effects of sulfur-containing radioprotective agents.

After analyzing the vasomotor effects in different animal species, we shall attempt to identify their common characteristics. In general, large doses of radioprotective substances induce lasting cardiovascular collapse, leading to a state of shock. The consequences of the latter, particularly the biochemical changes, are considered in a separate section. Also considered separately are the variations in vascular permeability, the effects on the ductless glands, nervous system, smooth muscles and the skin.

3.1

CARDIOVASCULAR EFFECTS

J. Lecomte

Liège, Belgium

3.1.1. ANALYSIS OF CARDIOVASCULAR REACTIONS INDUCED IN DIFFERENT SPECIES

3.1.1.1. FROG AND TORTOISE

Cystamine

In concentrations ranging from 1×10^{-5} to 1×10^{-2} g/l acting on the heart attached to a Straub canula, cystamine has no effect on the amplitude or rhythm of the contractions and does not affect myocardial excitability (Robbers, 1937; Della Bella and Bacq, 1953).

Cysteamine

Cysteamine (0.1 %) has no effect on isolated frog's heart or tortoise myocardium *in situ*. It exerts a slight atropinic effect which, in the tortoise, arrests the effects of vagal stimulation (Della Bella and Bacq, 1953).

3.1.1.2. CHICKEN

Cystamine

In certain individuals, a slight, short drop in arterial pressure is observed with 0.25 mg/kg, and this is proportional to the dose. Sometimes this drop is unexpectedly followed by a rise in pressure. The drop in pressure is suppressed by atropine while the rise in pressure can be suppressed by blocking the α-adrenergic receptors. Vasomotor changes are not affected by prior histamine depletion (Beaumariage *et al.*, 1966).

41

Cysteamine

The cardiovascular effects are qualitatively identical to those of cystamine (Beaumariage *et al.*, 1966).

3.1.1.3. MOUSE

DiStefano *et al.* (1962) have studied the cardiovascular effects of some radioprotective agents on mice C3H and C57B1 by recording the carotid pressure.

Cystamine

Doses of up to 16 mg/kg MEA produce no change in arterial pressure, but the pressure drops steadily with the injection of larger quantities. By intraperitoneal (i.p.) route, MEA raises the pressure slightly for at least 50 min (van der Meer *et al.*, 1960; DiStefano *et al.*, 1962).

Aminoethylisothiourea

Doses of from 8 to 16 mg/kg AET produce a slight drop in pressure, followed by a moderate and lasting rise. A similar arterial pressor effect is induced by i.p. injection. The myocardic norepinephrine stores are depleted (DiStefano and Klahn, 1966).

Aminopropylisothiourea

This produces more complex effects. From about 8 mg/kg injected intravenously (i.v.), the pressure drops, rises, falls again and then rises once more; finally a lasting depressor effect is established. By i.p. injection APT raises the pressure.

Aminopropyl-N'-methylisothiourea

This is depressive (4 mg/kg, i.v.). It exerts a pressor effect when injected into the peritoneal cavity.

By way of comparison DiStefano *et al.* (1962) also studied the properties of two iso-thiouronium derivatives devoid of radioprotective properties: 2-aminoethyl-N',N''-methylisothiouronium HBr (AEMMT) and 2,2'-bis (2 aminoethyl)-1,1'-ethylene-isothiouronium HBr (EbAET). Both exert depressor effects (50–300 mg/kg, i.v.). The consequent drop in arterial pressure often results in rapid collapse and death.

According to Rothe *et al.* (1963), the vasopressive activity of the amidines is not directly related to their radioprotective power, which depends on a lowering of the oxygen tension in the radiosensitive tissues.

Cystamine (5 mg/kg, i.p.) evokes an initial rise in arterial pressure, followed by a fall over 15 min (van der Meer *et al.*, 1960).

3.1.1.4. RATS

As the rat is used on a large scale for radiobiological research, the cardiovascular effects of radioprotective agents have been analyzed in greater detail (Heiffer *et al.*, 1962; Lecomte *et al.*, 1964).

3.1.1.4.1. *Cystamine*
Rapid i.v. administration

(a) With a dose range of 2.5–7.5 mg/kg the arterial pressure falls, this effect being immediate and proportional to the dose; recovery is rapid, and without tachyphylaxis.

(b) With 20–30 mg/kg, the preliminary drop in pressure is followed by a rise in arterial pressure varying with repetition of the injections according to the individual. The first three or four generally produce similar reactions to the initial injection, but subsequently the pressor effect drops progressively, finally resulting in a lowering of arterial pressure.

(c) With 50 mg/kg a lowering of pressure is observed; this is reproducible. Respiration slows down and in certain animals stops completely, the animal dying in apnea.

(d) With 100 mg/kg or more, the arterial blood pressure drops to zero; the animal dies in collapse. Sometimes a pink edematous fluid invades the trachea.

Continuous i.v. infusions of 1 mg/min

Cystamine infusions result in a significant drop in arterial pressure. Blood pressure remains at the minimum level throughout the perfusion process and does not recover when perfusion has stopped.

Intraperitoneal administration

Cystamine, in doses of from 50 to 200 mg/kg, produces a fall in arterial pressure proportional to the dose.

During the phase of lowered pressure, i.v. injection of cystamine itself (50–100 mg/kg) produces a distinct rise in pressure, from 30 to 60 mm Hg, lasting for 3 to 6 min. A significant fall in the catecholamine content in the adrenal medulla is brought about 30 min after the administration of 50–400 mg/kg cystamine. Blood catecholamine levels rise (Heiffer *et al.*, 1961).

Changes in the properties of certain pharmacodynamic agents

(a) Raised blood pressure and tachycardia due to the catecholamines (epinephrine, norepinephrine, 1–10 mcg/kg) are greatly reduced and sometimes completely suppressed by cystamine (150 mg/kg).

(b) Cystamine (20–100 mg/kg) does not modify the depressor effect of histamine (5–10 mcg/kg). However, it reduces the pressor effect of histamine to the extent of α-blocker proportions.

(c) Doses of 100 mg/kg of cystamine do not affect the depressor effects of 5-hydroxytryptamine (5-HT) (0.2–0.5 mcg).

Changes in the properties of cystamine itself

The arterial hypertension produced by cystamine is not affected by blocking sympathetic ganglion transmission, by blocking α-adrenergic receptors, or by bilateral adrenalectomy. Depletion of histamine stores and administration of antihistaminics oppose the fall of blood pressure induced by cystamine.

3.1.1.4.2. *Cysteamine*

This produces vasomotor effects qualitatively analogous to those of cystamine (Lecomte *et al.*, 1964).

Intravenous route

(a) Cysteamine produces an immediate fall in arterial pressure proportional to the dose; it is not subject to tachyphylaxis, and recovery is immediate. If the dose is increased (50–100 mg/kg), a rise in arterial pressure may follow the phase of lowered pressure, which is of shorter duration. The intensity of this raised pressure varies from 5 to 30 mmHg according to the animal. It diminishes gradually with successive injections. An initial injection of 20–40 mg MEA causes the pressure to drop completely, and cardiovascular collapse ensues, sometimes followed rapidly by death.

(b) Neither bilateral adrenalectomy nor blocking of the α-adrenergic receptors reduces the raised pressure produced by MEA.

(c) It reduces the raised pressure due to 0.1 mcg epinephrine and norepinephrine. Histamine depressor effect (1 to 2 mcg) is less marked, but lasts longer.

(d) Cysteamine is less toxic on the anesthetized rat than cystamine (100 and 200 mg/kg, i.v., respectively). Toxicity is increased by bilateral adrenalectomy.

Intraperitoneal route

Intraperitoneal administration of 200–500 mg/kg of MEA produces a progressive fall in arterial pressure, which—like cystamine—results in a state of collapse with cyanosis. Adrenalectomy aggravates the state of collapse, which is counteracted by epinephrine (Fischer *et al.*, 1955).

Perfusion of excised organs

Cysteamine (from 10 mg at a time) causes a reduction in the perfusion flow of the isolated hindquarters and perfused intestine (van der Meer *et al.*, 1960).

3.1.1.4.3. *Aminoethyl Isothiourea (AET), Mercaptoethylguanidine (MEG)*

This study was conducted by Lecomte and Bacq (1965) under conditions such that AET was immediately transformed into MEG (see p. 11).

Intravenous administration

Administration of small doses of MEG (2.5 mg/kg) produces a rise in arterial pressure in the rat, which increases with doses up to 10 mg/kg. This rise in pressure is reproducible and tachyphylaxis does not occur.

Administration of 5 mg/kg MEG causes a fall in arterial pressure— from 20 to 30 mmHg over a period of 2–3 min—in 10% of the rats studied.

When the arterial pressure is normal, a medium dose of MEG raises the pressure with an amplitude of 30–40 mmHg, lasting for 2–3 min, after a sharp, short initial drop (5–10 sec) due to bradycardia.

The rise in pressure is followed by a more lasting depressor effect (30–40 mmHg) over a period of 5–10 min. The pressure then becomes stabilized at the normal or at a slightly lower level. When the arterial pressure is low (about 50 mmHg), MEG initially causes a short drop, due to bradycardia, followed by a rapid increase in pressure, up to 80–100 mmHg, which is dissipated slowly, sometimes taking 10–15 min.

Repetition of an equal second dose of MEG reduces the initial brady-cardia, and this is accompanied by an increase in height and duration of the pressor effect.

Bilateral vagotomy suppresses the initial bradycardia, but does not prevent the depressor effect which demonstrates the intoxication of the rat.

Administration of 100 mg/kg MEG causes an immediate fall in pressure to zero. This cardiovascular collapse is usually irreversible. However, if artificial respiration is used and the thorax massaged, arterial pressure may be restored to normal. Soon afterwards, in 30–40% of animals, invasion of the tracheal passage by a pink fluid is observed, showing evidence of an acute pulmonary edema.

Intraperitoneal administration

In doses up to 500 mg/kg, MEG induces a slight rise in arterial pressure, reaching 10 or 20 mmHg. This rise starts within the first 3 min and continues for at least 30 min. With doses of 1000 mg/kg, a slight drop (10–20 mmHg) is seen. With 1500 mg/kg, the rat goes into cardiovascular collapse and dies in about 30 min.

Changes in the vasomotor effects of MEG

Pretreatment of the rat with guanethidine (20 mg/kg) increases pressor effect due to MEG. This effect is not modified by α-blockers, bilateral adrenalectomy, or hexamethonium (30 mg/kg, i.v.).

Synthetic antihistaminics administered peritoneally slightly modify some of the vasomotor effects of MEG. In the unusual cases of rats reacting to very small doses of MEG by a fall in pressure, antihistaminics reverse this effect, causing a pressure rise. The toxicity of MEG is not affected.

In animals treated with a specific anti-5-HT, MEG normally exerts a pressor effect.

Changes in the properties of certain pharmacodynamic agents

Doses of up to 200 mg/kg MEG modify the vasomotor effects of epinephrine; raising of arterial pressure becomes diphasic (raised pressure followed by lowered pressure) or is reversed. The lowered pressure is suppressed by dichloroisopropylnorepinephrine (DCI)—20 mg/kg. The raised pressure due to the norepinephrine is steadily reduced (by 40–50%) after 200 mg/kg of MEG.

A dose of 20 mg/100 g, i.p., MEG produces very moderate antihistaminic effects, but 250–500 mg/kg MEG, unlike MEA, increases postacetylcholine arterial pressor effects (Schliep and Michailov, 1965), and potentiates the pressor effects of 5-HT. This pressor effect is suppressed by phenothiazines but is not altered by adrenolytics (Schliep, 1965). Inversion of the depressor effects of 5-HT is not induced by other sulfur-containing radioprotective agents (Cession-Fossion *et al.*, 1968).

Action on the adrenal medulla

The catecholamine content of the adrenal medulla of rats treated with MEG (0.5–1 g/kg, i.p.) shows a slight increase (Cession-Fossion *et al.*, 1964).

Wang *et al.* (1971) have studied the cardiovascular responses of rats to radioprotective compounds. Their conclusions are the following:

"Heart rate and blood pressure were measured in anesthetized rats after i.p. administration of radioprotective doses of 5-HT, MEA, AET, and their mixtures. All of the chemicals produced a slowing of the heart in most of the animals. Both doses of 5-HT (7 and 14 mg/kg) consistently elicited a marked depressor response. While a low dose of AET (100 mg/kg) had little effect, higher doses (175 and 250 mg/kg) tended to increase blood pressure. On the other hand low doses of MEA (60 and 120 mg/kg) tended to lower blood pressure, while a high dose (165 mg/kg) produced no significant change. The blood pressure response after the administration of the mixtures of the chemicals appeared to be the resultant effect of the action of each component. The mixture of all three chemicals (7 mg/kg 5-HT, 100 mg/kg AET, 60 mg/kg MEA) elicited the most consistent response in all animals, slowing the heart rate by 20% and decreasing the blood pressure by 35%. The blood pressure reached its nadir 5 min after injection and remained relatively low for an additional 10 min. These conclusions are in close agreement with previous studies."

3.1.1.5. GUINEA-PIG

Intravenous injection of 0.5–2 g of cystamine causes changes in the electrocardiogram, which reveals excitation and conduction abnormalities (Kuna and Vokrouhlicky, 1967).

3.1.1.6. RABBIT

Cystamine

Cystamine (1 mg/kg, i.v., or more) results in a reproducible fall in arterial pressure. The animal can be kept in a state of permanent reduced pressure by repeated 15 mg/kg doses. With higher doses, the arterial depressor effect becomes irreversible, and the animal dies in acute collapse (Robbers, 1937; Lecomte, 1952a; Beaumariage *et al.,* 1966).

Lowered arterial pressure is accompanied by a vasodilatation, as is shown by perfusion of the excised ear (Pisemski's method). Increase in flow is observed at 1×10^{-5} and 1×10^{-4} g/l. The dilatory effects of cystamine oppose vasoconstriction due to epinephrine.

The coronary arteries are dilated *in vitro* in perfused hearts using Langendorf's method (Van de Berg, 1954). Cystamine (1×10^{-4} g/l) applied directly to the mesenteric vessels has no effect on their diameter (Lecomte, 1956).

Doses of from 50 to 200 mg/kg cystamine depress the activity of the sino-atrial node (sinus venosus) and the bundle of His. It causes the sudden appearance of ectopic beats, ventricular fibrillation, and finally, with large doses, preagonal bradycardia. These modifications of heart rhythm occur simultaneously with vascular collapse. They do not reappear after repeated administration of very small doses (Kuna and Vokrouhlicky, 1967).

Cysteamine

Less than 25 mg/kg MEA induces a slight lowering of blood pressure, from 10 to 15 mmHg, of short duration, followed by a sharp rise in pressure; this can reach 5 mmHg for 2–3 min. With 50 mg/kg MEA lowering of blood pressure is the most pronounced effect (Lecomte and Van de Berg, 1953; Beaumariage *et al.*, 1966).

The lowering of blood pressure due to sulfur-containing derivatives is not affected by atropine, antihistaminics, or histamine depletion. Aprotinin (Trasylol®) has no effect on the drop in arterial pressure (Beaumariage *et al.*, 1966).

Neither cystamine nor MEA has any atropinic or antihistaminic activity. Both slightly potentiate the epinephrine pressor effect (Lecomte and Van de Berg, 1953), but do not affect the first stages of the direct local allergic reaction of the Arthus type (Lecomte, 1956).

Aminoethylisothiourea

A single injection of AET administered to rabbits anesthetized by ethyl urethane causes a drop in arterial pressure, which is of short duration (Laborit *et al.*, 1959).

At 1×10^{-3} g/l, the amplitude of the contractions of the excised right auricle increases. The tonus of aortic strips is reduced (Laborit *et al.*, 1959).

3.1.1.7. CAT

Cystamine

Cystamine (15 mg/kg, i.v.) results in an immediate drop in arterial pressure of long duration, which is reproducible. The intensity is proportional to the dose, and there is a tendency to permanent lowered arterial pressure since re-establishment of the initial values is incomplete (Robbers, 1937; Lecomte, 1952a, b; Beaumariage *et al.*, 1966). Cystamine does not affect the performance of the Starling's heart–lung preparation; it has a coronary-dilating effect. However, *in situ*, the coronary flow always decreases in proportion to the reduction of arterial pressure. The same applies to cardiac output (Robbers, 1937).

Reduced arterial pressure varies according to the initial blood pressure value; the greater this is, the greater will be the drop in pressure. This drop, moreover, occurs together with a marked peripheral vasodilation, revealed by direct inspection of the terminal vascular beds or by plethysmographic exploration. Furthermore, direct measurement of muscular and cutaneous blood flow indicates a lowering of vascular resistance (Robbers, 1937).

The capillaries are simultaneously replenished, and when the lowered arterial pressure is established, the increase in flow diminishes.

According to Robbers (1937), all the cardiovascular effects of larger doses of i.v. administered cystamine depend essentially on a vasodilation which, by general lowering of arterial pressure and peripheral build-up of the blood volume, reduces the return venous flow, the coronary circulation, and finally the cardiac output.

These cardiovascular manifestations develop after a latent period following subcutaneous administration of cystamine. They do not occur with intrajejunal administration. Antihistaminics lessen the cardiovascular effects in an irregular manner; atropine has no effect (Beaumariage *et al.*, 1966).

Cysteamine

According to Robbers, MEA acts in a similar manner to cystamine. Its cardiovascular effects are always established more slowly. When the two compounds are given in equal quantities, the effects of MEA are less marked. These results are confirmed by Beaumariage *et al.* (1966).

Nevertheless, in the spinal cat, whose arterial pressure is low to begin with, MEA is hypertensive. Raised arterial pressure persists after bilateral adrenalectomy and ganglion blocking. It disappears after treatment with α-blockers. Cysteamine behaves like a weak sympathomimetic agent (Goffart, 1955).

Cystamine injected intra-aortically sometimes causes a rise in arterial pressure which results from direct stimulation of the chromaffin cells of the adrenal medulla (Lecomte, 1954; Goffart, 1955).

Aminoethylisothiourea

Administration of 2.5 mg/kg, i.v., AET causes a drop in arterial pressure which is prevented by vagotomy or by atropine. It is accompanied by bradycardia and apnea. In vagotomized animals, AET causes a rise in arterial pressure which persists after adrenalectomy and blockade of the α-adrenergic receptors (DiStefano *et al.*, 1956).

Administration of AET to the normal cat produces an initial fall in arterial pressure due to a vago-vagal reflex and a secondary rise of indeterminate origin (DiStefano and Klahn, 1966).

Aminopropylisothiourea

The cardiovascular effects of APT are identical with those of AET (DiStefano *et al.*, 1959).

Aminobutylisothiourea

This causes lowered arterial pressure, which is slower and of longer duration, and is not affected by vagotomy or atropine (DiStefano *et al.*, 1959).

Analysis of the effects of ABT isomers (DiStefano and Leary, 1959) shows that D-ABT sometimes produces biphasic responses consisting of an initial rise in arterial pressure followed by a fall.

Aminopropylmethylisothiourea

This (24 mg/kg or more) causes a slight rise in arterial pressure, but with small doses (4–16 mg/kg) this is sometimes preceded by a transitory lowering of the blood pressure.

The raised arterial pressure following APMT injection does not depend upon stimulation of the adrenergic system; APMT acts directly on the muscular fibers, causing them to contract (DiStefano *et al.*, 1961).

3.1.1.8. DOG

Cystamine

Intravenous cystamine causes an immediate fall in arterial pressure the intensity and duration of which are proportional to the amount injected, and this depressor effect is reproducible. It is potentiated by bilateral adrenalectomy (Robbers, 1937; Lecomte, 1952a; Mundy and Heiffer, 1960).

Cystamine has no toxic action on Starling's heart–lung preparation. Studies of the local flows performed with the Rein's *Thermostrohmuhr* show that the different vascular beds react like those of the cat. Cystamine causes vasodilatation, which is maximal at the level of the skin and striated musculature. This vasodilatation brings, apart from general lowered arterial pressure, a build-up of blood within the different organs. The volume of these organs increases, whilst the venous return and the cardiac output decrease (Robbers, 1937).

A similar direct vasodilatation appears during perfusion at constant pressure of the kidneys, the adrenals and the intestine transplanted in the neck, the vessels of which have been previously constricted by passing preheated blood (Barac, 1965a, b; Barac *et al.,* 1968).

The fall in arterial pressure induced by cystamine is decreased, but not completely prevented, by pretreatment of the dog with antihistaminics (Lecomte, 1952; Mundy *et al.*, 1963).

As cystamine has no direct excitatory effects on the adrenal medulla (Barac *et al.*, 1968), the rise in blood catecholamine levels following the fall in arterial pressure is due to a compensatory reflex of the adrenergic system (Mundy *et al.,* 1961).

These facts are interpreted by postulating that the cystamine directly dilates the vascular beds, in particular those of the tegument and of the striated musculature. This fall in local resistances explains the drop in the arterial pressure which, itself, reduces local blood flows. One part at least of the depressor action depends on the liberation of histamine induced by cystamine. Secretion of the catecholamines is due to homeostatic mechanisms.

Cysteamine

Cysteamine injected at the rate of 100 mg/kg in 5 min causes a drop in arterial pressure, which slowly recovers its initial level. In certain animals, recovery is transient, the arterial pressure subsequently falling until death. This depressor effect is accompanied by bradycardia, and the hematocrit value as well as the central venous pressure is increased.

Cardiac output decreases regularly after injection, reaching a minimum when the blood pressure is at its lowest (Mundy and Heiffer, 1960).

Catecholaminemia rises after administration of MEA. This rise, of central origin, depends on the drop in arterial pressure and on the concomitant anoxia (Mundy and Heiffer, 1960). Small doses (40 mg/kg) do not decrease the cardiac output (Charlier, 1954).

Local injection of MEA (0.037–0.3 mg) causes an increase in local vascular permeability (Mundy *et al.*, 1963).

Lowered arterial pressure and the increase in vascular permeability are reduced by synthetic antihistamines; it must be concluded that the release of endogenous histamine plays a part in the establishment of general arterial hypotension (Mundy *et al.*, 1963).

Aminoethylisothiourea

Aminoethylisothiourea (30 mg, i.v.) causes a sharp rise in arterial blood pressure. Perfusion at the rate of 12 mg/kg in 20 min results in an increase in the systolic/diastolic difference, as well as a slight rise in pressure. However, when injected into the circulation of the hind leg or the superior mesenteric system perfused at constant pressure, AET causes vasodilatation which is not modified by denervation. Furthermore, the cardiac output increases significantly (50–300%), as much after a single injection as after perfusion, and the cardiac rhythm is then slowed down. It increases the pressor effects of epinephrine as well as the duration of the epinephrine-produced reflex bradycardia (Laborit *et al.*, 1959). According to these authors, AET behaves essentially as a cardiotonic agent without sympathomimetic effect.

These results contradict those of Knott and Overman (1961) and Maxwell and Kneebone (1964). According to Knott and Overman (1961), AET (2–10 mg/kg/min) causes a rise in arterial pressure with tachycardia in the conscious animal, and bradycardia when anesthesia has been established. The cardiac output diminishes by about 50%.

The ECG shows that the QRS complex is depressed, and that the T-wave is negative. Extrasystoles with bigeminism are frequent. Intra-myocardiac conduction and mechanical efficiency are affected.

After rapid administration of 150 mg/kg AET the same phenomena appear, but the raised arterial pressure is rapidly followed by a lowering of blood pressure. The peripheral resistances are then steadily increased, even after blocking of ganglionic transmission.

Vagotomy has no effect on the bradycardia. The action of acetylcholine is antagonized by AET, thus AET exerts atropinic effects.

According to Maxwell and Kneebone (1964), AET (3.5 mg/kg) decreases the cardiac output, while the peripheral resistance increases with rise in arterial pressure. The coronary flow decreases but as the arterio-venous difference rises, the myocardic efficiency remains normal.

Pospíšil *et al.* (1966) have analyzed the ECG disturbances due to AET: ventricular extrasystoles, paroxysmal tachycardia with negative T-wave and flattening of the QRS complex are shown. Sinus activity is sometimes suppressed.

3.1.1.9. MAN

Cystamine

Intravenous administration of cystamine brings about a number of symptoms which in mild cases are characterized by cephalic congestion, facial erythema, and tachycardia. In the more severe cases dilatation of the facial vessels is more marked; arterial, systolic, and diastolic pressures undergo a transient fall, sometimes followed by raised pressure. These reactions are comparable with those clinically described as *nitritoid crisis*. It reveals, at least in part, the release of endogenous histamine. Indeed, intradermal injection of cystamine (0.1 ml at 1 %) causes the appearance of a typical urticarial wheal which may be prevented by prior treatment with synthetic antihistamines (Lecomte, 1952b; see Beaumariage, Chapter 3.2).

Cysteamine

Single i.v. injections of 50–100 mg of MEA produce no vasomotor reactions (Bacq, 1965).

Aminoethylisothiourea

Intravenous injection of AET produces an intense redness of the face, neck, and upper part of the thorax, frequently accompanied by nausea, vomiting and coughing.

When the dose of 25 mg/min for 30 min is exceeded, arterial hypotension can appear, which necessitates corrective administration of norepine-phrine (Condit *et al.*, 1958). This suggests the development of a nitritoid type crisis where endogenous histamine is probably involved. In human medicine, AET is contra-indicated (Pospíšil *et al.*, 1966).

3.1.2. GENERAL DISCUSSION

3.1.2.1. CYSTAMINE/MEA GROUP

Cystamine has a depressor effect, the drop in pressure being propor-tional to the amount injected; this effect is reproducible. It is not affected by atropine or suppressed by synthetic antihistamines. The drugs are not harmful to the excised heart and increase the coronary flow. They lower resistance to flow throughout all the perfused organs that have been investigated. They oppose the vasoconstrictive action of various agents. Finally, *in vivo*, they increase the blood flow throughout the cutaneous and muscular regions.

It is concluded, therefore, that cystamine is a vasodilator agent with a peripheral site of action. The vasodilatation is, for the most part, due to an action on vascular smooth muscle; to a lesser extent, especially in the cat and dog, release of histamine may contribute to the vasodilatation induced.

Peripheral vasodilatation affects the arterial and venous vascular beds so that the volume of the different organs increases. The circulating blood volume thus decreases. This, together with the increase in vascular permeability, i.e. passage of plasma fluids, through the endothelial layer results in a deficiency of right ventricular filling and a significant fall in cardiac output.

Lowered arterial pressure is thus explained by a fall in the peripheral resistances, and a decrease of systolic output. The lessening of perfusion pressure also causes reduction of blood flow in the different peripheral organs, which become anoxic. The arteriovenous oxygen difference increases, but remains insufficient to compensate for the reduction of blood flow. This particular circulatory situation is created especially when radioprotective doses are given.

In response to the lowered arterial pressure and central anoxia, sympathetic activity increases, demonstrated by the increase in blood catecholamine levels and a secondary increase in vascular resistances.

This increase aggravates tissue anoxia and its suppression by adrenalectomy favors collapse.

Cysteamine has two special classes of properties. The first class, to a certain extent, reproduces those of cystamine. This analogy is explained by the *in vivo* transformation of MEA into cystamine.

The other properties can be placed among the sympathomimetic effects. They are either direct (observed as a vasoconstriction suppressed by the α-blockers), or indirect, from the release of catecholamines from the adrenal medulla (Goffart, 1955).

As Robbers (1937) has already proposed, cystamine should be classified among the amines resulting from decarboxylation of the physiological amino acids. It approaches in character, among other substances, histamine and 5-HT. It is distinguished from them, however, by the persistence of its dilator effects after treatment by specific antagonists. Oxidation of MEA to cystamine strongly increases the cardiovascular effects.

3.1.2.2. ISOTHIOURONIUM DERIVATIVES

The derivatives of isothiouronium are in general substances with pressor effects; they increase the arterial pressure of the mouse, rat, and dog.

The interpretation of this result is a matter of dispute; according to Laborit *et al.* (1959), it depends essentially on a myocardial effect. The cardiac output rises due to inotropic properties in the presence of normal or slightly lowered vascular resistance.

According to DiStefano *et al.* (1961), part, at least, of the rise in pressure depends upon a vasoconstriction. This is not of an adrenergic nature, as it persists after blocking the peripheral sympathetic fibers or the α-receptors. Furthermore, there is no release of adrenal medullary amines because the arterial pressure remains stable or slightly raised. Reduced arterial pressure is a characteristic effect, in addition to the raised arterial pressure, of very weak doses. It depends either on vago-vagal reflex bradycardia suppressed by atropine, or on an incidental release of endogenous histamine.

This initial arterial pressure drop is not the same as the lasting fall characteristic of the acute or chronic intoxication which results from isothiouronium derivatives.

3.1.3. CONCLUSIONS

Tables 1 and 2 show that there is no relationship between the principal cardiovascular activities and the specific effects of the radioprotective agents; sometimes radioprotection develops simultaneously with a general lowering of arterial pressure, sometimes it occurs with a rise in blood

TABLE 1. PHARMACOLOGICAL ACTIONS OF I.P. RADIOPROTECTIVE AGENTS IN THE RAT

Radioprotective agent	Blood pressure	Histamine liberation	Concentration of catecholamines in blood
MEA ↓↑ Cystamine	Fall Precipitous fall	Weak Weak	Increased
AET ↓↑ MEG	Rise Rise	Weak Weak	Normal
5-HT	Fall	Weak	Increased

TABLE 2. VASOMOTOR AND RADIOPROTECTIVE ACTIVITY OF MEA IN DIFFERENT SPECIES

Species	Effect on blood pressure	Radioprotection
Mouse	Rise[a]	Active
Rat	Fall	Active
Dog	Fall	Active
Chicken	Fall	Not active

[a] Only after i.p. injection.

pressure. In contrast, lowered arterial pressure in the chicken is not sufficient to raise the resistance to X-rays.

No common characteristics are revealed by the comparative study of the most obvious cardiovascular manifestations of radioprotective agents. Perhaps some definite statements can be made if one considers the action of radioprotective agents on tissue perfusion, at the level of the microcirculation.

The local blood supply ($\mathring{Q}$) can be expressed by the equation:

$$\mathring{Q} = P/R$$

where P represents the head of the perfusion pressure relative to the general arterial pressure, and R is the peripheral resistance, dependent on the local vascular diameter.

In general it may be concluded that this perfusion decreases under the influence of radioprotective agents, perhaps because the arterial pressure undergoes a considerable drop (MEA, cystamine) or because the peripheral resistance increases directly (AET), or as a result of simultaneous adrenal medullary secretions.

Consequently, the tissues would each time be subjected to anoxia and acidosis, whatever the level of the general arterial pressure.

At present, techniques for investigating the mechanism of action of radioprotective agents at the level of tissue perfusion are not available. Measurements of the oxygen tension *in situ* are too uncoordinated for a general conclusion to be made.

REFERENCES

BACQ, Z. M. (1965) *Chemical Protection against Ionizing Radiation.* Charles C. Thomas. Springfield, Illinois, U.S.A., 328 pages.

BARAC, G. (1965a) Effets du sang chauffé et de la cystamine sur la circulation sanguine de l'intestin homotransplanté au cou chez le Chien. *C.R. Soc. Biol.* **159**: 1623–6.

BARAC, G. (1965b) Action vasodilatatrice rénale de la cystéamine et de la cystamine chez le Chien. *C.R. Soc. Biol.* **159**: 497–501.

BARAC, G., CESSION-FOSSION, A. and BACQ, Z. M. (1968) Effet direct de la cystamine sur le débit sanguin et la sécrétion de catécholamines des surrenales "au cou" chez le chien. *Arch. internat. Physiol. Bioch.* **76**: 154–6.

BEAUMARIAGE, M. L., VAN CANEGHEM, P. and BACQ, Z. M. (1966) Etude de certaines propriétés pharmacodynamiques de la cystamine et de la cystéamine chez diverses espèces animales. *Strahlentherapie* **131**: 342–51.

CESSION-FOSSION, A., VANDERMEULEN, R. and LECOMTE, J. (1964) Action de l'amino-éthylisothiouronium sur la médullosurrénale du rat. *C.R. Soc. Biol.* **158**: 1976–7.

CESSION-FOSSION, A., LECOMTE, J. and BACQ, Z. M. (1968) Sur les potentiateurs de l'hypertension artérielle post-sérotonine. *C.R. Soc. Biol.* **162**: 811–14.

CHARLIER, R. (1954) Effects of cysteamine and cysteine on cardiac output and oxygen content of venous blood. *Proc. Soc. Exptl. Biol. Med.* **86**: 290–5.

CONDIT, P. F., LEVY, A. H., VAN SCOTT, E. J. and ANDREWS, J. R. (1958) Some effects of β-aminoethylisothiouronium bromide (AET) in man. *J. Pharm. Exper. Ther.* **122**: 13A.

DELLA BELLA, B. and BACQ, Z. M. (1953) Action de la cystéamine sur le cœur isolé de grenouille et sur l'effet de l'excitation vagale chez la tortue. *Arch. f. exptl. Path. u. Pharmakol.* **219**: 366–70.

DISTEFANO, V. and KLAHN, J. (1966) Depletion of cardiac norepinephrine in the mouse and cat by mercaptoethylguanidine. *J. Pharmacol.* **151**: 236–41.

DISTEFANO, V. and LEARY, D. E. (1959) The pharmacological effects of D-II and L-2-aminobutylisothiouronium bromide and 3-aminopropyl-N'-methylisothiouronium bromide hydrobromide in the cat. *J. Pharmacol.* **126**: 304–10.

DISTEFANO, V., LEARY, D. E. and DOHERTY, D. G. (1956) The pharmacology of β-aminoethylisothiouronium bromide in the cat. *J. Pharmacol.* **117**: 425–33.

DISTEFANO, V., LEARY, D. E. and LITTLE, K. D. (1959) The pharmacological effects of some congeners of 2-aminoethylisothiouronium bromide (AET). *J. Pharmacol.* **126**: 159–63.

DISTEFANO, V., KORN, P. S. and LEARY, D. E. (1961) The blood pressure effects of 3-aminopropyl-N'-methylisothiouronium bromide hydrobromide in the cat. *J. Pharmacol.* **134**: 341–6.

DISTEFANO, V., KLAHN, J. J. and LEARY, D. E. (1962) The pharmacological effects of some radioprotective agents in mice. *Radiation Research* **17**: 792–800.

FISCHER, P., LECOMTE, J. and BEAUMARIAGE, M. L. (1955) Toxicité de la cystéamine après surrénalectomie. *Arch. internat. Physiol. Bioch.* **63**: 121–2.

GOFFART, M. (1955) Mode d'action de la cystéamine et de la cystamine au niveau de la médullo-surrénale. *Arch. internat. Physiol. Bioch.* **63**: 500–12.

HEIFFER, M. H., MUNDY, R. L. and MEHLMAN, B. (1961) Plasma catecholamine levels and adrenal ascorbic acid content following β-mercaptoethylamine (MEA) administration. *Endocrinology* **69**: 746–51.

HEIFFER, M. H., MUNDY, R. L. and MEHLMAN, B. (1962) The pharmacology of radioprotective chemicals. On some of the effects of beta-mercaptoethylamine (MEA) and cystamine in the rat. *Radiation Research* **16**: 165–73.

KNOTT, D. H. and OVERMAN, R. R. (1961) Cardiovascular effects of radioprotective compound beta-aminoethylisothiouronium Br-HBr (AET). *Am. J. Physiol.* **201**: 677–81.

KUNA, P. and VOKROUHLICKY, L. (1967) The influence of cystamine on the ECG. *Vojenske Zdravotnické Listy* **5**: 199–201.

LABORIT, H., BROUSSOLLE, B., JOUANY, J. M., NIAUSSAT, P., REYNIER, M. and WEBER, B. (1959) Etude pharmacologique du bromhydrate de 2-aminoéthylisothiouronium (AET). *Thérapie* **14**: 1116–35.

LECOMTE, J. (1952a) Propriétés pharmacodynamiques de la cystinamine. *Arch. internat. Physiol.* **60**: 179–80.

LECOMTE, J. (1952b) Sur la pathogénie du choc nitritoide bénin. *Arch. int. Pharmacodyn.* **92**: 241–51.

LECOMTE, J. (1954) Cystéamine et médullo-surrénale. *Arch. internat. Physiol.* **62**: 431–2.

LECOMTE, J. (1956) Contribution clinique et expérimentale à l'étude du rôle de l'histamine dans certains phénomènes anaphylactiques. Thèse d'Agrégation de l'Enseignement Supérieur. *Revue Belge Pathologie*, 1956, suppl. 11, 135 pages.

LECOMTE, J. and BACQ, Z. M. (1965) Propriétés vasomotrices de la MEG chez le rat. *Arch. int. Pharmacodyn.* **158**: 480–97.

LECOMTE, J. and VAN DE BERG, L. (1953) ß-mercaptoéthylamine, acétylcholine et histamine chez le lapin. *Arch. internat. Physiol.* **61**: 240–2.

LECOMTE, J., CESSION-FOSSION, A., LIBON, J. C. and BACQ, Z. M. (1964) Sur quelques effets pharmacodynamiques généraux de la cystamine chez le rat. *Arch. int. Pharmacodyn.* **148**: 487–510.

MAXWELL, G. and KNEEBONE, G. (1964) The effect of a radio-protective drug (S-(2-Amino ethyl) thiouronium bromide hydrobromide), upon the general and coronary haemodynamics and metabolism of the intact dog. *Austr. J. exp. Biol. med. Sci.* **42**: 601–6.

MEER, C. VAN DER, VALKENBURG, P. W., KUILE, C. A. TER and NEYHOFF, J. A. (1960) Farmacologische onderzoeking van cysteamine, cystamine, cysteine et AET, in verband met hun profylactische Werking tegen bestraling. In: *Medisch Biologisch Laboratorium RVO-TNO, MBL/1960/25.*

MUNDY, R. L. and HEIFFER, M. H. (1960) The pharmacology of radioprotectant chemicals. General pharmacology of β-mercaptoethylamine. *Radiation Research* **13**: 381–94.

MUNDY, R. L., HEIFFER, M. H. and MEHLMAN, B. (1961) The pharmacology of radioprotectant chemicals. Biochemical changes in the dog following the administration of beta-mercaptoethylamine (MEA). *Arch. int. Pharmacodyn.* **130**: 354–67.

MUNDY, R. L., HEIFFER, M. H. and MEHLMAN, B. (1963) Mechanism of beta-mercaptoethylamine-induced hypotension in the dog. *Am. J. Physiol.* **204**: 997–1000.

POSPÍŠIL, J., DIENSTBIER, Z. and KOTATKO, J. (1966) L'applicabilité d'une matière radioprotective, de l'aminoéthylisothiouronium Br HBr (AET). *Čas. Lèk. Čes.* **43**: 1165–71.

ROBBERS, H. (1937) Die pharmakologische Wirkung des Cystamins, einer blutdrucksenkenden Substanz. *Arch. f. exper. Path. u. Pharmakol.* **185**: 461–91.

ROTHE, W., GRENAN, M. and WILSON, S. (1963) Radioprotection by pressor amidines. *Science* **141**: 160–1.

SCHLIEP, H. (1965) Personal Communication to Z. M. Bacq.

SCHLIEP, H. J. and MICHAILOV, M. CH. (1965) The influence of AET and cysteamine on blood pressure responses to repeated acetylcholine and adrenaline test injections in rats. *Progr. biochem. Pharmacol.* **1**: 249–56.

VAN DE BERG, L. (1954) Cystéamine et débit coronaire du cœur isolé de lapin. *Arch. int. Pharmacodyn.* **99**: 346–67.

WANG, R., HOAG, W. and HASEGAWA, A. (1971) Cardiovascular responses to radioprotective compounds in rats. *Radiation Research* **45**: 355–63.

3.2

VASCULAR PERMEABILITY AND INFLAMMATORY PHENOMENA

M. L. Beaumariage

Liège, Belgium

3.2.1. CYSTAMINE–CYSTEAMINE INFLAMMATORY AGENTS

3.2.1.1. MAN

Cysteamine (MEA) (1 mg), injected intradermally, produces an erythema without urticarial papule, which usually disappears within 48 hr, but a local edema, occasionally with a slight necrosis, may persist for 24 hr (Lecomte, 1952a; Lecomte and Bohrenstayn, 1953). Injection of the same amount of MEA produces a typical Lewis triad, which may be eliminated by the administration of synthetic antihistaminics (e.g. mepyramine, promethazine) and local anesthetics (e.g. percaine, 0.1 ml of 1% solution). Repeated cystamine injection into the same cutaneous area causes the disappearance of the Lewis reaction.

3.2.1.2. DOG

Injection of cystamine (0.037–0.30 mg) in isotomic saline into the abdominal skin of the animal, following intravenous (i.v.) administration of Evans blue, results, within 2 min, in a blue coloration of the skin around the injection site. The reaction is similar to that observed after injection of histamine, and its concentration is proportional to the concentration of β-mercaptoethylamine (MEA) injected (Mundy *et al.*, 1963). Both the MEA reaction and the histamine reaction can be abolished by the antihistaminic pyrilamine maleate (10 mg/kg).

The same increase in vascular permeability may be observed in the peritoneum, where injection of radioprotective doses (100 mg/kg) of

MEA results in the exudation of a blood-stained, protein-rich fluid, which slowly coagulates at $4°C$. If Evans blue has previously been administered, the exudate is blue in color. It is considerably reduced if pyrilamine (5 mg/kg) and tripelennamine (10 mg/kg) are administered.

Aminoethylisothiourea (AET), 100 mg/kg, produces the same congestive and hemorrhagic effects, particularly in the central nervous system, bladder, and digestive tract. Hemorrhagic exudates collect in the cerebral ventricles and the peritoneal cavity (Benson *et al.*, 1961).

3.2.1.3. RABBIT

The transfer of trypan blue across the vascular walls is also observed after intradermal injection of cystamine (500 mcg–1 mg) (Lecomte, 1952a, b, 1956), and this increased permeability effect is also slowed down by prior injection of a synthetic antihistaminic. On the other hand, during local application of a solution of cystamine (10^{-4} M) in Zweifach liquid for 15 min to rabbit mesentery there is no local vascular alteration (Lecomte, 1956).

3.2.1.4. RAT

The injection of cystamine (500 mcg) into the plantar skin of the hind-paw of the rat has several effects, comprising a marked edema, and immediately following the injection, the temperature and blood pressure rise and increase regularly throughout the first hour, when they finally subside. The edema is macroscopically similar to that induced by dextran (Lecomte *et al.*, 1964). A synthetic antihistaminic (promethazine) and an anti-5-hydroxytryptamine (methysergide) reduce the severity of the edema, and accelerate its resorption. Cystamine (500 mcg in 0.1 ml) produces an increase in skin vascular permeability, shown by the passage of chlorazol blue into the interstitial spaces. The dye appears later if promethazine has been previously injected; corticotropin, cortisone, and adrenal cortical extracts have no effect (Van Cauwenberge and Lecomte, 1955).

3.2.1.5. MOUSE

Cysteamine (750 mcg), like its oxidized derivative, increases the vascular permeability of the plantar connective spaces of the mouse, so that i.v.

injected chlorazol blue will cross the capillary wall and stain the skin; the weight of paws, cut off at the tibio-tarsal joint, increases by about 25%. Sulfur-containing amines have a greater permeabilizing effect than histamine, 5-hydroxytryptamine (5-HT), and 48/80. Methysergide (10 mg/ kg, i.p.) and Aprotinin (Trasylol® 2000 UKI/kg, i.p.), a proteolytic enzyme inhibitor, prevent the cystamine inflammatory reaction, via a non-specific effect due to a decrease in the intercapillary hydrostatic pressure (Beaumariage *et al.*, 1966).

In about 60% of cases, injection of 750 mcg MEA under the skin of young mice causes a light spotty hemorrhage at the site of injection, which disappears without a trace (Beaumariage, 1968).

3.2.2. ACTION OF SULFUR-CONTAINING RADIOPROTECTIVE AGENT ON FACTORS AFFECTING INFLAMMATORY PHENOMENA

3.2.2.1. HISTAMINE

3.2.2.1.1. Histamine Release after Administration of Cysteamine–Cystamine

Dog

In 1937, Robbers observed that cystamine in the dog had similar vascular action to histamine. As cystamine is a diamine, its action could well be through histamine release (Lecomte, 1952b). Mundy *et al.* (1963) showed that blood histamine levels increased considerably during the fall in blood pressure which follows rapid i.v. injection of MEA (100 mg/kg) or cystamine (15–47 mg/kg). Cysteamine had a delayed action, probably because, in order to exert this effect, it must be converted to cystamine. This property of the sulfur-containing radioprotective agents is subject to tachyphylaxis. In dogs that have ceased to respond to 48/80, liberation of histamine by cystamine is still possible; the reverse situation has also been observed (Mundy *et al.*, 1967).

Rat

Lecomte and his coworkers (Lecomte, 1955; Lecomte and Franchimont, 1962; Lecomte *et al.*, 1964) showed that the amount of endogenous histamine in the skin, which exhibits an edematous reaction following local injection of cystamine, markedly decreases (from 29 mcg to 5.9 mcg per g of fresh tissue after 5 min). Subsequently, the histamine content increases to values a little above normal, when the edema is at its maximum; this may be due to the accumulation *in situ* of histamine-rich blood elements compensating for the initial loss of histamine.

Isolated rat hindquarters

The injection of 500 mcg of cystamine into an aortic canula which irrigates the rat hindquarters causes histamine liberation (Lecomte, 1955; Lecomte *et al.*, 1964), its mechanism of action being identical with that of other histamine liberators, such as 48/80. The early appearance of histamine in the perfusate may be verified, and it reaches its maximum concentration in less than 2 min; it then decreases progressively, the active material finally totally disappearing after 30 min. The further administration of the same quantity of cystamine is followed by a net reduction in the amount of histamine liberated; there is tachyphylaxis, which is "crossed" with tachyphylaxis due to other histamine liberators. Cystamine in this preparation is 20 times less active than "Labaz 1935".

Cells in peritoneal fluid

Treatment of these cells by cystamine liberates their endogenous histamine (Demaree *et al.*, 1964). The quantities measured in the supernatant, obtained by centrifugation following the incubation of the cells with the sulfur-containing radioprotective agent, increases as a function of the cystamine concentration in the medium (10^{-4} to 10^{-2} M), and as the length of incubation. The same effect may be observed with MEA, which is slightly less effective than the disulfur compound. It may also be seen that with concentrations above 10^{-3}M, the amount of histamine liberated sharply drops, probably because the enzyme responsible for the MEA–cystamine conversion is inhibited by a substrate excess, acting via a chelation mechanism.

Young mice

After cystamine injection (750 mcg, i.p.) the skin of young mice is still histamine-rich, and after 10 min there is a moderate rise in the histamine reserves. After 1 hr the situation reverts to normal (Beaumariage *et al.*, 1966). A significant reduction in cutaneous histamine is produced by 48/80 (30 mcg, i.p.) as early as $\frac{1}{2}$ hr after injection. The subcutaneous administration of either substance has identical results (Bacq *et al.*, 1961).

Chicken

Intravenous injection of cystamine (150 mg/kg) 10 min before the animal is sacrificed does not alter the histamine content of the lungs or small intestine, whereas polymyxine B (27.5 mg, three times) reduces the lung histamine content by half, without having any effect on that of the intestine (Beaumariage *et al.*, 1966).

3.2.2.1.2. *Histamine Release after Administration of MEG*

Some perfusates leaking from the hindquarters of the rat may contain histamine, following intra-aortic injection of MEG (Lecomte, 1964; Lecomte and Bacq, 1965). The kinetics of the liberation depend on the dose: up to 15 mg, the amount of histamine release reaches its maximum in 3 min following MEG injection; at higher doses, the maximum histamine concentration occurs 9–12 min after administration. Injection of MEG, a vasoconstrictor, results in a very considerable reduction in the volume of perfusate, thus affecting the elimination of the liberated histamine. It is 80 times less powerful than "Labaz 1935".

3.2.2.1.3. *Effect on Enzymatic Degradation of Histamine*

The addition of MEA to diamine oxidase or histaminase depresses the catabolism of histamine by that enzyme (De Marco *et al.*, 1962). The inhibition is temporary, since MEA is oxidized to cystamine, which is a substrate for the enzyme. This enzymatic inhibition could be due to the formation of a thiazolidine ring, inactive but dissociable between MEA and the aldehyde group of pyridoxal phosphate, which forms part of the structure of the enzyme. This property of MEA has been confirmed by Pany (1963), who showed moreover that cysteine and AET are equally effective inhibitors of histaminase.

3.2.2.1.4. *Modifications of the Pharmacodynamic Properties of Histamine*

Vasomotor properties

These have been described in Chapter 3.1.1.4.

Contraction of smooth muscle fibers

Isolated rabbit intestine. The addition of MEA (200–400 mcg/ml during 5–10 min) slightly reduces the contraction due to histamine (1–5 mcg/ml). This inhibition is reversible (Lecomte, 1955).

Guinea-pig ileum. According to Ackermann and Wasmuth (1939) and Edlbacher *et al.* (1937), high concentrations of cysteine suppress the histamine-induced contraction of the isolated ileum.

Lecomte (1955) showed that the presence of MEA in the bath in concentrations less than 50 mcg/ml moderately decreases sensitivity to histamine. As the dose is increased, the sensitivity of the intestine decreases regularly, this reduction being proportional to the concentration of MEA, and the duration of contact with it. If the intestine is incubated for 15 min with MEA(150mcg/ml)in an organ bath, it ceases to respond to histamine. According to Stepanović *et al.* (1963), MEA has an inhibitory effect at as low a concentration as 14.2 mcg/ml.

Cystamine produces the same variations in sensitivity to histamine as its reduced derivative.

Bronchospasm in the guinea-pig. When it is caused by inhalation from histamine-containing aerosols at varying concentrations, the broncho-spasm is not affected by i.p. injection of a 200 mcg/kg dose of MEA or cystamine (Lecomte, 1955). The latent period preceding the appearance of anoxemic convulsions is similar in the control and experimental animals (treated with sulfur-containing compounds).

3.2.2.2.   5-HYDROXYTRYPTAMINE (5-HT)

3.2.2.2.1.   *Liberation of 5-HT*

According to Varagić *et al.* (1965), there is no change in endogenous 5-HT of the rat ileum after injection of MEA (100 mg/kg, i.p.); the urinary excretion of 5-hydroxy-indolacetic acid is also unaffected (Deanović *et al.,* 1963).

Bioassay (guinea-pig ileum) of histamine in cystamine-containing perfusion fluids of isolated rat hindquarters showed that the antihistaminic mepyramine did not completely abolish the effect of the perfusate. A weak contraction remained, which could be inhibited by the later addition of anti-5-HT, BOL 148 (0.2 mcg/ml), to the water bath. This indicates simultaneous liberation of 5-HT with the histamine (Lecomte *et al.*, 1964). Similarly, hairless adult mice treated with a dose of 150 mg/kg, i.p., *in vivo* showed that a reduction in the 5-HT content (from 1 mcg/g to 0.5 mcg/g of fresh tissue) may be seen after extraction and bioassay on the uterus of the estrogenized female rat (Beaumariage *et al.,* 1966).

3.2.2.2.2.   *Alterations in the Pharmacodynamic Properties of 5-HT*

Vasomotor properties

These are dealt with in Chapter 3.1.1.4.

Contraction of smooth muscle fibers

The response of the isolated guinea-pig ileum to 5-HT is strongly inhibited by MEA. The smallest effective concentration is usually less than 3.8 mcg/ml (Stepanović *et al.*, 1963). The recovery of the ileum is slower relative to the concentration of MEA.

3.2.2.2.3. *Effect on Enzymatic Degradation of 5-HT*

Small doses of MEA increase the activity of brain and liver mitochondrial monoamine oxidase and oxidation of 5-HT is therefore accelerated (Rausa *et al.*, 1964). This stimulating effect is decreased and is followed by an inhibitory effect, if the dose of MEA is increased. This was also observed by De Marco *et al.* (1965), using spermidine in place of 5-HT as a substrate for monoamine oxidase. This team showed that the effect becomes reversible on oxidation of MEA to cystamine. It is possible that in this case, as with histaminase, the blocking of the enzyme takes place at the level of pyridoxal phosphate.

3.2.2.3. BRADYKININ AND KALLIDIN

3.2.2.3.1. *Formation of Bradykinin*

The treatment of kallikrein (an enzyme catalyzing the conversion of kininogens into kinins) with thiol compounds (e.g. cysteine, MEA, β-mercaptoethanol, and glutathione) decreases the intensity of the inflammatory reaction produced in guinea-pig skin by a subcutaneous injection of the enzyme (Davies and Lowe, 1966). It also decreases the permeabilizing effect of kallikrein on the capillaries. On the other hand, the incubation of bradykinin or histamine with the same thiol compounds does not alter their permeabilizing properties. The isolated rat uterus is very sensitive to bradykinin and contracts on addition of a mixture of kallikrein and kininogen. This response is less intense if the organ is pretreated with cysteine (Davies and Lowe, 1966). The process continues as though cysteine had inhibited the enzyme which activates the kininogen into kinin.

3.2.2.3.2. *Modification of the Pharmacologic Effects of Bradykinin and Kallidin*

Vasomotor properties

Guinea-pig. The i.p. injection of β-mercaptoethanol in the guinea-pig, before the administration of bradykinin or of kallidin, enhances the fall of blood pressure produced by the polypeptides (Erdös and Wohler, 1963). The action of MEA is much less marked.

Rat.   The fall of arterial pressure produced by bradykinin (10 mg/kg) is unmodified by prior injection of cystamine (Lecomte *et al.*, 1964).

Smooth muscles

According to Auerswald and Doleschel (1967), cysteine and MEA at a concentration of 10^{-3} M increase the response of guinea-pig ileum to the injection of bradykinin or of kallidin. The same effect is obtained with cysteine on the virgin rat uterus (Picarelli *et al.*, 1962). If the concentration of the sulfur-containing compound is increased, the contraction diminishes in intensity. While cysteine particularly increases the response to kallidin, MEA more selectively potentiates the action of bradykinin. β-Mercaptoethanol only slightly increases sensitivity to kinins.

The increase in the action of bradykinin under the influence of cysteine had been noticed by Cîrstea (1965). Thiols might break S—S bridges, and unmask a great number of bradykinin receptors. The potentiation of this effect would be due to an inhibition of the enzyme degrading kinins into inactive products (Auerswald and Doleschel, 1967).

3.2.2.4.   ANTIGEN–ANTIBODY REACTION

Compounds containing thiol groups inhibit the intensity of anaphylactic manifestations in the guinea-pig (Herberts, 1955). The same phenomenon is found *in vitro*: the addition of cysteine, reduced glutathione (G-SH), or β-mercaptoethanol in suitable quantities in a Tyrode bath containing fragments of guinea-pig lung strongly depresses the liberation of histamine normally produced by the addition of the specific antigen (Edman *et al.*, 1964). It seems that the antigen–antibody reaction needs the presence of free —SH groups, because *N*-ethylmaleimide, which is a powerful inhibitor of these functions, also inhibits histamine liberation. The presence of β-mercaptoethylamine, on the other hand, would increase the release of histamine, probably because it may be transformed into cystamine.

The agglutination of thrombocytes obtained *in vitro* by the addition of bacterial endotoxins is also inhibited by L-cysteine, β-mercaptoethanol and GSH (Jókay *et al.*, 1964a). At the same time a reduction in the liberation of histamine and 5-HT which accompanies agglutination is observed. Basing their experiments on passive anaphylactic reactions, such as the Prausnitz–Kustner test, Leddy *et al.* (1962) showed that the serum of allergic human subjects injected into normal subjects loses its sensitizing properties if it is previously incubated with β-mercaptoethanol, L-cysteine, or β-mercaptoethylamine. Antibodies with a high sedimentation constant (19S) are easily inhibited, while those with a lower sedimentation constant (7S) remain active after such treatment. It therefore seems that the existence of disulfide bridges, or of free —SH groups, may be absolutely necessary for γ-globulin mediation in the antigen–antibody reaction. According to Ishizaka *et al.* (1961), the blocking of the passive, sensitizing reactions can happen in the guinea-pig only if the antibodies are incubated with β-mercaptoethanol together with iodoacetate. According to these authors, sulfur-containing compounds break the S—S bonds of the antibody molecule, converting them into —SH; the altered antibody does not, however, lose its ability to fix itself in the tissue, nor to react with the antigen. It seems necessary for the unmasked —SH groups to be blocked by iodoacetate before antibodies become incapable of fixing themselves at the tissue level, so that an anaphylactic reaction can no longer be induced by the antigen. Precipitation reactions have shown that the antibody bearing an —SH group is still able to form a complex with the specific antigen, and that this complex can still fix complement.

Kiselev and Karpova (1965) have, in addition, studied the action of cysteine and denatured proteins on complement. The presence of free —SH causes inactivation of complement, which becomes incapable of taking part in the antigen–antibody reaction. Cystine and proteins deprived of thiol groups, on the other hand, do not act as anti-complement. These results have been confirmed *in vivo,* since an i.v. injection of cysteine (75–300 mg/kg) in guinea-pig caused a fall in the serum complement concentration. With stronger doses, this reduction remains even after 24 hr.

The action of sulfur-containing radioprotective agents on antibody synthesis has not, to our knowledge, been the subject of a systematic investigation. All that is known is that the injection of β-mercaptoethylamine or of MET 24 hr before administration of sheep red cells does not inhibit the formation of hemolysins in the rat (Simić *et al.,* 1960).

3.2.3.   ANTI-INFLAMMATORY ACTIONS

The effects of MEA and cystamine on the course of inflammatory phenomena appear in Table 1, and are compared with those of a synthetic antihistaminic, promethazine, and ACTH, or corticoids.

TABLE 1. SUMMARY OF THE ANTI-INFLAMMATORY PROPERTIES OF CYSTEINE AND ITS DERIVATIVES, WITH THE CORRESPONDING PROPERTIES OF ACTH AND OF A SYNTHETIC ANTIHISTAMINIC (Modified from Lecomte and Van Cauwenberge, 1957c)

Tests	Authors	Cysteine, MEA or cystamine	ACTH (corticoids)	Promethazine
Cutaneous Irritation (rat and rabbit)				
Histamine and histamine liberators	Lecomte, 1955	+	0	+
Chloroform	Lecomte and Bohrenstayn, 1953; Lecomte et al., 1953a	+	0	+
Formol	Mörsdorf et al., 1955	+	+	0
Croton oil (mouse)	Lecomte and Van Cauwenberge, 1957c	0	0	+
Allergic or Idiosyncrasic Reactions Subcutaneous injections of:				
Foreign protein (rabbit)	Lecomte and Van Cauwenberge, 1957c	+	0	+
Tuberculin (man)	Lecomte and Bohrenstayn, 1953	+		+
Tuberculin (guinea-pig)	Long, 1954	0		0
Mesentery (rabbit)	Lecomte, 1956	+		0
Anaphylactic shock (mouse)	Meyers and Burdon, 1960	+	+ +	+
Atopic edema (rat)	Lecomte et al., 1953b	+	+ +	+
Shwartzman phenomenon (rabbit)	Jókay et al., 1964b	—		
Permeability of Connective Tissue				
Hyaluronidase (rat)	Lecomte and Van Cauwenberge, 1957a	+	0	0
Synovial Permeability				
Fluoresceine (rabbit)	Lecomte and Van Cauwenberge, 1957b	+	0	0
Miscellaneous Inflammatory Reactions				
Cotton granuloma (rat)	Lecomte and Van Cauwenberge, 1957b	—		0
Kaolin arthritis (rat)	Coulon et al., 1954	+ +	+ +	0
Scalding (guinea-pig)	Davies and Lowe, 1966			0

+ = inhibition of the inflammatory reaction, 0 = no effect, — = increase.

3.2.3.1. TESTS SHOWING CHANGES IN VASCULAR PERMEABILITY
AND RESISTANCE

3.2.3.1.1. *Cutaneous Irritants*

Histamine and its liberators

In the rat i.p. injected with chlorazol blue, the increase in vascular permeability produced by an intradermal injection of histamine is reduced by prior i.p. injection of MEA or cystamine (50–1000 mg/kg) (Lecomte, 1955; Lecomte and Van Cauwenberge, 1957c). There is an increased latent period preceding the appearance of the blue coloration on the skin. Cystamine is more potent than MEA.

In the rabbit, the increased permeability effect of histamine and its liberators, such as 1935L and 48/80, is delayed, and reduced in intensity, by prior administration of MEA or cystamine (50 mg/kg) (Lecomte, 1955), the maximum inhibitory action occurring 10–15 min after the injection. Although the MEA effect decreases after 40 min, that of cystamine persists even after 60 min, illustrating its greater potency.

Chloroform

The same reduction of cutaneous permeability by MEA and cystamine can be demonstrated by the Ambrose and De Eds test in the rat and the rabbit. There is a marked reduction in the irritating effect of chloroform (Lecomte and Bohrenstayn, 1953; Lecomte *et al.*, 1953a).

Formol

Injection of formol (0.1 ml of 3% solution) under the plantar skin of the rat hind-paw causes a marked edema to develop, which may be considerably reduced if MEA (50 mg/kg) or cystamine (100 mg/kg) is injected subcutaneously 30 min before the irritating agent (Mörsdorf *et al.*, 1955). The anti-inflammatory effect of MEA is comparable to that of ACTH (2.5 U/kg, 4 times), or cortisone (50 mg/kg, twice), whereas that of cystamine is greater; but since the two sulfur-containing compounds were not injected in equimolecular quantities, the comparison may not be easily made.

Croton oil

In the mouse a dose of 50 mg/kg of MEA has no effect on cutaneous lesions produced in the animal by intracutaneous injection of croton oil. The number of petechiae and hemorrhages is the same in the control animals and the experimental animals treated with the sulfur-containing compounds. There is no effect on the edema or on the subcutaneous connective tissue edema (Lecomte and Van Cauwenberge, 1957c).

3.2.3.1.2.   *Inflammatory Reactions of Allergic or Idiosyncratic Origin*

Ovalbumin

In the rabbit sensitized with hen egg-white, the increase in vascular permeability resulting from intradermal injection of this foreign protein may be delayed by prior i.v. injection of cystamine (Lecomte, 1955). However, the course of the anaphylactic reactions of the mesentery is not affected *in vivo* by administration of MEA or cystamine 15 min before local application of the antigen. The delay in appearance of the thrombocyto-leukocytic emboli and the degree of rupture of the venous walls are identical in the experimental and control sensitized animals (Lecomte, 1956).

Intradermal reaction to tuberculin

In man, prior intradermal injection of MEA or cystamine in a dose indicated in Section 3.2.1.1 causes the Mantoux test to be weakened in 75% of cases (Lecomte and Bohrenstayn, 1953). Cysteamine, tested in BCG-sensitized guinea-pigs, has the same inhibitory effect when it is i.p. injected 6 hr prior to the intracutaneous administration of tuberculin (Long, 1954). The inhibition is very weak when MEA is injected simultaneously with the tuberculin, and does not occur in vitamin-C-deficient guinea-pigs; administration of GSH hinders the effect. The action of MEA is synergic with that of cortisone, when both are administered 6 hr before tuberculin; on the other hand, if the MEA is injected simultaneously with the tuberculin, it abolishes the anti-inflammatory action of the cortisone injected 6 hr earlier.

Anaphylactic shock in mice

Cysteine causes reduction in intensity of anaphylactic shock produced by ovalbumin in mice immunized either actively or passively against that protein (Meyers and Burdon, 1960). The best results are obtained when the sulfur-containing compound is injected 60 min before the trigger injection. It also reduces shock induced by the injection of the soluble fraction obtained from the formation of the antigen–antibody complex *in vitro*.

Shwartzman phenomenon

Jókay *et al.* (1964b) observed that the local Shwartzman phenomenon, elicited by endotoxin in the rabbit, has an increased duration and intensity if cysteine (200 mg/kg) is injected i.v. at the same time as the triggering injection of endotoxin. The subsequent leukopenia is similar in all the animals that show the sensitization reaction, but thrombopenia is less marked in rabbits treated with cysteine. In normal animals, the sulfur-containing compounds do not alter the number of platelets nor the leukocytosis. Cortisone (Marcus and Donaldson, 1952), ACTH, and antihistaminics (Rocha e Silva, 1955) protect animals against the Shwartzman phenomenon.

Eczema

De Gennes *et al.* (1956) drew attention to a favorable effect of MEA-treatment in causing regression of eczematous lesions (especially those induced by streptomycin) in man.

Atopic edema

Atopic edema, produced in the rat by the i.p. injection of egg-white, is strongly inhibited when radioprotective doses of cysteine and its derivatives are administered 1 hr before ovalbumin (Lecomte *et al.*, 1953b); cystamine is the most active compound.

3.2.3.2. TEST SHOWING ALTERATIONS IN THE PERMEABILITY OF CONNECTIVE TISSUE. DIFFUSION OF INDIA INK IN CONNECTIVE TISSUE

Hyaluronidase accelerates the dispersion of inert particles injected in the skin by depolymerizing hyaluronic acid, which is one of the constituents of connective tissue. In the rat, MEA (100 mg/kg) slightly inhibits intradermal diffusion of India ink diluted with hyaluronidase, while an equimolecular dose of cystamine sharply prevents the passage of particles of India ink in connective spaces (Lecomte and Van Cauwenberge, 1957a).

3.2.3.3. TEST SHOWING MODIFICATION IN THE PERMEABILITY OF CONNECTIVE TISSUE AND OF THE VASCULAR WALLS. MODIFICATION OF THE PERMEABILITY OF THE SYNOVIA

Although MEA does not affect the permeability of rabbit talotarsal synovia, cystamine inhibits the absorption of fluorescein injected into the middle of the joint cavity, and delays its appearance in the urine (Lecomte and Van Cauwenberge, 1957b).

3.2.3.4. MISCELLANEOUS INFLAMMATORY REACTIONS

3.2.3.4.1. *Abscess Induced by Foreign Bodies*

Cysteamine and cystamine (100 mg/kg) administered continuously over 10 days do not slow down the development of experimental abscesses produced by the subcutaneous insertion of a cotton pellet (Lecomte and Van Cauwenberge, 1957b). On the contrary, these substances increase the inflammation severity.

3.2.3.4.2. *Kaolin Arthritis*

The severity of inflammatory reactions produced in rats by the injection of 10% kaolin under the aponeurosis of the tibio-tarsal joint is considerably reduced if MEA (50 mg/kg/day, i.p.) is administered (Coulon *et al.*, 1954). Treatment given before injecting kaolin is ineffective.

3.2.3.4.3. *Edema Caused by Scalding*

In the guinea-pig, MEA, cystamine, and β-mercaptoethanol strongly inhibit edema produced by scalding if they are injected i.v. at a dose of 25 mg/kg, 10 min before the animal is placed in hot water (Davies and Lowe, 1966). Synthetic antihistaminics (Wilhelm and Manson, 1958) and ACTH (Selye, 1951) are equally effective.

3.2.4. DISCUSSION

3.2.4.1. CAN LIBERATION OF VASOACTIVE SUBSTANCES EXPLAIN THE VASCULAR AND PERMEABILIZING PROPERTIES OF SULFUR-CONTAINING RADIOPROTECTIVE AGENTS?

Changes of blood pressure

The importance of histamine liberation varies strongly between species, as is shown by bioassay of the histamine content of different tissues in different animal species. In dogs and in rats it is important, whereas in mice and chickens it is non-existent. Sensitivity to histamine also varies according to the animal species: the dog is very sensitive; the rat and the mouse are very resistant. The blood pressure reaction is not identical for all sulfur-containing radioprotective compounds: MEA is less hypotensive than cystamine, and MEG is hypertensive or provokes diphasic reactions. Consequently if histamine put in the circulation can play a role in shock induced by sulfur-containing radioprotective agents in the dog, it should only weakly influence the vascular reaction in the rat, and have no effect at all in tension reactions observed in the mouse and chicken. The use of synthetic antihistaminics confirms this view. Undoubtedly the blocking of the diamine oxidase can potentiate the effects of histamine, but this observation made *in vitro* with MEA, cysteine, and AET has not been realized *in vivo*.

Participation of 5-HT in the vasomotor effects of sulfur-containing radioprotective agents appears to be negligible in the rat and the mouse: the quantities of 5-HT released are small, urinary excretion of 5-hydroxy-indolacetic acid is unchanged, and anti-5-hydroxytryptamine is unable to alter the effects of cystamine or MEG.

Vasoactive polypeptides, such as bradykinin and kallidin, cannot participate in the tension effects of MEA, since the latter, both *in vivo* and *in vitro*, blocks the kallikrein needed for the formation of kinins, but nothing is known of their possible eventual participation in shock caused by cystamine.

Alterations in capillary permeability

The role of histamine and of 5-HT in alterations in capillary endothelia permeability induced by MEA and by cystamine is established, since previous liberation of endogenous histamine and also use of antihistaminics (especially in dogs), or an anti-5-hydroxytryptamine, causes a reduction in the edema and intensity of the inflammatory reaction which occurs with the application of sulfur-containing compounds.

3.2.4.2. HYPOTENSION AND THE ANTI-INFLAMMATORY EFFECT OF MEA AND CYSTAMINE

Cysteamine and cystamine inhibit inflammatory phenomena when the effect of increasing vascular permeability predominates, but they do not affect or potentiate those characterized by a pronounced alteration of the capillary endothelium (e.g. cutaneous purpura induced by croton oil, Shwartzman phenomenon, anaphylactic reaction of the mesentery), or those which depend on complex tissue reactions (granuloma against foreign bodies). It is the drop in arterial pressure that plays the major role in the depression of edema formation, whether cutaneous, articular, or general, induced by histamine liberators, formol, chloroform, certain sensitizing agents, scalding, or kaolin. In reducing the blood pressure in the arterial capillaries, cystamine, and probably MEA, reduce the passage of fluid across the endothelium, and inhibit fluid accumulation in the interstitial connective tissue. The reduction in the permeability of the intact synovia to fluoresceine proves that this is the real mechanism.

Doubtless, other factors than hypotension contribute to the anti-edematous action. Among these we can put the following: the reduction in the histamine and 5-HT content of certain tissues; adrenal cortex stimulation; epinephrine release; inhibition of complement; and possible damage to the antibody-binding sites in the tissue.

Lesions in the venous and capillary walls are unchanged or sometimes increased by prior or simultaneous injection of —SH-bearing compounds. According to Jókay *et al.* (1964b), the destruction of the vascular walls that would result from their infiltration by leucocytes and the development of microthrombi of leucocytes and platelets would be due to —SH-bearing leucocyte proteases, which cysteine is able to activate.

REFERENCES

ACKERMANN, D. and WASMUTH, W. (1939) Zur Wirkungsweise des Histamines. *Z. Physiol. Chem.* **267**: 28–31.

AUERSWALD, W. and DOLESCHEL, W. (1967) On the potentiation of kinins by sulfhydrylic compounds. *Arch. int. Pharmacodyn.* **168**: 188–99.

BACQ, Z. M., BEAUMARIAGE, M. L. and RADIVOJEVIĆ, D. V. (1961) Protection chimique locale et générale contre l'épilation par le rayonnement X. *Bull. Acad. Roy. Méd. Belg.* VIIth series **1**: No. 6: 519–50.

BEAUMARIAGE, M. L. (1968) Contribution à l'étude de la radioprotection du système pileux du souriceau contre le rayonnement X. *Thèse de Licence en Sciences Nucléaires.* Liège, pp. 174.

BEAUMARIAGE, M. L., VAN CANEGHEM, P. and BACQ, Z. M. (1966) Etudes de certaines propriétés pharmacodynamiques de la cystamine et de le cystéamine chez diverses espèces animales. *Strahlentherapie* **131**: 342–51.

BENSON, B. E., MICHAELSON, S. M., DOWNS, W. L., MAYNORD, K. F., SCOTT, F. K., HODGE, H. C. and HOWLAND, J. W. (1961) Toxicological and radioprotection study on S. β-aminoethylisothiouronium bromide (AET). *Rad. Res.* **15**: 561–72.

CÎRSTEA, M. (1965) Potentiation of some bradykinin effects by thiol compounds. *Brit. J. Pharmacol.* **25**: 405–10.

COULON, R., CHARLIER, R. and VANDERSMISSEN, L. (1954) Action de la cystéinamine sur une arthrite expérimentale. *Arch. int. Pharmacodyn.* **99**: 474–80.

DAVIES, G. E. and LOWE, J. S. (1966) Inhibitory effects of thiol compounds on kallikrein and on experimental burns in guinea-pigs. *Brit. J. Pharmacol.* **27**: 107–13.

DEANOVIĆ, Z., SUPEK, Z. and BULAT, M. (1963) Effect of chemoprotection by cystamine on urinary excretion of 5-hydroxyindolacetic acid in X-irradiated rats. *Int. J. Rad. Biol.* **7**: 109–11.

DE GENNES, J. L., LAROCHE, CL. and DELTOUR, G. (1956) Effets de la cystamine dans différentes affections allergiques. *Semaine des Hôpitaux de Paris* **32**: 2850–3.

DE MARCO, C., MONDOVI, B. and CAVALLINI, D. (1962) Temporary suppression of diamine oxidase (histaminase) activity by cysteamine. *Biochem. Pharmacol.* **11**: 509–14.

DE MARCO, C., COLETTA, M. and BOMBARDIERI, G. (1965) Inhibition of plasma monoamine oxidase by cysteamine. *Nature* **205:** 176.

DEMAREE, G. L., MUNDY, R. L. and HEIFFER, M. H. (1964) *In vitro* histamine release from rat peritoneal cells by beta-mercaptoethylamine and cystamine. *J. Pharmacol.* **144:** 380–4.

EDLBACHER, S., JUCKER, P. and BAUR, H. (1937) Die Beeinflussung der Darmreaktion des Histamins durch Aminosäuren. *Z. Physiol. Chem.* **247:** 63–4.

EDMAN, K. A. P., MONGAR, J. L. and SCHILD, H. O. (1964) The role of SH and SS groups and oxygen in anaphylactic reaction of chopped guinea-pig lung. *J. Physiol.* **170:** 124–37.

ERDÖS, E. G. and WOHLER, J. R. (1963) Inhibition of the *in vivo* enzymatic inactivation of bradykinine and kallidin. *Life Sci.* **2:** 270–4.

HERBERTS, G. (1955) Proteolytic activity in organ extracts after anaphylactic shock with special regard to the action of thiols. *Acta Soc. Med. Upsalien.* **60:** 246–69.

ISHIZAKA, K., ISHIZAKA, T. and SUGAHARA, T. (1961) Molecular bases of passive sensitization. 1. Role of disulfide linkages in γ-globuline molecule. *J. Immunol.* **87:** 548–54.

JÓKAY, I., KASSAY, L. and KISS, A. (1964a) Inhibition of endotoxin induced platelet agglutination, histamine, and serotonine release *in vitro* by thiol-compounds. *Experientia* **20:** 315–16.

JÓKAY, I., KISS, A. and KASSAI, L. (1964b) Effect of cysteine on local Shwartzman phenomenon. *Acta Microbiol. Acad. Sci. Hung.* **11:** 29–33.

KISELEV, P. N. and KARPOVA, E. V. (1965) Role of sulfhydryl groups of proteins in blocking and fixation of complement. *Fed. Proc.* **24:** 1073–5.

LECOMTE, J. (1952a) Propriétés pharmacodynamiques de la cystinamine. *Arch. internat. Physiol.* **60:** 179–80.

LECOMTE, J. (1952b) Sur la pathogénie du choc nitritoide bénin. *Arch. int. Pharmacodyn.* **92:** 241–51.

LECOMTE, J. (1955) Propriétés antihistaminiques des dérivés décarboxylés de la cystéine (cystéamine et cystamine). *Arch. internat. Physiol. Bioch.* **63:** 291–304.

LECOMTE, J. (1956) Contribution clinique et expérimentale à l'étude du rôle de l'histamine dans certains phénomènes anaphylactiques. *Thèse d'Agrégation de l'Enseignement Supérieur.* DUCULOT, J. (ed.), Gembloux, pp. 92 and 95.

LECOMTE, J. (1964) Activité histamino-libératrice du *S*, 2-amino éthylisothiouronium (AET) chez le rat. *Arch. internat. Physiol. Bioch.* **72:** 510–13.

LECOMTE, J. and BACQ, Z. M. (1965) Propriétés vasomotrices de la 2-mercaptoéthylguanidine (MEG) chez le rat. *Arch. int. Pharmacodyn.* **158:** 480–97.

LECOMTE, J. and BOHRENSTAYN, C. (1953) Action anti-inflammatoire de la cystéamine et de la cystamine. *C.R. Soc. Biol.* **147:** 359–62.

LECOMTE, J. and FRANCHIMONT, P. (1962) Histamine endogène et pathogénie de l'œdème par cystamine. *C.R. Soc. Biol.* **156:** 1951–3.

LECOMTE, J. and VAN CAUWENBERGE, H. (1957a) Inhibition de la diffusion hyaluronidasique par les dérivés décarboxylés de la cystéine. *C.R. Soc. Biol.* **151:** 1032–5.

LECOMTE, J. and VAN CAUWENBERGE, H. (1957b) Les dérivés de la cystéine sont-ils des anti-inflammatoires? *C.R. Soc. Biol.* **151:** 609–11.

LECOMTE, J. and VAN CAUWENBERGE, H. (1957c) Sur l'activité anti-inflammatoire des dérivés décarboxylés de la cystéine. *Semaine des Hôpitaux* (Semaine Thérapeutique) **33:** 906–10.

LECOMTE, J., VAN CAUWENBERGE, H. and GOBLET, J. (1953a) Action anti-inflammatoire chez le rat de la cystéinamine et de son dérive oxydé la cystinamine. *C.R. Soc. Biol.* **147:** 1121–4.

LECOMTE, J., VAN CAUWENBERGE, H., GOBLET, J. and VLIERS, M. (1953b) Action inhibitrice comparée de la cystéinamine et de ses dérivés sur l'œdème au blanc d'œuf chez le rat. *Ann. Endocr.* **14:** 123–7.

LECOMTE, J., CESSION-FOSSION, A., LIBON, J. CL. and BACQ, Z. M. (1964) Sur quelques effets pharmacodynamiques généraux de la cystamine chez le rat. *Arch. int. Pharmacodyn.* **148**: 487–510.

LEDDY, J. P., FREEMAN, G. L., LUZ, A. and TODD, R. H. (1962) Inactivation of the skin-sensitizing antibodies of human allergy by thiols. *Proc. Soc. Exp. Biol. Med.* **111**: 7–12.

LONG, D. A. (1954) Influence of cysteinamine on tuberculin sensitivity in guinea-pigs. *Brit. J. Pharmacol.* **9**: 118–20.

MARCUS, S. and DONALDSON, D. M. (1952) Suppression of Shwartzman phenomenon by adrenocorticotropic hormone and cortisone. Quantitative aspects. *J. Immunol.* **69**: 101–8.

MEYERS, W. M. and BURDON, K. L. (1960) Inhibition of anaphylaxis in mice by pre-treatment with cysteine, lysine ethyl ester and tyrosine ethyl ester. *Experientia* **16**: 52–4.

MÖRSDORF, K., STENGER, E. G., THEOBALD, W. and DOMENJOZ, R. (1955) Der Einfluss von Cystinamin und Cysteinamin auf das Formalioedem und der Gehalt der Nebenniere an Cholesterin und Ascorbinsäure bei der Ratte. *Arzneimittel Forschung* **5**: 314–15.

MUNDY, R. L., HEIFFER, M. H. and MEHLMAN, B. (1963) Mechanism of beta-mercapto-ethylamine induced hypotension in the dog. *Amer. J. Physiol.* **204**: 997–1000.

MUNDY, R. L., DEMAREE, G. E., JACOBUS, D. P. and HEIFFER, M. H. (1967) Beta-mercapto-ethylamine and cystamine-induced histamine release in the dog. *Arch. int. Pharmacodyn.* **165**: 64–70.

PANY, J. E. (1963) The influence of sulfur-containing radiation protection materials on the metabolism of histamine. I. The action of SH— and disulfide compounds on the enzymes of histamine decomposition. *Z. ges. Exptl. Med.* **137**: 609–18.

PICARELLI, Z. P., HENRIQUES, O. B. and OLIVEIRA, M. C. (1962) Potentiation of bradykinine action on smooth-muscles by cysteine. *Experientia* **18**: 77–9.

RAUSA, L., PALAZZOADRIANO, M. and CANNIZZARO, G. (1964) Influenza della β-mercap-toetilamina sulla velocita di ossidazione della serotonina. *Arch. int. Pharmacodyn.* **149**: 444–53.

ROBBERS, H. (1937) Die pharmakologische Wirkung des Cystamins, einer blutdrucksen-kenden Substanz. *Arch. exp. Path. Pharmakol.* **185**: 461–91.

ROCHA E SILVA, M. (1955) *Histamine. Its Role in Anaphylaxis and Allergy.* Charles C. Thomas, Springfield, Illinois, U.S.A. p. 170.

SELYE, H. (1951) 1st Annual Report on Stress. *Acta Inc. Medical Publ.,* Montreal, p. 441.

SIMIĆ, M. M., SLIJIVIĆ, V. S. and PETKOVIĆ, M. Z. (1960) Antibody formation in X-irradiated rats protected with β-mercaptoethylamine and β-ethylisothiouronium. *Bull. Boris Kidrich Inst. Nucl. Sci.* **10**: 149–61.

STEPANOVIĆ, S., VARAGIĆ, V. and HAJDUKOVIĆ, S. (1963) The effect of cysteamine on the responses to biologically active substances of the isolated guinea-pig ileum taken from normal and gamma-irradiated animals. *Bull. Boris Kidrich. Int. Nucl. Sci.* **14**: 163–74.

VAN CAUWENBERGE, H. and LECOMTE, J. (1955) Introduction à l'étude, chez l'animal, du déterminisme des propriétés anti-inflammatoires du salicylate de soude. *Bull. Acad. Roy. Méd. Belg.* IInd series **III**: No. **7**: 1–75.

VARAGIĆ, V., KRSTIĆ, M., STEPANOVIĆ, S. and HAJDUKOVIĆ, S. (1965) The effect of gamma-radiation and cysteamine on the amount of 5-hydroxytryptamine in the rat ileum in the course of 12 hours after irradiation. *Int. J. Rad. Biol.* **9**: 153–5.

WILHELM, D. L. and MANSON, B. (1958) Rational of antihistaminic therapy in thermal injury. An experimental evaluation in the guinea-pig. *Brit. Med. J.* **2**: 1141–3.

3.3

SHOCK AND BLOOD COMPOSITION

P. Van Caneghem

Liège, Belgium

3.3.1. CYSTAMINE AND CYSTEAMINE

Cysteamine (MEA) and even more cystamine injected at doses generally used for radioprotective action provoke a non-specific shock as do other "aggressions". These substances have pharmacological effects favoring the appearance of a state of shock. They cause a significant and long-lasting fall in blood pressure, which Robbers (1937) studied while doing pharmacological research on cystamine. They are, furthermore, tissue irritants, provoking local vasodilatation, increase of the vascular permeability and interstitial edema (Lecomte *et al.*, 1964; Beaumariage *et al.*, 1966) (see Chapters 3.1 and 3.2).

It is known that states of shock are accompanied by various metabolic changes due to a restriction of the exchanges between the intracellular and extracellular compartments and alterations of permeability. These changes affect the concentrations of different substances in the blood, the time of their appearance depending on their localization in the pathologic and metabolic cycles. They are in no way specific, but are definitely related to the severity of the shock and to its causes.

For all reactions mentioned in this chapter cystamine and MEA were administered at radioprotective doses, that is 100–150 mg/kg.

3.3.1.1. CARDIOVASCULAR COLLAPSE

Cysteamine and cystamine show a significant hypotensive effect (Robbers, 1937; Lecomte *et al.*, 1964), accompanied by hypothermia (Liébecq-Hutter and Bacq, 1958) and a reactional discharge of

epinephrine (Mundy *et al.*, 1961). These effects have been studied in
Chapter 3.1 to which we refer. The hypotensive action of cystamine is more
important than that of MEA (Lecomte *et al.,* 1964; Beaumariage *et al.,*
1966). Cystamine provokes a tissue vasodilatation (Robbers, 1937).
This phenomenon is more important with cystamine than with MEA,
since the vascular resistance on perfusion of an organ, such as the isolated
rabbit ear or the liver, by these substances is decreased more by cystamine
(Van Caneghem and Beaumariage, unpublished results) than by MEA.

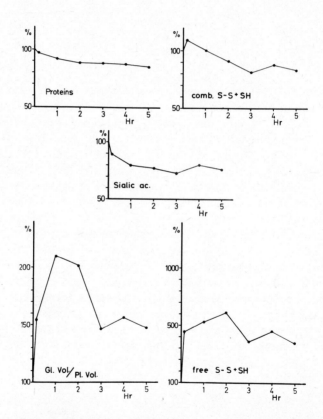

FIG. 1. Ratio of cells to plasma volumes, of the concentration of proteins, of —SS—
and —SH groups combined with proteins, of free —SS— and —SH groups, and of
sialic acid in the rat plasma after injection of cystamine (100 mg/kg) (Van Caneghem
and Stein, 1967). Ordinate: ratio of the cells to plasma volumes, concentrations
expressed in % of the initial values. Abscissa: time (hr) after injection of cystamine.

3.3.1.2. MODIFICATION OF THE BLOOD COMPOSITION

Hemoconcentration
Following intraperitoneal (i.p.) injection of cystamine into the rat a significant increase in hematocrit values is to be observed (Fig. 1). This hemoconcentration occurs soon after the injection as shown by Table 1. It varies according to the way cystamine is administered (see also Table 2). It is less important with MEA (Van Caneghem, 1969).

Plasma Cations
Cystamine causes a significant increase of K^+ and Mg^{2+} in the plasma after i.p. injection (Fig. 2), lasting several hours. Since these ions are normally located in the intracellular space this indicates a change in permeability of the cell membranes. The Na^+ concentration remains unchanged. The noted decrease of Ca^{2+} is not statistically significant under our experimental conditions (Van Caneghem *et al.*, 1967). These effects are similar to those found with other forms of shock (Henrotte *et al.*, 1967).

TABLE 1. RATIO OF BLOOD CELLS AND PLASMA VOLUMES AFTER I.P. AND I.V. INJECTIONS OF CYSTAMINE AND MEA (100 mg/kg) IN THE RAT (From Van Caneghem, 1969)

Substances	Methods	Delay (min)	n^a	Vol. cells / Vol. plasma
NaCl	—	3	10	0.95 ±0.08
Cystamine	i.p.	3	10	1.16 ±0.05
		10	10	1.94[b] ±0.09
		25	10	2.32[b] ±0.28
	i.v.	3	10	1.43[b] ±0.09
		10	10	1.25 ±0.11
		25	10	1.22 ±0.08
MEA	i.p.	3	10	1.09 ±0.07
		10	10	1.22 ±0.06
		25	10	1.13 ±0.07
	i.v.	3	10	1.10 ±0.06
		10	10	1.15 ±0.07
		25	10	1.17 ±0.08

[a] n indicates the number of animals.
[b] The observed difference is highly significant with respect to the control value (NaCl).

TABLE 2. SAMPLES OF RAT BLOOD TAKEN 3 HR AFTER INJECTION OF CYSTAMINE (100 mg/kg), UNDER DIFFERENT CONDITIONS (From Van Caneghem and Stein, 1967)

Methods[a]	n	Vol. cells / Vol. plasma	Plasma proteins (g %)	Plasma sialic acid (mg %)	Combined plasma —SS— and —SH (mcg/ml)	Free plasma —SS— and —SH (mcg/ml)	Albumins (g %)	α-Globulins (g %)
NaCl, i.v.	6	0.93 ±0.05	6.28 ±0.05	86 ±4.8	763 ±34	9.9 ±1.1	2.79 ±0.15	1.39 ±0.06
NaCl, i.p.	6	1.06 ±0.08	6.27 ±0.09	85 ±3.9	687 ±51	9.6 ±1.6	2.56 ±0.08	1.34 ±0.12
NaCl, i.v. +An.	6	0.98 ±0.04	6.13 ±0.09	89 ±2.7	780 ±40	12.6 ±0.9	2.75 ±0.10	1.36 ±0.04
NaCl, i.p. +An.	6	0.91 ±0.03	6.14 ±0.08	93 ±6.2	723 ±46	10.1 ±0.9	2.52 ±0.10	1.37 ±0.05
Cyst., i.v.	6	0.98 ±0.06	5.31[b] ±0.13	70[b] ±3.3	625[a] ±23	17.0[b] ±2.5	2.29[a] ±0.10	1.16[a] ±0.05
Cyst., i.p.	6	1.37[b]±0.10	5.01[b] ±0.11	62[b] ±4.4	607[b] ±42	34.9[b] ±4.7	2.14[b] ±0.02	1.15[a] ±0.08
Cyst., i.v. +An.	6	1.07 ±0.07	5.71[b] ±0.07	79 ±2.5	683[c] ±27	18.8[b] ±1.4	2.41[b] ±0.10	1.24 ±0.08
Cyst., i.p. +An.	6	1.44[b] ±0.14	5.44[b] ±0.09	76[c] ±6.5	612[c] ±23	24.3[b] ±3.4	2.27[b] ±0.13	1.19[c] ±0.05
Cyst. +Epin., i.p.	6	1.47[b] ±0.08	5.33[b] ±0.14	58[b] ±5.6	625[c] ±33	25.5[b] ±1.3	2.17[c] ±0.04	1.21[c] ±0.07
NaCl +Epin., i.p.	6	1.13 ±0.07	6.13 ±0.11	75[c] ±8.9	626[c] ±28	12.7 ±1.7	2.39[c] ±0.13	1.58[c] ±0.14

[a] Epin. = epinephrine, 1 mg/kg, i.p.; An. = ether anesthesia.

[b] The difference is highly significant with respect to the controls.

[c] The difference is statistically significant.

n indicates the number of measurements. The results of the analysis of the —SS— and —SH groups are expressed in mcg cysteine.

Plasma Proteins

In the rat and rabbit cystamine causes hypoproteinemia, a decrease of sialic acid (characterizing the glycoproteins) and of the —SS— and —SH groups combined with proteins (characterizing proteins rich in sulfur) (Fig. 2). These effects are more obvious after i.p. injection of cystamine than after intravenous (i.v.) injection, being amplified by the vasoconstriction caused by epinephrine (Table 2). There is a correlation between the decrease of sialic acid and the thiol and disulfide groups bound to proteins on the one hand and the hypoproteinemia on the other. Amongst the proteins, albumin decreases less than the globulins. Contrary to what is observed in some states of shock, after injection of cystamine there is no tendency to inversion of the albumin/globulin ratio (Van Caneghem and Stein, 1967). For comparison we show the changes observed in the same strain of rats after burning (Table 3).

After injection of MEA the drop in the concentration of sialic acid is not significant, which suggests that the shock is less intense. Twenty-four hours after injection of cystamine the concentration of sialic acid has again increased and becomes higher than its original value (Van Caneghem and Stein, unpublished experiments). This later elevation of the sialic

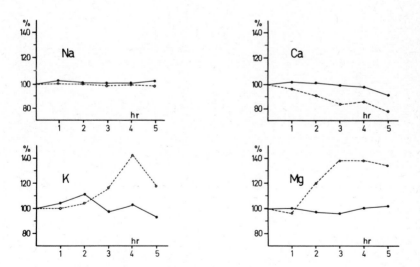

FIG. 2. Concentration of Na^+, K^+, Ca^{2+}, and Mg^{2+} in the rabbit plasma after i.p. injection of cystamine (100 mg/kg) (Van Caneghem *et al.*, 1967). Ordinate: cation concentration expressed in % of the initial value. Abscissa: time; ——: control animals injected with NaCl 0.85%;----: animals injected with cystamine.

TABLE 3. SAMPLES OF RAT BLOOD TAKEN 4 HR AFTER BURNING THE HIND QUARTER AT 60°C FOR 15 SEC
(Van Caneghem and Stein, 1967)

	n	$\dfrac{\text{Vol. cells}}{\text{Vol. plasma}}$	Plasma sialic acid (mg %)	Plasma proteins (g %)	Plasma combined —SS— + —SH (mcg cysteine/ml)	Plasma free —SS— + —SH (mcg cysteine/ml)	Albumins (g %)	α-Globulins (g %)
Controls	10	1.07±0.03	88.8±1.14	6.23±0.06	766.67±16.12	8.38±0.28	3.05±0.08	1.22±0.07
Burnt animals	10	1.70±0.08	78.1±0.95	5.04±0.05	596.72±20.47	12.24±0.69	2.17±0.11	1.22±0.04
Significance		$P<0.001$	$P<0.001$	$P<0.001$	$P<0.001$	$P<0.001$	$P<0.001$	$0.95>P>0.90$

n indicates the number of measurements.

TABLE 4. SAMPLES OF RAT BLOOD TAKEN AFTER I.P. INJECTION OF CYSTAMINE (100 mg/kg) (Van Caneghem, 1968)

Delay	n^a	Vol. cells / Vol. plasma	Serum proteins (g %)	Blood pyruvic acid (mcm/100 ml)	Plasma aldolase (Un/ml)	Esterified plasma fatty acids (mval/100 ml)
0	10	1.37 ±0.04	6.52 ±0.09	12.91 ±2.23	12 ±1.21	0.662 ±0.035
25 min	10	4.92[b] ±0.38	5.32[b] ±0.10	23.61[b] ±2.33	19 ±4.71	0.594 ±0.048
3 hr	10	4.42[b] ±0.40	5.52[b] ±0.09	18.79 ±1.64	54[b] ±4.71	0.627 ±0.041
24 hr	10	1.42 ±0.08	5.59[b] ±0.16	12.31 ±2.07	47[b] ±7.79	0.803[c] ±0.030

[a] n indicates the number of measurements.
[b] The difference is highly significant with respect to the controls (time 0).
[c] The difference is statistically significant.

acid concentration corresponds to the reactional hyperglycoproteinemia described in different forms of shock (Owen, 1961). It is a sign of an inflammatory reaction which takes about 10 days to disappear.

Enzyme Liberation

After injection of cystamine or MEA liberation of different enzymes and other metabolic products into the blood can be observed, as in other forms of shock (Back *et al.,* 1968; Harvengt and Jeanjean, 1966; Migone, 1962), indicating an increased catabolic activity (Table 4). There is an early elevation of pyruvic acid concentration (suggesting an increase in glycolysis) and of the aldolase, corresponding to tissue damage. There is also a definite increase of the cathepsic activity of the serum (Table 5). Plomteux *et al.* (1967) have shown that the β-glycuronidase in the plasma increases after injection of cystamine. The increase in concentration of these two enzymes points to the labilization or destruction of lysosomes as found in other forms of shock and in anoxia (Janoff *et al.,* 1962). This increase in proteolytic activity is accompanied by the decrease in the antitryptic power of the serum (Table 5) which is observed in traumatic shock (Fürstenberg, 1962), in the shock caused by epinephrine and after burning (Van Caneghem, 1968).

Along with a liberation of lysosomic enzymes the liberation of enzymes of mitochondrial and cytoplasmic origin (GOT, LDH, MDH, GDH) has also been observed (Plomteux *et al.,* 1967; Barnes *et al.,* 1968) (Fig. 3).

Effects on Glycemia and Lipemia

Sokal *et al.* (1959) and Mundy *et al.* (1961) have found an early hyperglycemia in the dog, due to secretion of epinephrine into the blood. Thus as we have said above, there is an increase in glycolysis (Sokal *et al.,* 1959) (Table 4). As in other kinds of shock (Harvengt and Jeanjean, 1966),

TABLE 5. SAMPLES OF RAT BLOOD TAKEN AT VARIOUS TIMES AFTER INJECTION OF CYSTAMINE (100 mg/kg). THE ACTIVITIES ARE MEASURED IN THE SERUM (Van Caneghem, 1968)

Time after injection	n^a	Cathepsic activity (arbitrary units)	n^a	Trypsic inhibition power ($\%$)
0	10	13.1 ± 1.8	20	44.0 ± 2.8
25 min	10	12.9 ± 1.5	20	$34.6^b \pm 2.1$
3 hr	10	$40.7^b \pm 6.0$	20	$32.7^b \pm 2.3$
24 hr	10	19.8 ± 2.3	20	$36.6^c \pm 2.3$

[a] *n* indicates the number of measurements.
[b] The difference is highly significant with respect to the controls (time 0).
[c] The difference is statistically significant.

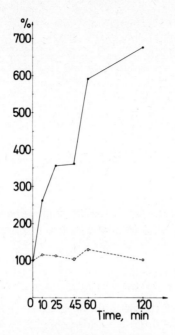

FIG. 3. Concentration of malic dehydrogenase (MDH) in the plasma of the rat after i.p. injection of MEA or mercaptoethanol (Plomteux *et al.*, 1968). Ordinate: MDH concentration expressed as % of the initial value. Abscissa: time (min); —— : MEA 1.3×10^{-3} M/kg; - - - - : mercaptoethanol 1.3×10^{-3} M/kg.

a hyperlipemia can be found in the rat after i.p. injection of cystamine (Table 4). The serum can become milky 24 hr after injection and remain so for several days.

Alteration in Blood Coagulation

With the help of a thrombograph we have studied the action of an i.p. injection of cystamine on the blood coagulation of the rat (Table 6). There is evidence of hypocoagulability. Praga *et al.* (1966) showed that 2-aminoethylisothiourea (AET) also interferes with the mechanism of coagulation.

The results obtained with compounds carrying —SS— and —SH groups oppose those yielded by other forms of shock, as for instance burning or hemorrhagic shocks. In these cases one finds hypercoagulation of the blood (see Shoemaker, 1967).

There may be a connection between the decreased clotting ability and the high content of substances carrying—SH groups in the blood.

TABLE 6. SAMPLES OF RAT BLOOD TAKEN 2 HR AFTER I.P. INJECTION OF CYSTAMINE
(100 mg/kg)

	n	Latency (in min)	Height (mm)	Surface (cm²)
Controls	5	4.0 ± 0.4	62 ± 16	189 ± 67
Cystamine	5	3.8 ± 1.6	12 ± 2	33 ± 25

n stands for the number of measurements; latency for clotting time; height is connected with the formation of blood clot; surface represents the integral between the curve and the coordinates during 30 min.

This may also be observed after administration of 4- and 5-mercapto-pyridoxine, as well as after mixing rat blood with MEA.

3.3.2. OTHER THIOLATED SUBSTANCES

Sodium mercaptoethane sulfonate ($SH-(CH_2)_2-SO_3Na$) though injected at a higher dose does not produce hemoconcentration, but a certain degree of hypoproteinemia and a decrease of sialic acid (Table 7). This decrease may be due, partly at least, to the abundance of injected —SH groups. Such substances are known to be capable of splitting proteins into smaller fractions by breaking the disulfide bridges (Lorber *et al.*, 1964). Mercaptoethanol, although chemically related to MEA, is without shock-producing property and does not produce a liberation of β-glycuronidase (Plomteux *et al.*, 1968). 5-Mercaptopyridoxine does produce liberation of β-glycuronidase, while 4-mercaptopyridoxine does not (Fig. 4) (Plomteux *et al.*, 1970); only the former shows radioprotective properties (Koch and Schmidt, 1960; Braun and Koch, 1968).

TABLE 7. SAMPLES OF RAT BLOOD TAKEN 4 HR AFTER I.P. INJECTION OF 1.28 G/KG OF
SODIUM MERCAPTOETHANE SULFONATE (Van Caneghem and Stein, 1967)

	n	Vol cells / Vol. plasma	Proteins (g %)	Sialic acid (mg %)
Controls	10	0.95 ± 0.07	5.30 ± 0.09	82.9 ± 2.62
Mercaptoethane	10	0.94 ± 0.05	4.75 ± 0.08	73.25 ± 2.39
Significance		$0.99 > P > 0.98$	$0.01 > P > 0.001$	$0.02 > P > 0.01$

n indicates the number of measurements.

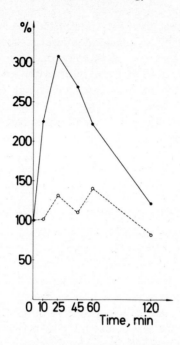

FIG. 4. Concentration of malic dehydrogenase (MDH) in the plasma of the rat after i.p. injection (125 mg/kg) of 5-mercaptopyridoxine and 4-mercapto-pyridoxine (Plomteux *et al.*, 1969). Abscissa: time (min); ——— : 5-mercaptopyridoxine; ---- : 4-mercaptopyridoxine.

3.3.3. CONCLUSIONS

Administration of MEA and cystamine to the animal rapidly produces non-specific shock, causing alterations in the metabolism which affect the blood composition: hemoconcentration, hypoproteinemia, increase of K^+ and Mg^{2+}, enzymatic liberations, drop in antitrypsic power. The same modifications can be found with other forms of shock and under prolonged anoxia. The activity of these amines does not depend on their thiol groups, since it can be reproduced by injection of non-thiolated substances (histamine, epinephrine), but on the other hand substances with thiol groups which are incapable of shock production do not cause the above-mentioned changes in blood composition. Only a few modifications, for instance some modifications of the plasma proteins, may be attributed to the presence of —SH groups.

The catecholamines liberated after injection of cystamine may also be concerned with the phenomena in question, since epinephrine can on the one hand reproduce and enhance certain effects of cystamine and on the other be liberated after injection of these amines (Mundy *et al.,* 1961). Cystamine provokes a more intense and lasting shock than MEA, its pharmacological action being stronger, although it has been demonstrated that the —SS— group of cystamine can be rapidly reduced in the organism (see Bacq, 1965). The action of cystamine is more intense after i.p. injection, especially without anesthesia, than after i.v. injection.

The state of shock observed after the injection of cystamine is followed by a reaction, similar to that observed in inflammatory states and after other conditions of shock, which is characterized by an increased sialic acid concentration in the blood.

The liberation in the blood of enzymes of mitochondrial or lysosomal origin by injection of substances carrying —SS— or —SH groups seems essentially due to a non-specific effect in connection with the slowing down of the blood circulation and the anoxia caused by it, rather than to a direct action of these substances on the organelles. Indeed, if a number of thiols and above all disulfides (with exclusion of penicillamine) favor the swelling of the rat mitochondria *in vitro* (Neubert and Lehninger, 1962), a study covering a wider range of these substances on the fragilization of the rat lysosomes *in vitro* should show that substances carrying a thiol group exercise rather a stabilizing effect, while disulfides have a fragilizing effect, but this last effect does not appear clearly unless these substances carry aromatic groups enabling them to form mixed disulfides of particular stability (Van Caneghem, 1972). It seems that injected MEA can be found in the rat cell mostly in its reduced form, that is, in a form which should stabilize the lysosomes or at least be inactive on their membranes (Filippovich *et al.,* 1970).

REFERENCES

BACK, N., WILKENS, H. and STEGER, R. (1968) Proteinases and proteinase-inhibitors in experimental shock states. *Ann. N.Y. Acad. Sci.* **146:** 491–516.

BACQ, Z. M. (1965) *Chemical Protection against Ionizing Radiation.* Charles C. Thomas, Springfield, pp. 328.

BARNES, J. H., LOWMAN, D. M. R., BAUTISTA, S. C., DE LA CRUZ, B. and LANSANGAN, L. (1968) Further studies on plasma transaminase of irradiated mice. *Int. J. Radiat. Biol.* **14:** 417–25.

BEAUMARIAGE, M. L., VAN CANEGHEM, P., and BACQ, Z. M. (1966) Etude de certaines propriétés pharmacodynamiques de la cystamine et de la cystéamine chez diverses espèces animales. *Strahlentherapie* **131:** 342–51.

BRAUN, H. and KOCH, R. (1968) Untersuchungen über einen biologischen Strahlenschutz. 86. Mitteilung: Veränderungen der Mitochondrien nach strahlenschützenden Sulfhydrylkörpern bzw. nicht schützenden Homologen. *Strahlentherapie* **135**: 628–31.

FILIPPOVICH, I., KOSHCHEENKO, N. and ROMANTZEV, E. (1970) The mechanism of "Biochemical shock"—I The correlation between the accumulation of some thiol radioprotectors in rat tissues and biochemical changes induced by them. *Biochem. Pharmacol.* **19**: 2533–40.

FÜRSTENBERG, H. (1962) Blutveränderungen in den ersten Stunden des traumatischen Schocks. *Langenbecks Arch. klin. Chir.* **301**: 114–17.

HARVENGT, C. and JEANJEAN, M. (1966) The hyperlipemia and other metabolic disorders in the burned rat. *Med. Pharmacol. exp.* **15**: 233–40.

HENROTTE, J. G., TROQUET, J. and COLINET-LAGNEAUX, D. (1967) Variation de l'ionogramme plasmatique chez le lapin en état de choc anaphylactique. *Arch. internat. Physiol. Bioch.* **75**: 77–89.

JANOFF, A., WEISSMANN, G., ZWEIFACH, B. and THOMAS, L. (1962) Pathogenesis of experimental shock. IV. Studies of lysosomes in normal and tolerant animal subjected to lethal trauma and endotoxemia. *J. Exp. Med.* **116**: 451–66.

KOCH, R. and SCHMIDT, U. (1960) Untersuchungen über einen biologischen Strahlenschutz. Weitere Untersuchungen zur Strahlenschutzwirkung SH-Gruppen-tragender Vitamin B_6-Derivate. *Strahlentherapie* **113**: 89–99.

LECOMTE, L., CESSION-FOSSION, A., LIBON, J. and BACQ, Z. M. (1964) Sur quelques effets pharmacodynamiques généraux de la cystamine chez le rat. *Arch. int. Pharmacodyn.* **148**: 487–510.

LIÉBECQ-HUTTER, S. and BACQ, Z. M. (1958) Température interne de la souris après injection de radioprotecteurs. *Arch. internat. Physiol. Bioch.* **66**: 469–71.

LORBER, A., PEARSON, G., MEREDITH, W. and GANTY-MANDELL, L. (1964) Serum sulfhydryl determination and significance in connective tissue diseases. *Ann. Int. Med.* **61**: 423–34.

MIGONE, L. (1962) Metabolische Aspekte des Schocks, pp. 85–104. In: *Schock Pathogenese und Therapie*. BOCK, K. (Ed.). Springer-Verlag, Berlin.

MUNDY, R., HEIFFER, M. and MEHLMAN, B. (1961) The pharmacology of radioprotectant chemicals. Biochemical changes in the dog following the administration of β-mercaptoethylamine (MEA). *Arch. int. Pharmacodyn.* **130**: 354–67.

NEUBERT, D. and LEHNINGER, A. (1962) The effect of thiols and disulfides on water uptake and extrusion by rat liver mitochondria. *J. Biol. Chem.* **237**: 952–8.

OWEN, J. (1961) Effect of injury on plasma proteins, pp. 1–41. In: *Advances in Clinical Chemistry*, vol. 9, SOBOTKA, H. and STEWART (Eds.). Academic Press, New York.

PLOMTEUX, G., BEAUMARIAGE, M. L., BACQ, Z. M. and HEUSGHEM, C. (1967) Variations enzymatiques dans le plasma du rat après injection d'une dose radioprotectrice de cystéamine. *Biochem. Pharmacol.* **16**: 1601–7.

PLOMTEUX, G., BEAUMARIAGE, M. L., BACQ, Z. M. and HEUSGHEM, C. (1968) Influence du β-mercaptoethanol sur certains enzymes plasmatiques du rat. *Biochem. Pharmacol.* **17**: 1998–2002.

PLOMTEUX, G., BEAUMARIAGE, M. L. and BACQ, Z. M. (1969) Radioprotective thiol compounds and some plasma enzymes. *2nd International Symposium on Radiosensitizing and Radioprotective Drugs, Rome,* p. 84.

PLOMTEUX, G., BEAUMARIAGE, M. L., BACQ, Z. M. and HEUSGHEM, C. (1970) Mercaptopyridoxines, hypoxia and plasma enzymes. *Bioch. Pharmacol.* **19**: 2799–803.

PRAGA, C., JEAN, G. and FERRONE, S. (1966) Effet du bromure de 2-aminoéthylisothiouronium (AET) sur la coagulation sanguine. *Throm. Diath. Haemorrh.* **15**: 131–42.

ROBBERS, H. (1937) Die pharmakologische Wirkung des Cystamins, einer blutdrucksenkenden Substanz. *Arch. exper. Path. Pharmakol.* **185**: 461–91.

SHOEMAKER, W. (1967) *Shock.* Charles C. Thomas, Springfield.

SOKAL, J., SARCIONE, E. and GERSZI, K. (1959) Glycogenolytic action of mercaptoethylamine. *Amer. J. Physiol.* **196:** 261–4.

VAN CANEGHEM, P. (1968) Influence de l'état de choc provoqué par la cystamine et l'adrénaline sur le pouvoir antitrypsique du sérum chez le rat. *C.R. Soc. Biol.* **162:** 2331–3.

VAN CANEGHEM, P. (1969) Vergleich der Strahlenschutzwirkung von Cystamin und Cysteamin auf die Haut. *Strahlentherapie* **137:** 231–7.

VAN CANEGHEM, P. (1972) Influence of substances with thiol functions and of their reagents on the fragility of lysosomes. *Biochem. Pharmac.* **21:** 2417–24.

VAN CANEGHEM, P. and STEIN, F. (1967) Influence de l'injection de cystamine et de divers états de choc sur les protéines plasmatiques du rat, du lapin, et du poulet. *Arch. internat. Physiol. Bioch.* **75:** 769–786.

VAN CANEGHEM, P., HENROTTE, J. G. and BACQ, Z. M. (1967) Modification de la concentration plasmatique des cations après injection de cystamine chez le lapin. *Arch. internat. Physiol. Bioch.* **75:** 469–73.

3.4

ENDOCRINE GLANDS

M. L. Beaumariage

Liège, Belgium

3.4.1. HYPOTHALAMO–PITUITARY–ADRENAL SYSTEM

3.4.1.1. ADRENAL GLANDS

3.4.1.1.1. *Adrenal Medulla*

Direct action

Lecomte (1954) has shown that a single intra-aortic injection of 10–50 mg/kg of cysteamine (MEA) produces a blood pressure rise of medullo-adrenal origin in cats and dogs, repeated injections being followed by disappearance of the pressor response. Following up this study in cats, Goffart (1955) confirmed the nicotinic action of MEA and also observed with smaller doses competitive ganglionic blocking of splanchnic–medullo-adrenal. Although MEA has a direct stimulating effect on the adrenal medulla this is sometimes difficult to demonstrate, since adrenalectomy does not always prevent the pressor response to 5–10 mg injected into the celiac trunk.

In the dog, the addition of cystamine to blood perfused through adrenals, transplanted in the neck, directly causes an increase in the blood flow and secretion of catecholamines (Barac *et al.*, 1968). Perfusion with cystamine immediately followed by complete ischemia does not prevent a considerable discharge of catecholamines when circulation is re-established and the arterial pressure of the perfused dog increases. These denervated, transplanted adrenals remain capable of synthesizing catecholamines and of converting a considerable amount of nor-epinephrine into epinephrine.

91

TABLE 1. EFFECT OF ADMINISTRATION OF 100 mg/kg OF MEA ON THE PERIPHERAL PLASMA EPINEPHRINE AND NOREPINEPHRINE VALUES OF DOGS ANESTHETIZED WITH SODIUM PENTOBARBITAL (36 mg/kg i.v.) (Mundy *et al.*, 1961)

Period	n	Epinephrine (mcg/l)			Norepinephrine (mcg/l)		
		Mean ± S.E.	t	P	Mean ± S.E.	t	P
Control	15	0.55 ± 0.19			2.38 ± 0.91		
Normotension	7	1.57 ± 0.40	2.318	0.05	4.33 ± 1.20	1.291	0.30
Hypotension	14	48.25 ± 16.69	2.856	0.01	12.11 ± 2.24	4.022	0.001
One hour post-administration	10	6.92 ± 3.22	2.441	0.05	9.02 ± 2.38	2.598	0.02
Two hours post-administration	6	8.13 ± 2.74	2.762	0.02	9.72 ± 4.85	1.286	0.30

Indirect action

In dogs and rats, the intravenous (i.v.) or intraperitoneal (i.p.) injection of MEA or cystamine in doses used for radioprotective tests produces an increase in the epinephrine and norepinephrine content of the blood, 10 min after injection (Table 1) (Heiffer *et al.*, 1961; Mundy *et al.*, 1961). In dogs this increase in catecholamines occurs simultaneously with the fall in blood pressure resulting from injection of the sulfur-containing compound. Adrenalectomy, vagotomy and diphenhydramine (a ganglion blocker) prevent or reduce the rise in blood catecholamine levels.

In rats, the emptying of the adrenal medulla occurs within $\frac{1}{2}$ hr of injection of the sulfur-containing substance, without sufficient compensatory neosynthesis of catecholamines (Cession-Fossion *et al.*, 1962; Debijadji *et al.*, 1962; Libon *et al.*, 1963; Lecomte *et al.*, 1964). Mercaptoethylguanidine (MEG), which has little effect or may increase the arterial pressure in rats, produces a slight increase in the catecholamine content of the adrenals (Cession-Fosson *et al.*, 1964; Lecomte and Bacq, 1965). This liberation of catecholamines may be responsible for the hyperglycemia observed after administration of MEA and its derivatives (Section 4.2) and may contribute to the anti-inflammatory effects of these drugs. According to Willoughby and Spector (1960), the sympathetic nerve endings of a region of skin injured by scalding liberate an anti-inflammatory adrenergic amine which is destroyed by monoamine oxidase.

The toxicity of MEA is greatly increased by bilateral adrenalectomy; it is restored to normal by a previous i.p. injection of epinephrine (Fischer *et al.*, 1955).

3.4.1.1.2. *Adrenal Cortex*

In rats and mice, cystamine stimulates the activity of the adrenal cortex; histochemical alterations may be seen (Bronzetti *et al.*, 1958), and a decrease in ascorbic acid content (Van Cauwenberge *et al.*, 1953; Van Cauwenberge, 1956; Mörsdorf *et al.*, 1955). Dehydro-ascorbic acid appears in the adrenals (Polikarpova, 1965) while the concentration of ascorbic acid in the blood increases (Bacq *et al.*, 1952). On the other hand, glandular cholesterol considered as the precursor of active steroids shows only a negligible reduction, sometimes delayed and preceded by an increase, contrary to that observed after the administration of adrenocorticotropic hormone (ACTH) (Van Cauwenberge *et al.*, 1953; Van Cauwenberge, 1956; Mörsdorf *et al.*, 1955). Despite the non-depletion of cholesterol (classically observed in all types of stress) there is an increase

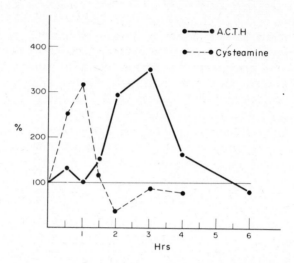

FIG. 1. Changes in 17-hydroxycorticosteroid content in the blood of rats after the injection of ACTH or cysteamine. The increase observed after cysteamine injection is more rapid but not as persistent as that seen after ACTH (Van Cauwenberge, 1956).

in the 17-hydroxycorticosteroids in the circulating blood (Van Cauwenberge, 1954, 1955, 1956; Flemming and Geierhaas, 1967). This phenomenon appears much earlier than after injection of ACTH (Fig. 1), and is inhibited by adrenalectomy (Van Cauwenberge, 1956). Secretion of cortisol and corticosterone by adrenals acutely transplanted in the neck of dogs is about doubled by perfusion with blood containing 0.3% cystamine (Robaye *et al.*, 1970). Davison and Hofmann (1954), studying the influence of different sulfur-containing compounds on the synthesis of formaldehydrogenic deoxycorticosteroids of the deoxycortico type by slices of adrenals *in vitro*, observed an increase in steroid production after the addition of MEA, but not after cystamine. According to these authors, this stimulation could be related to the formation of coenzyme A, of which MEA is a constituent.

Cysteine does not affect cholesterol levels and barely alters the adrenal ascorbic acid of the rat (Van Cauwenberge, 1954) although depletion of these chemical constituents is more intense after strong doses of reduced glutathione (GSH) in the rat and the guinea-pig (Carey *et al.*, 1951).

Cysteine and GSH are actively taken up by adrenal glands, as can be demonstrated by giving ^{35}S-labeled molecules to the rat (Goldzieher *et al.*, 1953); they reduce the synthesis of steroids *in vitro* (Davison and Hofmann,

1954). The mechanism of this inhibitory action of cysteine and of GSH is not clear. The synthesis of steroids depends, according to Davison and Hofmann (1954), on enzymes whose activity is modified by the presence of sulfhydryl groups, as this is supported by the considerable reduction in the production of steroids in adrenal slices under the influence of iodoacetate and the complete inhibition by suitable doses of *N*-ethyl-maleimide, a specific inhibitor of the —SH group.

After aminoethylisothiourea (AET) administration, the corticosteroid content of adrenal venous blood is somewhat increased in rats, but no histological or histochemical changes in the structure of the glands are observed (David *et al.*, 1965).

Other tissue and metabolic stress alterations are also found in small rodents after administration of MEA. An increase in the number of pycnotic cells in the thymus cortex is visible 6 hr after injection of MEA (Tanaka and Rixon, 1965), while the weight of the organ is reduced to 65–75% of the initial value 4 days after the administration of MEA, as is the case with cystamine (Beaumariage, unpublished observation). Selye (1950) drew attention to the fact that disintegration of thymus cells occurred soon after an injection of ACTH or of cortisone, while the involution of the thymus initially masked by edema does not become apparent until after 48 hr. The weight of the spleen remains unchanged (Beaumariage, unpublished observations). Eosinopenia is seen after administration of MEA in rats conditioned not to give stressful reactions due to the injection (Beaumariage, 1959) but if this precaution is not taken the results are more irregular and the eosinopenia is barely significant (Van Cauwenberge *et al.*, 1953; Van Cauwenberge, 1956). According to Innes and Nickerson (1965), eosinopenia can be the result of a direct effect of epinephrine on eosinophils. In rats, after a single injection of cysteine, eosinopenia is slight (Beaumariage, 1959) or non-existent (Van Cauwenberge, 1956), but repeated daily oral administration of cysteine for a week lowers the number of eosinophils in the skin, the duodenum and the colon, as does prolonged treatment with ACTH (Holsti and Rytoemaa, 1965).

Dienstbier *et al.* (1968) observed in rats injected i.p. with AET a significant fall in the number of circulating erythrocytes, leukocytes, and especially lymphocytes; when the bone-marrow becomes particularly rich in cells of the erythrocyte and myeloid series, the number of eosinophils also increases greatly. Return to normal occurs during the third week. A marked hypereosinophilia in bone-marrow has been noted in the literature in patients treated with ACTH or cortisone (Rosenthal *et al.*, 1950).

Repeated administration of MEA in man affected with chronic lymphatic leukemia in certain cases brings about regression of adenopathy and hypertrophy of the spleen and reduces the number of circulating leucocytes, particularly lymphocytes, while the polynuclear neutrophils are practically unchanged (Bacq *et al.*, 1952). A significant eosinopenia is occasionally observed, but the doses injected (6–7 mg/kg) are much smaller than those administered in animals (100–150 mg/kg). The reduction in the ratio uric acid/creatinine, very occasionally observed under these conditions, has not been studied in the normal animal.

While ACTH causes an increase in hepatic glycogen, MEA or cystamine causes a decrease when injected into the normally fed rat and mouse (Bacq and Fischer, 1953; Van Cauwenberge, 1956); on the other hand, no change occurs in the fasting animal (Fischer, 1954). Certain antiinflammatory properties of these compounds have been described by Mörsdorf *et al.* (1955) and by Lecomte and Van Cauwenberge (1957) that may depend, at least in part, on the hypercorticism initiated by the injection of these substances (Section 3.2.3).

Certain phenomena (drop in adrenal cholesterol, eosinopenia, rise in liver glycogen) regularly produced in the rat by the injection of ACTH may be absent after giving sulfur-containing radioprotective agents; the increase in the level of blood corticoids occurs earlier after MEA than after ACTH injection (Fig. 1). Thus it was thought that sulfur-containing radioprotective agents might act directly on the adrenals, like cyanide, and not via the hypothalamus and adenohypophysis (Van Cauwenberge, 1956). This hypothesis should be abandoned, because hypophysectomy inhibits the fall in adrenal ascorbic acid after MEA administration (Heiffer *et al.*, 1961); this fact suggests that ACTH may be a necessary intermediate step.

3.4.1.2. NEUROHYPOPHYSEAL SYSTEM

Duchesne *et al.* (1968) have shown that, in the rat, MEA and cystamine (at a dose of 10 mg/kg, i.p.) stimulate within 10 min the movement of the neurosecretion of the hypothalamus and posterior hypophysis, which is seen in the form of Gomori-positive grains in axons and round the vessels (Figs. 2 and 3). The reaction is more pronounced after the injection of cystamine. Analogous modifications, though appearing later, are observed under the influence of cysteine (Heckmann *et al.*, 1963) and of AET (Künkel and Heckmann, 1966). Three days after the injection of AET, the neurosecretory depletion of the posterior hypophysis of the rat is still more marked than after irradiation with 1000 r.

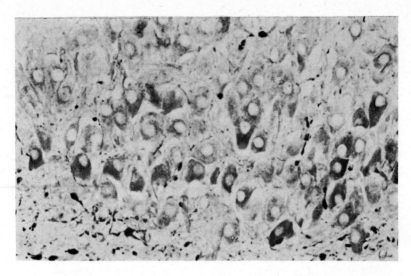

FIG. 2. Supraoptic nucleus of control rat. Normal amount of intra- and extracellular material. Aldehyde-fuchsin stain (×410) (Duchesne *et al.*, 1968).

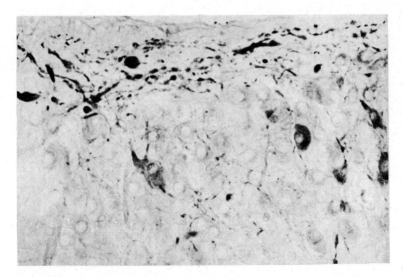

FIG. 3. Supraoptic nucleus after cysteamine. Same picture as after irradiation: intracellular depletion and axonal increase of neurosecretory material (×350) (Duchesne *et al.*, 1968).

3.4.2. PANCREAS AND REGULATION OF CARBOHYDRATE METABOLISM

In the rat MEA and cystamine, injected i.p. (100–200 mg/kg) or given p.o. (200–400 mg/kg), produce a considerable decrease in hepatic glycogen and hyperglycemia (Fig. 4), which is accompanied by an increase in lactic and pyruvic acid in the blood and urine (Fischer, 1956; Van Caneghem, 1968) and by a rise in blood catecholamine levels. Hyperglycemia is also observed in the dog and persists in spite of administration of insulin, disappearing after medullo-adrenalectomy, treatment with an α-blocker such as dihydroergotamine (Fig. 4), or diphenhydramine (Sokal *et al.*, 1959; Mundy *et al.*, 1961). The action of the latter, according to Mundy *et al.* (1961), is probably due to ganglion blocking and perhaps also to inhibition of the action of epinephrine on carbohydrate metabolism. Sokal *et al.* (1959) have confirmed the hepatic glycogenolytic effect of MEA and especially of cystamine in the rat; they both decrease muscle glycogen content. Hepatic glycogenolysis persists after pancreatectomy and medullo-adrenalectomy, which seems to exclude the action of the

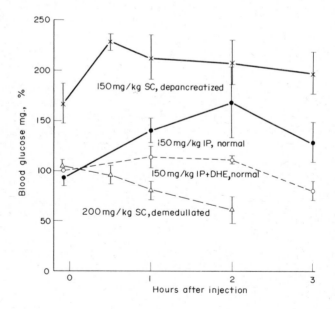

FIG. 4. Blood glucose levels after mercaptoethylamine injection in 4 normal, 4 dihydro-ergotamine treated, 4 adrenomedullated and 2 pancreatectomized rats. Vertical lines represent standard errors (Sokal *et al.*, 1959).

adrenal medulla and of the α cells of the pancreas which secrete glucagon. MEA therefore seems to act directly on the hepatic cell. On the other hand, adrenalectomy, but not pancreatectomy, inhibits hyperglycemia after MEA administration, which indicates a predominant if not exclusive participation of the adrenal medulla and its secretion in the control of this metabolic change. Hyperglycemia is also observed in the rabbit after injection of *N*-acetylcysteamine, but not after *N-S*-diacetylcysteamine (Kuhn and Quadbeck, 1951). Cysteine and GSH in quantities equimolecular to the effective doses of MEA have no effect on hepatic glycogen (Bacq and Fisher, 1953). In the rat, AET produces temporary hyperglycemia, followed by hypoglycemia (due to insulin release as well as hepatic glycogenolysis and lactacidemia (Zins *et al.*, 1958, 1959). These actions depend on the adrenal medulla, since in the alloxan diabetic rat, AET rapidly produces hyperglycemia, which is abolished by adrenalectomy and reduced by ergotamine. A slight hypoglycemia is observed in man after AET administration (Jouany and Weber, 1961).

We also note an alteration in the enzymatic reactions that control the metabolism of carbohydrates (Chapter 6.4). It is possible that stimulation of adrenal medulla and pancreatic secretions are usual homeostatic reactions tending to re-establish a biochemical equilibrium which is seriously threatened.

3.4.3. THYROID

The antithyroid properties of thiourea, a moderate radioprotective agent, are well known, but the action of cysteine derivatives on the thyroid is still poorly defined.

The work of Foster *et al.* (1953) on cysteine and that of Vittorio *et al.* (1961) on MEA show that a single injection of these substances in the rat decreases the fixation of radioiodine by the thyroid gland. After MEA administration (130 mg/kg, i.p.), the amount of serum protein combined with iodine declines. The antithyroid action of MEA has also been pointed out by Lomonos and Pivanova (1966). On the other hand, Eldjarn and his coworkers observed that MEA and cystamine (30 mg/kg, s.c.), which accumulate in significant amounts in the thyroid gland (Eldjarn and Nygaard, 1954), increase its capacity to concentrate radioiodine, whose speed of elimination increases (Nygaard and Eldjarn, 1954). Wolff and Rall (1965) have drawn attention to the fact that MEA and cystamine in a single injection temporarily increase the capacity of the thyroid gland to accumulate ^{131}I; however, they have a moderate antithyroid action, probably by preventing the transformation of molecular iodine into organic iodine, *in vivo* as well as *in vitro*. Administered over a period of time, MEA and cystamine are deprived of goitrogenic action, both in rat (Wolff and Rall, 1965) and in man (Bacq *et al.*, 1952a), probably because they are too rapidly metabolized; histological examination shows no sign of decreased functioning of the thyroid follicles in the rat.

According to Vittorio *et al.* (1960, 1961) AET (200 mg/kg, i.p.) diminishes the concentration of iodine by the thyroid in the rat and lowers the amount of serum proteins combined with iodine. Its effects last longer than do those of MEA. If both sulfur-containing protective agents are injected simultaneously, their effects are additive. In addition, Maruyama (1963) observed that the thyroid depression is stronger after administration of MEG than with AET (250 mg/kg, i.p.) but he did not verify any important alterations in the mechanisms that lead to iodination of organic compounds, nor any change in the biological period of the radio-elements in the thyroid of the normal rat; in animals treated with thyreostimulin, treatment with AET slows down, to some extent, the release of thyroid hormones. There was no significant change in the amount of serum proteins that had combined with radioactive iodine. Finally, when administered over a long period of time, there were no macroscopic or microscopic indications of hypofunctioning of the thyroid. These facts would tend to eliminate direct antithyroid action of AET, which would perhaps depend on extrathyroid factors of cardiovascular, renal, or neuroendocrine origin.

3.4.4. CONCLUSIONS

1. Cysteamine and cystamine liberate adrenal catecholamines into the blood. This secretion is probably due to the setting into motion of usual homeostatic mechanisms of arterial pressure, caused by the hypotension produced by these substances, since MEG, which only slightly alters or increases the arterial pressure, does not affect the adrenal catecholamines. Cysteamine and cystamine have, in addition, a synapse-blocking action affecting the splanchnic–medullo-adrenal transmission; only MEA has a nicotinic effect.

2. The administration of sulfur-containing radioprotective agents produces a stimulation of the hypothalamo–hypophyso–adrenal axis as shown by the escape of the neurosecretion in the hypothalamus and the

posterior hypophysis, and the increase in corticoidemia. In the present state of our knowledge, it is impossible to say whether the stress reaction observed is induced by the sulfur-containing radioprotective agent itself, or by its effect of increasing the circulating level of epinephrine.

3. Cysteamine, cystamine, and AET do not appear to exercise any direct effect on the pancreas. The hyperglycemia that follows their injection would be due to epinephrine, which produces a secondary hypoglycemia by secretion of insulin. Hepatic glycogenolysis is due to a direct effect of the sulfur-containing radioprotective agents on hepatic glycogen reserves. The muscular glycogenolysis appears to be linked to the secretion of epinephrine.

4. The study of the action of sulfur-containing radioprotective compounds on the thyroid gland has given results from which it is difficult to draw definite conclusions, because of the numerous different techniques used and the diversity of the parameters studied. In a single injection, the compounds studied affect the thyroid function only slightly. Cysteamine and cystamine appear to act by a different mechanism from that of AET and of MEG; all of them lose antithyroid activity if repeated doses are given.

REFERENCES

BACQ, Z. M. and FISCHER, P. (1953) The action of cysteamine on liver glycogen. *Arch. internat. Physiol.* **61**: 517–18.

BACQ, Z. M., BERNARD, J., RAMIOUL, H. and DELTOUR, G. (1952a) La mercaptoéthylamine dans le traitement des leucémies chroniques. *Bull. Acad. Roy. Méd. Belg.*, VIIth series, **17**: 460–82.

BACQ, Z. M., FISCHER, P. and PIROTTE, M. (1952b) Métabolisme de la cystéamine et de la cystamine chez le lapin. *Arch. internat. Physiol.* **60**: 535–8.

BARAC, G., CESSION-FOSSION, A. and BACQ, Z. M. (1968) Effet direct de la chlorpromazine, de la cystamine et de la phénoxybenzamine sur le débit sanguin et la sécrétion de catécholamines des surrénales "au cou" chez le chien. *Agressologie* **9**: 449–55.

BEAUMARIAGE, M. L. (1959) Action de la cystéamine sur le taux des éosinophiles sanguins du rat. *Arch. int. Pharmacodyn.* **118**: 146–54.

BRONZETTI, P., PIZZAGALLI, G. and VIVIANI, C. (1958) Sulle modificazioni topografiche e quantitative della reazione di Giround–Leblond–Sosa per la determinazione istochimica dell'acido ascorbico nella ghiandola surrenale del ratto dopo trattamento con cisteamina. *Radiol. Latina* **1**: 280–96.

CAREY, M. M., VOLLMER, E. P., ZWEMER, R. L. and SPENCE, D. L. (1951) Decrease of adrenal ascorbic acid and cholesterol in rat and guinea pig following large doses of glutathione. *Amer. J. Physiol.* **164**: 770–3.

CESSION-FOSSION, A., LECOMTE, J. and FRANCHIMONT, P. (1962) Mécanisme de l'action antiinflammatoire de la cystamine. *C.R. Soc. Biol.* **156**: 1196–9.

CESSION-FOSSION, A., VANDERMEULEN, R. and LECOMTE, J. (1964) Action de l'aminoéthylisothiouronium sur la médullo-surrénale du rat. *C.R. Soc. Biol.* **158**: 1976–7.

DAVID, G., FAREDI, L. and TANKA, D. (1965) About the change of suprarenal function in acute radiation injury. *Radiobiol. Radiotherap.* **6**: 405–12.

DAVISON, CL. and HOFMANN, F. G. (1954) Influence of sulphydryl compounds on *in vitro* steroid production by the rat adrenal gland. *Endocrinology* **54**: 654–8.

DEBIJADJI, R., VARAGIĆ, V., ELČIĆ, S. and DAVIDOVIĆ, J. (1962) Adrenergic blocking action of cysteamine. *Experientia* **18**: 32–3.

DIENSTBIER, Z., ARIENT, M., POSPÍŠIL, J. and KOURILEK, K. (1968) On the question of toxic and radioprotective effects of AET. *Panel on Radiation Damage to the Biological Molecular Information System, with Special Regard to the Role of SH-Groups.* Vienna, 21–25 October, PL-3III/7, 36 pages.

DUCHESNE, P. Y., HAJDUKOVIĆ, S., BEAUMARIAGE, M. L. and BACQ, Z. M. (1968) Neurosecretion in the hypothalamus and posterior pituitary after irradiation and injection of chemical radioprotector in the rat. *Rad. Res.* **34**: 583–95.

ELDJARN, L. and NYGAARD, O. (1954) Cysteamine–cystamine: Intestinal absorption, distribution among various organs and excretion. *Arch. internat. Physiol.* **62**: 476–86.

FISCHER, P. (1954) Glycogène hépatique, rayons X et cystéamine. *Arch. internat. Physiol.* **62**: 134–6.

FISCHER, P. (1956) Elimination urinaire d'acides organiques après administration de cystéamine, cystamine et cyanure. *Arch. internat. Physiol. Bioch.* **64**: 130–2.

FISCHER, P., LECOMTE, J. and BEAUMARIAGE, M. L. (1955) Toxicité de la cystéamine après surrénalectomie. *Arch. internat. Physiol. Bioch.* **63**: 121–2.

FLEMMING, K. and GEIERHAAS, B. (1967) Radiation effects and adrenal cortex. III. Inhibition of corticosteroid increase by cysteamine after whole-body irradiation. *Int. J. Rad. Biol.* **3**: 13–19.

FOSTER, W. C., WASE, A. W. and REPPLINGER, T. E. (1953) Effect of sulfhydryl compounds on the formation of tissue protein-bound radioactive iodine in the thyroid, adrenal and pituitary glands. *Fed. Proc.* **12**: 44.

GOFFART, M. (1955) Mode d'action de la cystéamine et de la cystamine au niveau de la médullo-surrénale. *Arch. internat. Physiol. Bioch.* **63**: 500–12.

GOLDZIEHER, Y. W., RAWLS, W. R. and GOLDZIEHER, M. A. (1953) The uptake of sulfhydryl compounds by rat adrenal, liver and muscle measured by an improved amperometric technic. *J.B.C.* **203**: 519–26.

HECKMANN, U., KLEIVERT, H. and KUNKEL, H. A. (1963) Die Beeinflussbarkeit der Wirkung von Ganz-körperbestrahlungen auf das Zwischenhirnhypophysensystem der Ratte durch Cystein. *Naturwissenschaften* **50**: 732–3.

HEIFFER, M. H., MUNDY, R. L. and MEHLMAN, B. (1961) Plasma catechol amine levels and adrenal ascorbic acid content following β-mercaptoethylamine (MEA) administration. *Endocrinology* **69**: 746–51.

HOLSTI, L. R. and RYTOEMAA, T. (1965) Tissue eosinophils of rat under the influence of cysteine, lysine and X-irradiation. *Acta Physiol. Scand.* **63**: 370–6.

INNES, J. R. and NICKERSON, M. (1965) Drugs acting on postganglionic adrenergic nerve endings and structures innervated by them (sympathomimetic drugs). *The Pharmacological Basis of Therapeutics.* GOODMAN, L. S. and GILMAN, A. (Eds.), 3rd ed., The Macmillan Company, New York, pp. 477–520.

JOUANY, J. M. and WEBER, B. (1961) Substances de réveil. Pharmacologie succincte et utilisations cliniques de l'AET (Aminoéthylisothiouronium). *Agressologie* **2**: 30–7.

KUHN, R. and QUADBECK, G. (1951) Darstellung und Wirkungen von Acetyl-Derivaten des Cysteamins. *Chem. Berichte* **84**: 844–7.

KÜNKEL, H. A. and HECKMANN, U. (1966) Wirkung von Aminoathylisothiuronium auf die strahleninduzierten Veränderungen im Zwischenhirn-Hypophysensystem der Ratte. *Naturwissenschaften* **53**: 110–11.

LECOMTE, J. (1954) Cystéamine et médullo-surrénale. *Arch. internat. Physiol.* **62**: 431–2.

LECOMTE, J. and BACQ, Z. M. (1965) Propriétés vasomotrices de la 2-mercaptoéthylguanidine (MEG) chez le rat. *Arch. int. Pharmacodyn.* **158**: 480–97.

LECOMTE, J. and VAN CAUWENBERGE, H. (1957) Sur l'activité anti-inflammatoire des dérivés décarboxylés de la cystéine. *Semaine des Hôpitaux* (*Semaine thérapeutique*) **10**: 906–10.

LECOMTE, J., CESSION-FOSSION, A., LIBON, J. C. and BACQ, Z. M. (1964) Sur quelques effets pharmacodynamiques généraux de la cystamine chez le rat. *Arch. int. Pharmacodyn.* **148**: 487–510.

LIBON, J. C., LECOMTE, J. and CESSION-FOSSION, A. (1963) Sur les propriétés cardio-vasculaires de la cystéamine chez le rat. *C.R. Soc. Biol.* **157**: 685–7.

LOMONOS, P. I. and PIVANOVA, P. S. (1966) Function of rat thyroid gland during repeated irradiation and mercamine injection. *Radiobiologiya* **6**: 246–9. (Russian.)

MARUYAMA, Y. (1963) The effect of AET (β-aminoethylisothiuronium) on thyroid function in the rat. *Rad. Res.* **19**: 538–50.

MÖRSDORF, K., STENGER, E. G., THEOBALD, W. and DOMENJOZ, R. (1955) Der Einfluss von Cystamin und Cysteinamin auf das Formalinoedem und der Gehalt der Nebenniere an Cholesterin und Ascorbinsäure bei der Ratte. *Arzneimittel Forschung* **5**: 314–15.

MUNDY, R. L., HEIFFER, M. H. and MEHLMAN, B. (1961) The pharmacology of radioprotectant chemicals. Biochemical changes in the dog following the administration of beta-mercaptoethylamine (MEA). *Arch. int. Pharmacodyn.* **80**: 354–67.

NYGAARD, O. and ELDJARN, L. (1954) Cysteamine–cystamine: Effect on uptake and biological halflife of radioactive iodine in the thyroid gland of rats. *Arch. internat. Physiol.* **62**: 528–34.

POLIKARPOVA, L. I. (1965) Metabolism of ascorbic acid in adrenal gland irradiated with or without mercamine and cystamine protection. *Radiobiologiya* **5**: 896–8. (Russian.)

ROBAYE, B., BOURDON, V., RENSON, J., BACQ, Z. M. and BARAC, G. (1970) Effet direct de la cystamine sur la sécrétion des glycocorticoides des surrénales au cou, chez le chien. *Arch. internat. Pharmac. Therap.* **186**: 199–200.

ROSENTHAL, R. L., WALD, N., JAGER, A. and LITWINS, J. (1950) Effects of cortisone and ACTH therapy on eosinophils of the bone marrow and blood. *Proc. Soc. Exp. Biol. Med.* **75**: 740–1.

SELYE, H. (1950) Stress. Textbook of Endocrinology. *Acta Endocrinologica,* University of Montreal, Montreal, Canada, pp. 45β–6.

SOKAL, J. E., SARCIONE, E. J. and GERSZI, K. E. (1959) Glycogenolytic action of mercaptoethylamine. *Amer. J. Physiol.* **196**: 261–4.

TANAKA, Y. and RIXON, R. H. (1965) Protection of lymphocytes in the thymus of X-irradiated rats by cysteamine. *Nature* **206**: 418–19.

VAN CANEGHEM, P. (1968) Influence de l'état de choc provoqué par la cystamine et l'adrénaline sur le pouvoir antitrypsique du sérum chez le rat. *C.R. Soc. Biol.* **162**: 2331–3.

VAN CAUWENBERGE, H. (1954) Influence de l'ACTH, du salicylate de sodium et de la cystéamine sur les 17-hydroxycorticoides sanguins chez le rat. *C.R. Soc. Biol.* **148**: 1297–1300.

VAN CAUWENBERGE, H. (1955) Cystéamine et 17-hydroxycorticostéroides sanguins chez le rat. *C.R. Soc. Biol.* **149**: 605–9.

VAN CAUWENBERGE, H. (1956) Contribution à l'étude de la réactivité surrénalienne du rat. *Thèse d'Agrégation de l'Enseignement Supérieur.* Imprimerie Ste Catherine, Bruges, pp. 61–3.

VAN CAUWENBERGE, H., ROSKAM, J., HEUSGHEM, C., FISCHER, P., DELTOUR, G. and BACQ, Z. M. (1953) Action de la mercaptoéthylamine sur la teneur en acide ascorbique des glandes surrénales du rat. *Arch. internat. Physiol.* **61**: 124–7.

VITTORIO, P. V. and ALLEN, J. M. (1960) The effect of 2-aminoethylisothiouronium Br-HBr (AET) on thyroid activity in non-irradiated and X-irradiated rats. *Rad. Res.* **13**: 256–62.

VITTORIO, P. V., ALLEN, M. J. and SMALL, D. L. (1961) The effects of some radioprotective agents on thyroid activity in non-irradiated and X-irradiated rats. *Rad. Res.* **15**: 625–31.

WILLOUGHBY, D. A. and SPECTOR, W. G. (1960) *Adrenergic Mechanisms*. Ciba Foundation Symposium. J. A. Churchill Ltd., London, pp. 466–8.

WOLFF, J. and RALL, J. E. (1965) Thyroidal iodide transport. VII. Acute stimulation of thyroidal iodine concentrating ability by cystamine and cysteamine. *Endocrinology* **76**: 949–57.

ZINS, G. R., SEIDEL, D. M. and RAYMUND, A. B. (1958) Some mechanisms involved in the hyperglycemic and glycogenolytic effects of AET in alloxan-diabetic rats. *Univ. USAF, Rad. Lab. Quart. Report* No. **28**: 150.

ZINS, G. R., SEIDEL, D. M. and DUBOIS, K. P. (1959) Effect of β-aminoethylisothiuronium (AET) on glucose metabolism. *Fed. Proc.* **18**: 463.

3.5

NERVOUS SYSTEM AND RECEPTORS

M. L. Beaumariage

Liège, Belgium

3.5.1. CENTRAL NERVOUS SYSTEM AND GENERAL SYMPTOMATOLOGY

We shall attempt to explain the action of sulfur-containing radio-protective agents on the central nervous system (CNS), by describing the neurological changes observed in alert animals and their modification by anesthetics.

3.5.1.1. DOG

Cysteamine–Cystamine (Mundy and Heiffer, 1960)

Slow intravenous (i.v.) injection of 100 mg/kg of cysteamine (MEA) is followed by a group of characteristic manifestations. Salivation increases during the injection, followed by nausea and violent repeated vomiting. The animal is agitated; tonic and clonic convulsions occur after about 20–30 min. During the crises the animal is unable to remain standing, and the pupils are dilated, but react to light. After $1\frac{1}{2}$ hr ataxia occurs, the animal is depressed, it no longer reacts to painful stimuli, and it suffers anoxia and bloody diarrhea. These manifestations persist for several hours. The rhythm and depth of the respiratory movements increase during the injection, but subsequently become very irregular during the bouts of convulsions; this is followed by alternate acceleration and depression. Anesthesia prevents vomiting and convulsions.

Aminoethylisothiourea (AET) (Benson *et al.*, 1961; Newsome *et al.*, 1962)

A few minutes after intraperitoneal injection of AET (100 mg/kg) the dog shows intense agitation accompanied by hyperpnea, nausea with vomiting, tenesmus and defecation, intense salivation and anorexia. There is mydriasis, and the nictitating membranes are relaxed. After 30–60 min, lethargy sets in, with slight muscular tremor and ataxia when the animal lifts itself up and tries to move about. Respiratory activity slackens and these manifestations gradually die away. This phase of depression, during which one sees lowered powers of perception and only sluggish conscious response to any stimulus, may persist up to 18–24 hr. Administration of 160 mg/kg i.p., or 125 mg i.v., is necessary to produce severe tonic and clonic convulsions and intermittent opisthotonos particularly pronounced in the presence of external stimuli. There are myosis, nystagmus and diarrhea. With 160 mg/kg, death follows in 40–52 hr. A pneumographic recording and a spirometric study show that the anesthetized dog has constant strong ventilatory excitation, with increased respiratory output after 30 mg of AET, followed by hypoventilation, a probable consequence of hypocapnia (Laborit *et al.,* 1959). The respiratory depression induced by barbiturates is said to be counteracted by AET.

3.5.1.2. CAT

Cystamine (Robbers, 1937)

In the alert animal, after 105 mg/kg of cystamine anorexia and abundant salivation are observed. As much as 135 mg/kg must be administered subcutaneously in order to see (after 1 hr) unrest and acceleration of respiration. There is mydriasis, the cat no longer moves spontaneously, and convulsions appear and increase in intensity. Occasionally there is redness of the oral cavity, the tongue and the nose. Recovery occurs after 24 hr. If the dose is increased to 200 mg/kg, the hind-quarters become paralyzed and death is caused by respiratory failure.

AET (DiStefano *et al.,* 1956)

In an anesthetized cat, i.v. injection of 15 mg/kg produces convulsive movements of the fore-limbs. If the dose is increased to 25 mg/kg convulsions become general and the animal dies. With 2.5–10 mg/kg immediately after injection there is momentary apnea, which is abolished by sectioning the vagus nerves but not by the injection of atropine (0.1 mg/kg).

3.5.1.3. RABBIT

Cysteamine

According to Arbusow (1959), latency of the spinal reflexes increases regularly after injection of 70–100 mg/kg of mercaptoethylamine, some animals being sensitive even to doses of 40–50 mg/kg. The action of MEA is in any case less rapid than that of narcotics, which immediately modifies the flexor reflex. The hypnotic effect and narcosis of phenobarbitone, cycloheptenylethylmalonylurea, and pentothal are reinforced by their association with the sulfur-containing protective agent, whereas the latter reduces the depressive action of pentothal on the respiratory center (Benigno and Palazzoadriano, 1964).

Aminoethylisothiourea

According to Laborit *et al.* (1959) and Jouany and Weber (1961), i.v. injection of 1–250 mg/kg into an alert animal produces high voltage slow waves in the EEG; they flatten and accelerate secondarily. The depths of anesthesia and of the barbituric depression on the respiratory center are slightly decreased by AET. According to these authors, AET excites the respiratory center, whereas according to DiStefano *et al.* (1956) severe apnea follows an injection of AET. As in the case of the cat, it is inhibited by bivagotomy. Jouany and Weber (1961) have not noted any epileptoid crisis with the doses used.

3.5.1.4. GUINEA-PIG

Cystamine (Robbers, 1937)

The symptomatology of intoxication by cystamine is less characteristic than in cats, rats or mice. When an animal is injected with 300 mg/kg subcutaneously (s.c.), it drips, becomes apathetic and curls up in a corner of its cage. Its hind-limbs tremble and appear paralyzed. Death follows rapidly owing to respiratory failure, but is not always preceded by convulsions as in other species.

3.5.1.5. RAT

Cysteamine–Cystamine

After i.v. injection of 100–200 mg/kg of MEA, rats show a slower rate of breathing. Convulsions occur early after 200 mg, later after 100 mg. With high doses, the animals breathe spasmodically, they suffocate and froth appears around the nostrils (van der Meer *et al.*, 1960). Similar symptoms are observed after i.p. injection. If MEA is s.c. injected, the convulsions are of shorter duration and are preceded by a phase of unrest (van der Meer *et al.*, 1960).

Arbusow (1959) says that small doses of MEA (1–3 mg *per animal*) lower the excitability of the cerebral cortex and the sub-cortical layers. Inhibition increases with the dose of MEA; 25 mg causes ataxia. As in the rabbit, β-mercaptoethylamine increases the soporific action of cyclo-heptenylethylmalonylurea, the narcotic effect of nembutal® and of pentothal® ; it prolongs the depressive effect caused by injection of phenobarbitone® , whereas the latter used in inactive dose reinforces the deconditioning action of MEA (van der Meer *et al.*, 1960; Benigno and Palazzoadriano, 1964). The action of MEA on the neurohypophysis of the rat has been described in Chapter 3.4.1.2.

After i.v. injection of 100 mg/kg of cystamine, the manifestations are very rapid and severe (Lecomte *et al.*, 1964). A few seconds after injecting, the animal becomes agitated, it makes repeated uncontroled jumps and then lies on its side and its breathing slows down, sometimes even stopping completely for 1–3 min. Respiration gradually picks up, laboriously and slowly and the animal remains cyanotic and exhausted. Its behavior gradually returns to normal. In heavier doses, the apathetic animal experiences brief convulsive fits and death can occur through respiratory failure.

The behavior of the rat, after s.c. injection with different doses of cystamine, has been described by Robbers (1937). About ¼ hr after receiving 200 mg/kg, the animal rolls on to its side, is extremely apathetic and returns to normal only on the following day; if the dose is increased to 300–350 mg/kg, its sleepiness is disturbed by fits of convulsions, respiration is disturbed, cyanosis appears and death occurs due to respiratory failure after 30–60 min.

Aminoethylisothiourea (Laborit *et al.*, 1959)

The symptoms that follow injection of a 300–400 mg/kg dose are characterized by a more speedy agitation, followed by clonic crises, closely followed by death. Ocular hemorrhage is common.

3.5.1.6.   MOUSE

Cysteamine–Cystamine

According to Hulse (1963), an i.p. dose of 100 mg/kg of MEA renders the animals irritable and hypertonic. They must be given a dose of 350 mg/kg (LD_{50}) to induce severe fits of convulsions which may be initiated by an unusual noise or stimulation. The convulsions may cause death. If the animal survives, the fits stop after 4 hr, but muscular rigidity continues to some extent for a further 2 hr.

With 150 mg/kg, the rectal temperature drops from 36.5° to 33° after 1 hr (Bacq *et al.*, 1965). More than 200 mg must be injected in order to obtain after 3 min a slight reduction in conditioned reflexes, which are abolished 3 hr later (Bacq, 1965). Cystamine is more toxic than MEA but the symptomatology observed was similar. With doses of 4–200 mg/kg, there is no significant effect on the respiratory rhythm (DiStefano *et al.*, 1962).

Aminoethylisothiourea

This is two or three times less toxic to mice than β-mercaptoethylamine. Death occurs if the dose is sufficiently heavy (Doherty and Burnett, 1955). In an anesthetized mouse, DiStefano *et al.* (1962) observed that an i.v. dose of less than 16 mg/kg increases the extent of respiratory movement. With about 16 mg, respiratory activity decreases; hypothermia is deeper after AET than after MEA (Locker and Pany, 1964).

3.5.2. LOCAL ANESTHETIC POWER OF MEA
(Goffart and Piret, 1955)

SENSITIVE FIBERS OF THE LUMBAR PLEXUS IN FROG

Sollmann's method, adapted by Bülbring and Wajda (1945), shows that 2% of MEA in Ringer's liquid shortens by 54% the time during which *Rana temporaria* with brain removed responds by a flexor reflex to the chemical stimulation of the skin of the lower limb. Total block of conduction in sciatic nerves occurs in 60 min. But the disappearance of the defence reflex by anesthesia of the plexus takes place usually within 22 min. It therefore seems probable that MEA has a greater affinity with pain and tactile fibers than with motor fibers.

SENSITIVE CUTANEOUS ENDINGS IN THE GUINEA-PIG

Intradermal injection of MEA diluted in physiological liquid decreases cutaneous sensitivity in the guinea-pig. The anesthetic effect is observed only in the papula area of the injection; it starts after 5 min and lasts for more than $\frac{3}{4}$ hr. There is a linear relationship between the percentage of negative response and the logarithm of the MEA concentration between

0.25 and 1%. No linear relationship has been verified for higher concentrations. Cysteamine therefore acts more rapidly on the sensitive terminations of the skin than on the nerve plexus, the connective sheath of which it slowly crosses. It is less active than procaine.

CORNEA OF RABBITS

This test is to establish whether MEA is active as a superficial anesthetic. Cysteamine (2–4%) is an irritant if dropped in a rabbit's eye, following the technique of Sinha (1936). It causes a brief blepharospasm and slight conjunctival vasodilatation. For $\frac{1}{2}$ hr after application of the drops, anesthesia of the cornea is slight or nil.

3.5.3. MOTOR NERVE AND MOTOR END-PLATE

3.5.3.1. SCIATIC NERVE OF *Rana temporaria*
(Goffart and Della Bella, 1954)

Application of a wad of cottonwool dipped in 2% MEA to the sciatic nerve of the frog (myelinated motor fibers with a diameter 5–14 μ results in disturbance of conduction within 30 min. The block is complete after only 1 hr. Application of 1% MEA does not inhibit conduction even after contact for 1 hr, whereas under the same conditions 1% procaine produces partial block in 20 min and complete block in 40 min.

3.5.3.2. NEURO-MUSCULAR JUNCTION

ANTERIOR TIBIALIS MUSCLE OF THE CAT
Cysteamine (Goffart and Della Bella, 1954) (Fig. 1)

Close intra-arterial injection into the tibial artery of 4–10 mg MEA may in less than 10 sec lower the isometric response of the *anterior tibialis* to isolated stimuli (slightly supramaximal) of the nerve, without affecting its response to direct stimulation. The dose may be reduced to 250 mcg if the arterial circulation is interrupted for 10–30 sec. Allowing for the weight of the muscle and the extent of the extracellular muscular space, it may be said that neuromuscular blockade occurs with concentrations of MEA of the order of 1×10^{-4} to 1×10^{-3} M. The duration of blockade is a function of the dose of MEA and the length of time it is in contact with the muscle. Blockade of the neuromuscular junction is probably due to a competitive process because MEA inhibits the action of acetylcholine on the motor end-plate; its effect is added to those of *d*-tubocura-

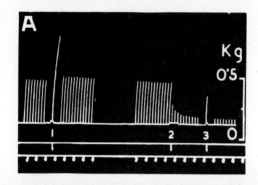

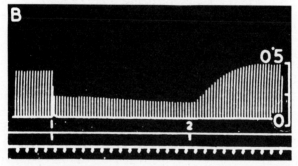

Fig. 1. (A) Cat, 2.25 kg; chloralose anesthesia. Isometric contractions of anterior tibialis stimulated every 10 sec by maximal shocks to the nerve. Time 30 sec. In 1 and 3: close intra-arterial injection of 1 mcg acetylcholine; in 2: intra-arterial injection of 2 mg MEA. (B) Cat, 3.6 kg; in 1: intra-arterial injection of 500 mcg MEA. Muscle circulation stopped for 10 sec. In 2: 500 mcg prostigmine, i.v. (Goffart and Della Bella, 1954.)

rine and is antagonized by a depolarizing substance, such as decamethonium. Neuromuscular blockade by MEA can be prevented by a tetanus, injection of potassium, epinephrine and prostigmine. These processes either potentiate or have no effect on neuromuscular blockade by decamethonium.

Cystamine (Goffart and Della Bella, 1954)

This has the same curarizing properties as MEA, but in double the doses. It has no action on the contraction of directly stimulated muscle.

Cysteine, Reduced Glutathione and Ethanolamine (Goffart and Della Bella, 1954)

Although these substances have no effect on the contraction of the curarized muscle, they cause contracture of the muscle together with a decrease of the effects of nervous stimulation when they are injected intra-arterially into the tibialis muscle. Ethanolamine has no effect on muscular contraction or neuromuscular transmission.

Aminoethylisothiourea, Aminopropylisothiourea (Tables 1 and 2)*

Contraction of the anterior tibialis muscle stimulated by its nerve is scarcely affected by i.v. injection of small doses of AET, and slightly increased by doses of 15–20 mg/kg which are close to lethal doses (Di-Stefano *et al.*, 1956). Laborit *et al.* (1959) find that AET also increases the neuromuscular excitability, having less effect on muscle than on nerve. Among the thiouronium compounds derived from AET (DiStefano *et al.*, 1963) AEMMT and AEMT potentiate the paralyzing effect of *d*-tubocurarine (0.2 mg/kg) without having any intrinsic curariform activity. EbAET in 4 mg/kg doses causes a temporary blockade of the neuromuscular junction of the anterior tibialis muscle and considerably potentiates the effects of *d*-tubocurarine.

Aminopropylisothiourea has the same effect as AET on the neuro-muscular junction, but three derivatives of this molecule act on the striped musculature. EbAPT (8 mg/kg) has a very slight paralyzing effect on the muscles. APMMT (4 mg/kg) has no direct effect on muscle, but poten-tiates the block of the motor end-plate induced by *d*-tubocurarine. ABMT has been shown to be the most powerful neuromuscular blocking agent of the compounds studied. In a dose of 1 mg/kg, it blocks the effects of indirect stimulation of the tibialis muscle. Blocking of the neuromuscular junction caused by 2 mg/kg of ABMT is neutralized by 0.3 mg of *d*-tubocurarine or gallamine. Edrophonium (0.8 mg/kg) and decametho-nium intensify the neuromuscular depression caused by ABMT, in doses of 1.2 and 1.4 mg/kg. ABMT and probably EbAET would behave like acetylcholine by causing depolarization; this would overflow the motor end-plate and reach the muscle, interrupting transmission between the motor end-plate and the muscle. This mechanism of action differs from that of MEA, which is curariform.

PHRENIC NERVE DIAPHRAGM OF THE RAT
(Goffart and Della Bella, 1954)

Cysteamine added to an organ-bath containing Tyrode solution (concentration of $3–5 \times 10^{-4}$M) reduces the maximal muscular contrac-tions produced by stimulation of the phrenic nerve by 50%. In a second

---

* The meaning of the abbreviations AEMT, AEMMT, etc., will be found in Chapter 1 on pp. 2–3 of this volume.

...TABLES OF VARIOUS COMPOUNDS OBTAINED BY SUBSTITUTIONS IN THE AET MOLECULE

(DiStefano et al., 1963) (Doses in boxes refer to lowest dose at which an unequivocal response was obtained)

$$\left[\begin{array}{c} H \quad H \quad N-R_1 \\ R-C-C-S-C \\ \quad NH_2 \ H \quad N \stackrel{R_2}{\scriptstyle R_3} \end{array} \right]$$

Substitution	Name	Vagal	Gut	B.P.	Gang. X	S.N.S. X	Curar.	Rad. prot. (mice)
$R, R_{1,2,3} = H$	AET	+ / 2 mg/kg	+ / 2 mg/kg	←↑↓→ / 2 mg/kg	+ / 12 mg/kg	+ / 12 mg/kg	−	+++
$R = C_2H_5$ $R_{1,2,3} = H$	2-ABT	−	+ / 4 mg/kg	←→ / 1 mg/kg	−	+ / 4 mg/kg	+ / 4 mg/kg	+++
$R = C_2H_5$ $R_2 = CH_3$ $R_{1,3} = H$	ABMT	−	+ / 2 mg/kg	→ / 1 mg/kg	−	+ / 2 mg/kg	++ / 1 mg/kg	++
$R_2 = CH_3$ $R, R_{1,3}$	AEMT	−	+ / 8 mg/kg	→↑ / 4 mg/kg	+ / 4 mg/kg	−	+ / 8 mg/kg	+
$R_{1,2} = CH_3$ $R_3 = H$	AEMMT	−	+ / 4 mg/kg	→ / 2 mg/kg	+ / 4 mg/kg	−	+ / 4 mg/kg	+
$R_{2,3} = CH_3$ $R_1 = H$	AEdiMT	−	+ / 4 mg/kg	←↑ / 8 mg/kg	+ / 4 mg/kg	−	+ / 4 mg/kg	++
$R_2 = CH_2CH_2AET$ $R_{1,3} = H$	EbAET	−	+ / 4 mg/kg	→ / 1 mg/kg	+ / 2 mg/kg	−	++ / 4 mg/kg	0

Vagal—initiation of vagus-mediated chemoreflex. Gut—production of gut contractions. B.P.—blood pressure. Gang. X—ganglionic blockade. S.N.S. X—sympathetic blockade. (Blockade of nictitating membrane contractions evoked by stimulation of the postganglionic nerve from the superior cervical ganglion.) Curar.—(+) indicates potentiation of curare activity, (++) indicates skeletal muscle blocking activity. Rad. prot.—(+++) 100% radiation protection at 900 r, (++) 50 to 70% protection at 900 r, (+) below 50% protection at 900 r, − no response.

TABLE 2. PHARMACOLOGICAL PROPERTIES OF VARIOUS COMPOUNDS OBTAINED BY SUBSTITUTIONS IN THE APT MOLECULE
(DiStefano et al., 1963) (Doses in boxes refer to lowest dose at which an unequivocal response was obtained)

Substitution	Name	Vagal↑	Gut↑	B.P.	Gang. X	S.N.S. X	Curar.	Rad. prot. (mice)
$R, R_{1,2,3} = H$	APT	+ 2 mg/kg	+ 2 mg/kg	↓↑↓ 2 mg/kg	+ 15 mg/kg	+ 12 mg/kg	−	+++
$R_2 = CH_3$ $R_{1,3} = H$	APMT	−	+ 16 mg/kg	↑ 2 mg/kg	−	−	−	+++
$R_{2,3} = CH_3$ $R_1 = H$	APdiMT	−	+ 4 mg/kg	↑↓ 8 mg/kg	−	−	−	++
$R_{1,2} = CH_3$ $R_3 = H$	APMMT	−	+ 4 mg/kg	→ 1 mg/kg	+ 4 mg/kg		+ 4 mg/kg	0
$R_2 = CH_2CH_2OH$ $R_{1,3} = H$	APMHET	−	+ 4 mg/kg	→ 4 mg/kg	+ 4 mg/kg		−	++
$R_2 = CH_2CH_2APT$ $R_{1,3} = H$	EbAPT	−	+ 1 mg/kg	→ 1 mg/kg	+ 1 mg/kg	−	++ 8 mg/kg	+++ (i.p.)

Vagal—initiation of vagus-mediated chemoreflex. Gut—production of gut contractions. B.P.—blood pressure. Gang. X—ganglionic blockade. S.N.S. X—sympathetic blockade. (Blockade of nictitating membrane contractions evoked by stimulation of the postganglionic nerve from the superior cervical ganglion.) Curar.—(+) indicates potentiation of curare activity. (+ +) indicates skeletal muscle blocking activity. Rad. prot.—(+ + +) 100% radiation protection at 900 r, (+ +) 50 to 70% protection at 900 r, (+) below 50% protection at 900 r, — no response.

test carried out after washing, MEA has only a very slight curariform effect. This preparation is not suitable for studying the curariform activity of MEA, because its effects are almost irreversible.

ISOLATED RECTUS ABDOMINIS OF RANA TEMPORARIA
(Goffart and Della Bella, 1954)

This muscle is the standard preparation for evaluating the influence of a drug on the nicotinic effects of acetylcholine. The technique used shows the action of acetylcholine on certain slow muscle fibers of a particular type, but the results obtained can be transposed to rapid fibers.

A concentration of 1×10^{-6}M MEA in a Ringer bath does not prevent contraction of the rectus abdominis induced by adding 0.5–1 mcg/ml of acetylcholine. A concentration of 4×10^{-5}M MEA in contact with the muscle lowers the muscular response to acetylcholine by about 50%. The latter is reduced to 10% of its original value if the concentration of MEA in the bath is doubled. Simultaneous injection of acetylcholine and MEA into the Ringer bath shows that MEA acts instantaneously. If the sulfur-containing substance is added to the bath during the acetyl-choline-induced contraction of the muscle, the contraction ceases during its development. These facts indicate that MEA enters into competition with acetylcholine on the numerous motor end-plates of each slow muscle fiber of the rectus abdominis. On the other hand, acetylcholine appears to protect the motor end-plate against MEA. Cysteamine at 2×10^{-4}M only very slightly reduces the response of the rectus to potassium, whereas at this concentration it completely nullifies the effects of acetylcholine. At a concentration four times stronger than that at which acetylcholine desensitizes the muscle, MEA does not cause the muscle to contract.

3.5.4. AUTONOMIC NERVOUS SYSTEM

3.5.4.1. GANGLIONIC SYNAPSES

SUPERIOR CERVICAL GANGLION
Cysteamine (Goffart and Paton, 1955) (Fig. 2)

In cats, close intra-arterial injection (external carotid) of 100–250 mcg MEA into the superior cervical ganglion during preganglionic stimulation causes relaxation of the nictitating membrane. A further injection of 0.5–5 mg of the same substance a few minutes later leaves it completely relaxed for 20 min: this effect is reversible. It adds to the effects of *d*-tubocurarine, tetraethylammonium, or hexamethonium. During block-

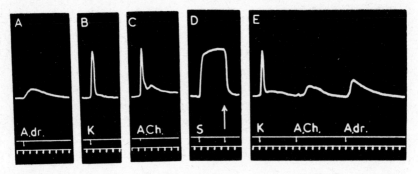

Fig. 2. Cat, 2.3 kg; chloralose anesthesia. Isotonic contractions of the nictitating membrane. Time 30 sec. (A) 25 mcg epinephrine, i.v. (B) Close intra-arterial injection in the superior cervical ganglion of 1 mg KCl. (C) 50 mcg acetylcholine. (D) Stimulation of sympathetic preganglionic fibers 2/sec; close intra-arterial injection of 2 mg MEA. (E) 1 mg KCl as in (B); 50 mcg acetylcholine as in (C), 25 mcg epinephrine, i.v. (Goffart and Paton, 1955.)

ing of the effects of preganglionic stimulation, the nictitating membrane responds normally to stimulation by post-ganglionic fibers, and to the i.v. injection of epinephrine. This synaptic block is removed by preganglionic stimulation at high frequency and by injection of eserine. This is a case of blocking by competition, since the ganglionic cells are desensitized to the acetylcholine normally released by preganglionic nerve endings. At the same time, the ganglionic cells retain their sensitivity to potassium.

The preganglionic cervical sympathetic nerve must be surrounded by a solution of 2% MEA to prevent nervous conduction in the preganglionic fibers and thereby suppress the release of acetylcholine. In this case, MEA blocks the ganglionic transmission by a double mechanism of the procaine type.

GANGLIONIC STIMULANT

If 0.5–5 mg MEA is injected into the artery of the superior cervical ganglion, the nictitating membrane contracts and synaptic transmission is subsequently blocked. This action is subject to tachyphylaxis. It is lessened by previous i.v. administration of 1 mg/kg hexamethonium, or 200 mcg cocaine intra-arterially and suppressed by atropinization of the cat with a dose of 1 mg/kg. This effect is certainly of ganglionic origin, because the excitatory action of MEA persists when the preganglionic fibers have degenerated, but disappears if the cervical ganglion is removed. The nicotinic excitation effect is followed by a synaptic blocking, possibly by depolarization, which is followed by competitive blocking, as in the case of nicotine. In some cases there is a further period during which MEA causes increased response of the ganglion to acetylcholine, possibly through a very slight anticholinesterase action.

Cystamine (Goffart and Paton, 1955)

Cystamine has similar effects on ganglia as MEA, but in order to achieve the same quantitative effects, double the quantity of cystamine must be injected. At the same time, cystamine never has a "nicotinic excitatory" effect; it easily inhibits nervous conduction in the sympathetic preganglionic axons. It is probable that the ganglion blocking activity of cystamine is due to MEA being formed *in vivo* from the disulfide.

Cysteine, Glutathione, Ethanolamine (Goffart and Paton, 1955)

Cysteine (4 mg) brings about slight blocking; the same dose of ethanolamine (a molecule of similar structure to MEA but without —SH) causes approximately 50% blocking; glutathione (4 mg) has no effect.

Aminoethylisothiourea, Aminopropylisothiourea, and Derivatives (Table 1)

According to DiStefano *et al.* (1956), contraction of the nictitating membrane induced by preganglionic stimulation is slightly lessened by 10 mg/kg of AET and considerably reduced by 12.5 mg/kg, i.v.

After a dose of 15 mg/kg the effects of pre- and post-ganglionic stimulation are blocked, but the preganglionic inhibition is more intense and lasts longer.

Contraction of the nictitating membrane is suppressed by APT, partly due to inhibition of ganglion transmission and partly to direct effect on the nictitating membrane. The same effects were observed with similar doses of AET (DiStefano *et al.*, 1959). The same group of researchers (DiStefano *et al.*, 1963) studied the effects of substitution in AET and APT molecules. They showed that AEMT (4 mg/kg), AEMMT (4 mg/kg), AEdiMT (4 mg/kg), EbAET (2 mg/kg), APMMT (4 mg/kg), APMHET (4 mg/kg) and EbAPT (1 mg/kg) induce a certain degree of ganglion blocking; 2-ABT, APMT, APdiMT and ABMT do not have this property. However, ABMT reduces very significantly the effects of pre- and post-ganglionic stimulation (Tables 1 and 2).

3.5.4.2.   THE ADRENAL MEDULLA (Goffart, 1955)

Cysteamine

In the eviscerated cat, with both vagi cut and under artificial respiration, injection of 500 mcg MEA into the celiac trunk does not cause hypertension, or excitation of the adrenal medulla, but desensitizes the medullary cells to acetylcholine and splanchnic nerve stimulation. Synaptic blocking with small doses of MEA is of a purely competitive nature and is reversible. However, although MEA does not affect the sensitivity of neurons of the superior cervical ganglion, to an injection of KCl, it slightly lowers the discharge of sympathomimetic amines produced by potassium at the level of the adrenal medulla. Increasing the dose of MEA (1–20 mg) causes hypertension, and contraction of the nictitating membrane due to a discharge of adrenal medullary hormones followed by blocking of transmission of the preganglionic nerve stimulation. But increased blood pressure and contraction of the nictitating membrane are not simple nicotinic effects of MEA because they persist in spite of bilateral adrenalectomy and blockade of sympathetic ganglia. In large doses, MEA has sympathomimetic properties; hypertensive response is reversed by phentolamine (4 mg/kg), tolazoline (8 mg/kg) and 933 F (2 mg/kg).

Cystamine

In doses of 500 mcg, cystamine reduces the nicotinic action of 10–25 mcg acetylcholine on the adrenals by 40–80% and the effects of splanchnic stimulation by 50–80%. At the same time, it has no nicotinic effect.

Cysteine, Glutathione and Ethanolamine

These substances have neither ganglion blocking action, nor nicotinic effect on the adrenals.

3.5.4.3. PARASYMPATHETIC SYSTEM AND ACETYLCHOLINE

TORTOISE CERVICAL VAGUS (Della Bella and Bacq, 1953)

The nerve should be steeped in a 2% solution of MEA to obtain complete local blocking of the excitation in 20–30 min. This effect is slowly reversible after frequent washing with Ringer solution. Cysteamine (1%) does not affect nervous conduction even after having been in contact with the nerve for 1 hr.

CAT VAGUS (Goffart and Della Bella, 1954)

This consists of fine myelinated fibers (4.5–1.5μ) and unmyelinated fibers. Cysteamine (2%) determines a conduction block; it is rapidly initiated and is complete in 16 min. This phenomenon is reversible.

TORTOISE POSTGANGLIONIC VAGAL FIBERS
(Della Bella and Bacq, 1953)

If one stimulates electrically the right auricle at a slightly higher frequency than that of the spontaneous contraction, one stimulates the postganglionic vagal fibers (Fredericq, 1936). Cysteamine reduces the effect of this vagal stimulation, but this action is usually slower and weaker than the reduction of preganglionic stimulation effects.

ACETYLCHOLINE RECEPTORS
Cysteamine

The action of acetylcholine on the isolated frog heart is inhibited by preventive treatment with MEA (Della Bella and Bacq, 1953). If the concentration of acetylcholine is weak, a concentration of 2×10^{-5}M MEA is sufficient to counteract it, but if the concentration of acetylcholine is sufficient to cause the heart to stop beating, at least 1×10^{-3}M is necessary; inhibition is not complete. This atropinic action of MEA is rapid; it persists 10–20 min after repeated washing and is reversible. The atropinic action of MEA (7.6 mcg/ml) is also conspicuous in the isolated guinea-pig ileum, which it renders less sensitive to acetylcholine (Stepanović *et al.,* 1963). However, β-mercaptoethylamine (17.5 mg/kg) and cystamine (50 mg/kg) do not neutralize the hypotensive effect of acetylcholine on the nembutal anesthetized rabbit (Van de Berg and Lecomte, 1953). On the other hand, atropine prevents the fall in blood pressure which immediately follows injection of 10 mg/kg of MEA into a cat or chicken, whereas bilateral section of the vagus has no such effect (Beaumariage *et al.,* 1966). The depressive effect of the same dose of MEA in the cat is not affected by previous atropinization.

Aminoethylisothiourea

The hypotensive action of acetylcholine in dogs (0.5 mg/kg) seems to be increased by AET, whereas the hypertensive action of AET (30 mg) is potentiated by atropine (1 mg) (Laborit *et al.,* 1959).

In cats, atropinization (0.1 mg/kg) prevents or reduces the brief fall in blood pressure, bradycardia, apnea and intestinal contraction that follows injection of 2.5 mg/kg of AET, but whereas the first two also disappear after bilateral vagotomy, apnea and intestinal stimulation are unaffected (DiStefano *et al.,* 1956).

3.5.4.4. ADRENERGIC SYSTEM AND CATECHOLAMINES

CATECHOLAMINE RECEPTORS
Cysteamine–Cystamine

In rats, a dose of 100–120 mg/kg MEA completely blocks the hypertensive effects of epinephrine (0.2 mcg) and norepinephrine (0.3 mcg), as well as the fall in blood pressure caused by i.v. injection of isoprenaline (Debijadji *et al.*, 1962). Cystamine (5–15 mg/kg) considerably reduces and sometimes even totally suppresses the blood pressure raising and tachycardiac effects of catecholamines (1–10 mcg/kg). These are also less intense in rats treated with MEA (Lecomte *et al.*, 1964). Hyperglycemia caused by epinephrine in rabbits (Debijadji *et al.*, 1962) and acceleration of the rabbit isolated atrium are also blocked by MEA, whereas the response to calcium remains intact (Varagić *et al.*, 1963). An adrenergic blocking effect of MEA can be observed on the rabbit uterus; the curve representing the percentage of reduction of the response of the uterus to epinephrine (2 mcg) is a straight line proportional to the MEA concentration; the response is completely abolished at 15.3 mcg/ml.

MEA does not change the inhibitory action of epinephrine on the rabbit duodenum. MEA potentiates the response of the isolated guinea-pig terminal ileum to epinephrine (Varagić *et al.*, 1963) and the inhibitory effect of this amine on the non-pregnant cat uterus (Goffart and Grévisse, 1960). Cystamine has no regular effect on this last test. The α-blockers reverse the hypertensive action of MEA (20 mg) i.v. administered to the spinal cat whose ganglions are blocked by hexamethonium (Goffart, 1955).

Aminoethylisothiourea

Although in dogs a small dose of AET increases the intensity and duration of hypertension after i.v. injection of epinephrine and norepinephrine (Laborit *et al.*, 1959), the injection of a large dose of the sulfur-containing compound abolishes the *secondary* fall in blood pressure that follows administration of catecholamine (Laborit *et al.*, 1967). This β-blocking effect is also obtained with cysteine and reduced glutathione. In addition, 200 mg/kg of mercaptoethylguanidine (MEG) administered to the rat in divided doses alters the vasomotor effects of epinephrine: arterial hypertension is replaced by a diphasic or hypotensive reaction (Lecomte and Bacq, 1965). The hypertension following norepinephrine is also reduced.

CATECHOLAMINE CONTENT OF SOME ORGANS

The catecholamine content of adrenals of rats killed 30 min after injection of MEA or cystamine (50–400 mg/kg) is significantly reduced, whereas it remains unchanged after treatment with AET (see Chapter 3.4.1.1). Although the norepinephrine content of the myocardium remains unchanged in rats killed shortly after injection with cystamine (Lecomte *et al.*, 1964), slow depletion of cardiac catecholamines after MEG is observed in mice and cats (DiStefano and Klahn, 1966). This phenomenon is already detectable 1 hr after injection with the sulfur-containing substance; at that moment increased contractile strength of the isolated atrium is observed. The depletion after MEG injection is maximal after 4 days whereas the effect of guanethidine reaches a maximum after 24 hr. Mercaptoethylguanidine has no effect on the norepinephrine of the brain.

3.5.5. CHEMO- AND PRESSOR-RECEPTORS (Tables 1 and 2)

The triple effect following i.v. administration to the cat of 2.5 mg/kg of AET (hypotension, bradycardia and apnea) is associated with an effect on the chemosensitive regions (DiStefano *et al.*, 1956). The bradycardia in the rat responsible for the initial drop in blood pressure that marks the administration of a weak dose of MEG probably depends on the same mechanism (Lecomte and Bacq, 1965). Administration of APT in small doses (2.5 mg/kg) is also followed by a drop in blood pressure and apnea. Bilateral vagotomy reduces hypotension, and abolishes apnea (DiStefano *et al.*, 1959). On the other hand, none of the AET or APT derivatives elicit any chemoreflex response mediated via the vagus nerve (DiStefano *et al.*, 1963).

The sensitivity of the pressor-receptors does not seem to be altered by AET, because hypertension following bicarotid occlusion in dogs is not affected (Laborit *et al.*, 1959).

3.5.6. CONCLUSIONS

3.5.6.1. CENTRAL NERVOUS SYSTEM

The agitation and convulsions that appear soon after injection of MEA, cystamine, or AET occur even more rapidly depending on how quickly the drug passes into the circulation and the size of the dose injected. These symptoms are often accompanied by nausea and vomiting. Such manifestations are of central origin because they can be prevented by general anesthesia. It seems likely that this is a direct effect of the sulfur-containing radioprotective agents on the cortical and subcortical structures and not the result of reaction of these nervous structures to anoxia. In fact, they can occur immediately following injection of the drug as is the case in rats.

Salivation, anorexia, defecation, changes in respiratory rhythm, rise in blood epinephrine content (Chapter 3.4.1.1), mydriasis, hyperglycemia (Chapter 3.4.2) can arise from several mechanisms: (a) interrelation between the bulbar centers, the cortical and subcortical structures (such as hypothalamus); (b) reflex originated from the pressor and chemo-sensitive regions (hypotension, bradycardia and apnea following injection of AET); (c) direct effect of the sulfur-containing compounds on certain smooth muscular receptors (intestine, sphincter and iris), or on the sympathetic and parasympathetic ganglionic synapses. Proof of stimulation of the hypothalamic centers has been found by Duchesne *et al.* (1968), who showed that in rats MEA and cystamine stimulate the neuro-secretion of the posterior hypophyseal and hypothalamic cells (Chapter 3.4.1.2). In any species of animal, MEA, and cystamine in small doses, have very little effect on the respiratory center; in large doses it becomes depressed and the animal dies in apnea. However, with convulsions, respiration can become spasmodic. On the other hand, the effect of AET seems to vary according to the type of animal. In dogs (Laborit *et al.,* 1959), it stimulates respiration, whereas in cats and rabbits (DiStefano *et al.,* 1956) it causes a very temporary apnea due to a chemoreflex whose afferent receptors are situated in the lungs or heart. Manifestations of nervous hyper-excitability are generally followed by a period of depression; this may result from fatigue of the neurons, an accumulation of waste from catabolism, reduction of basic energy or elements essential to cellular metabolism, or even to depletion of the stock of potential transmitters. This depression is seen as a state of sleepiness which could also be the result of release of the integrating control of the reticular formation. Reactions to painful stimuli and conditioned reflexes may be abolished; the depression is interrupted by periods of convulsions probably due to hypoxia following hypotension caused by high doses of MEA, cystamine, or AET. There may also be signs of hypertonia, muscle tremor and ataxia; these symptoms may be explained in part by loss of cortical control on the central gray nuclei, whose functioning may be altered by the drug, and also by reduced cerebellar control. Whereas the depressive effect of MEA potentiates that of the barbiturates, AET slightly lowers the intensity of anesthesia and respiratory depressive action of these drugs.

3.5.6.2. LOCAL ANESTHETIC ACTION

The local anesthetic action of MEA is less than that of procaine. The sensitive endings of the skin are much more sensitive to the anesthetic effect of MEA than are the myelinated fibers. The concentration of MEA necessary to produce anesthesia is smaller than that required to block conduction in the nerve fibers and the delay shorter. The appearance of an edematous papule on the site of injection following release *in situ* of chemical mediators of inflammatory reaction such as histamine and 5-hydroxytryptamine, under the action of MEA, could involve squeezing of the nerve endings that would raise the threshold of tactile or painful stimuli. This local anesthesia can scarcely be observed on the cornea.

3.5.6.3. MOTOR NERVE AND NEUROMUSCULAR JUNCTION

Cysteamine competitively blocks the neuromuscular junction by inhibiting the action of acetylcholine on the motor end-plate. It potentiates the effects of *d*-tubocurarine and antagonizes a substance like decamethonium that "curarizes" by depolarization, but, contrary to what is observed when several successive doses of curare are injected, the repeated injection of MEA produces progressively less intense results. It further differs from curare since the effective concentration of MEA on the sympathetic ganglion is smaller than the curarizing concentration on the motor end-plate. This curarizing action is weak, as the i.v. dose of MEA which produces the neuromuscular block is lethal to the cat being treated.

These properties are due to the association in the molecule of an $-NH_2$ function and an $-SH$ function; replacing the sulfhydryl group by an hydroxyl renders the curarizing effect insignificant.

Cystamine has similar but weaker effects than MEA: it probably acts by transforming itself into MEA. Cysteine and reduced glutathione have a powerful "excitatory nicotinic" action on the tibialis muscle of the cat, which is rarely found and is always weak, with MEA. Although MEA blocks nervous conduction only in strong concentrations following prolonged contact with the nerve, it is not excluded that this mechanism participates in determination of the neuromuscular block; it could prevent the nervous impulse from going through the unmyelinated motor nerve endings and thus from reaching the neuromuscular junction and releasing acetylcholine.

Although AET has no effect on the neuromuscular junction, most of its derivatives (2-ABT, AEMT, AEMMT, AEdiMT, EbAET) potentiate the paralyzing action of curare on striated muscle, or block transmission of the nerve impulse as is the case with EbAET and above all ABMT. The latter blocks the motor end-plate by depolarization like decamethonium and its action is reversed by *d*-tubocurarine. In the APT series, only two derivatives show any effect: EbAPT has a curariform effect, whereas APMMT facilitates the effect of *d*-tubocurarine.

3.5.6.4. AUTONOMIC NERVOUS SYSTEM

Small doses of MEA administered intra-arterially to the superior cervical ganglion of the cat do not prevent the release of acetylcholine by preganglionic stimulation, but they desensitize the neurons to acetylcholine, without changing their excitability to potassium. It is known that acetylcholine receptors have thiol groups that can be inactivated by —SH inhibitors, such as mono-iodoacetate and *p*-chloromercuribenzoate (Halász *et al.*, 1960); thus it is possible that certain compounds with thiol or disulfide functions capable of forming mixed disulfides may cause inhibition of these receptors.

If the doses of MEA are increased, transmission of the nerve impulse in the preganglionic fibers is blocked and the release of acetylcholine prevented. This phenomenon, in addition to acetylcholine desensitization of the ganglionic cells, reflects a procaine-type block. A third mechanism of the synaptic block by large doses of MEA could be envisaged: MEA like cysteine could block synthesis of acetylcholine by formation of *S*-acetylcysteamine, thus utilizing up all available acetyl-coenzyme A (Smith and Weiskopf, 1967). However, this possibility is highly improbable, because, according to Perry (1953), the reserves of acetylcholine in the ganglion are sufficient to allow frequent stimulation without recourse to new synthesis. In addition to its synaptic blocking effect in small doses, MEA has in moderate doses a ganglion excitatory effect, probably through acting on the same cellular receptors as acetylcholine, as is shown by reduction or suppression of the excitatory effect of hexamethonium, cocaine, and atropine. The ganglion blocking activity of MEA, like its curariform effect, is due to the association of the —NH$_2$ and —SH functions in the same molecule. Replacement of the sulfhydryl group by a hydroxyl decreases the synaptic blocking action. Cystamine has less marked blocking properties than MEA, and has no excitatory nicotinic effect on the superior cervical ganglion.

Cysteine and glutathione have a negligible ganglion blocking effect.

Aminoethylisothiourea and APT, which lessen the effects of pre- and postganglionic stimulation on contraction of the nictitating membrane, act partly at least by reducing ganglionic transmission. Most of the other derivatives of AET also have a certain ganglion blocking activity. ABMT causes severe blocking of the effects of pre- and postganglionic stimulation, without altering synaptic transmission in the superior cervical ganglion. Three APT derivatives (APMMT, APMHET and EbAPT) have moderate ganglion blocking properties.

In the tortoise, excitation of the cervical vagus (preganglionic fibers) is inhibited much more rapidly and severely than is excitation of the postganglionic fibers. Synaptic transmission of parasympathetic ganglia has not been studied, but it is likely that they are affected by the sulfur-containing radioprotective agents, in a similar manner to the sympathetic ganglia.

Acetylcholine receptors of the striated muscles and the ganglia of the autonomic system are not the only areas where inhibition by some sulfur-containing radioprotective agents occurs; there are other receptors situated in smooth muscles (isolated ileum of the guinea-pig, vessels of the cat and chicken) and in the frog's heart which can be blocked by MEA. However, MEA is incapable of abolishing the hypotensive effect of acetylcholine in rabbits, whereas atropine does not invert the hypotension due to cystamine in cats. It is possible that the sensitivity of certain cholinergic receptors remains unchanged after the administration of a sulfur-containing radioprotective substance. The hypertensive action of AET potentiated by atropine (Laborit *et al.,* 1959) perhaps results from the abolition of the Bezold-Jarisch reflex as noted by DiStefano *et al.* (1956). Cysteamine, cystamine and AET have multiple effects; some among them could prevent or counteract certain muscarinic actions of acetylcholine.

The same applies to the sympathetic nervous system, where epinephrine-like substances are released under the influence of acetylcholine. In radioprotective doses MEA, cystamine and AET have certain α- and β-blocking actions; this can be observed in the vessels of the rat and the isolated atrium and uterus of the rabbit.

Nevertheless, the sensitivity of certain adrenergic receptors appears to be maintained (isolated duodenum of the rabbit), or even increased (ileum of the guinea-pig, uterus of the virgin cat). A small dose of AET (0.6 mg) potentiates the hypertensive action of epinephrine in dogs.

Cysteamine and cystamine bring about sudden depletion of the adrenal catecholamines by a homeostatic mechanism tending to re-establish the blood pressure level; AET, which is not hypotensive, does not cause such changes but empties the reserves of cardiac norepinephrine. This action, however, is much slower than that of guanethidine.

3.5.6.5. CHEMO- AND PRESSOR-RECEPTORS

The sensitivity of the chemo- and pressor-sensitive endings of the aortic branch, the carotids and the lungs is not affected by the administration of sulfur-containing radioprotective agents; the rise in blood pressure following bicarotidian occlusion is not affected in dogs; injection of AET or APT is followed by a Bezold-Jarisch reflex.

REFERENCES

ARBUSOW, S. J. (1959) Die Schutzwirkung einiger pharmakologischer Mittel bei Strahlenschäden. *Arch. exp. Path. Pharmak.* **236**: 265–72.

BACQ, Z. M. (1965) *Chemical Protection against Ionizing Radiation.* Charles C. Thomas. Springfield, Illinois, p. 64.

BACQ, Z. M. and ALEXANDER, P. (1961) *Fundamentals of Radiobiology.* Pergamon Press, London, p. 464.

BACQ, Z. M., BEAUMARIAGE, M. L. and LIÉBECQ-HUTTER, S. (1965) Relation entre la radioprotection et l'hypothermie induite par certaines substances chimiques. *Int. J. Rad. Biol.* **9**: 175–8.

BEAUMARIAGE, M. L., VAN CANEGHEM, P. and BACQ, Z. M. (1966) Etude de certaines propriétés pharmacodynamiques de la cystamine et de la cystéamine chez diverses espèces animales. *Strahlentherapie* **131**: 342–51.

BENIGNO, P. and PALAZZOADRIANO, M. (1964) Sur la potentialisation des effets de barbituriques par la cystéamine (β-mercaptoéthylamine). *Arch. int. Pharmacodyn.* **151**: 86–92.

BENSON, R. E., MICHAELSON, S. M., DOWNS, W. L., MAYNARD, E. A., SCOTT, J. K., HODGE, H. C. and HOWLAND, J. W. (1961) Toxicological and radioprotection studies on S,β-aminoethylisothiouronium bromide (AET), *Radiation Res.* **15**: 561–72.

BÜLBRING, E. and WAJDA, I. (1945) Biological comparison of local anesthetics. *J. Pharmacol. exp. Therap.* **85**: 78–84.

DEBIJADJI, R., VARAGIĆ, V., ELČIĆ, S. and DAVIDOVIĆ, J. (1962) Adrenergic blocking action of cysteamine. *Experientia* **18**: 32–3.

DELLA BELLA, D. and BACQ, Z. M. (1953) Action de la cystéamine sur le cœur isolé de grenouille et sur l'effet de l'excitation vagale chez la tortue. *Arch. f. exper. Path. u. Pharmakol.* **219**: 366–70.

DISTEFANO, V. and KLAHN, J. J. (1966) Depletion of cardiac norepinephrine in the mouse and cat by mercaptoethylguanidine. *J. Pharmacol. exp. Therap.* **151**: 236–41.

DISTEFANO, V., LEARY, D. E. and DOHERTY, D. G. (1956) The pharmacology of β-aminoethylisothiouronium bromide in the cat. *J. Pharmacol. exp. Therap.* **117**: 425–33.

DISTEFANO, V., LEARY, D. E. and LITTLE, K. D. (1959) The pharmacological effects of some congeners of 2-aminoethylisothiouronium bromide (AET). *J. Pharmacol exp. Therap.* **126**: 158–63.

DISTEFANO, V., KLAHN, J. J. and LEARY, D. E. (1962) The pharmacological effects of some radioprotective agents in mice. *Rad. Res.* **17**: 792–800.

DISTEFANO, V., KORN, P. S. and LEARY, D. E. (1963) A comparison of the pharmacological effects of some compounds related to 2-aminoethylisothiouronium bromide hydrobromide (AET). *Rad. Res.* **18**: 177–85.

DOHERTY, D. G. and BURNETT JR., W. T. (1955) Protective effect of S,β-aminoethylisothiouronium Br, HBr and related compounds against X-irradiation death in mice. *Proc. Soc. exp. Biol. Med.* **89**: 312–14.

DUCHESNE, P. Y., HAJDUKOVIĆ, S., BEAUMARIAGE, M. L. and BACQ, Z. M. (1968) Neurosecretion in the hypothalamus and posterior pituitary after irradiation and injection of chemical radioprotector in the rat. *Rad. Res.* **34**: 583–95.

FREDERICQ, H. (1936) La nature cholinergique des fibres postganglionnaires du pneumogastrique cardiaque de la tortue. *Arch. internat. Physiol.* **43**: 212–18.

GOFFART, M. (1955) Mode d'action de la cystéamine et de la cystamine au niveau de la médullo-surrénale. *Arch. internat. Physiol. Bioch.* **63**: 500–12.

GOFFART, M. and DELLA BELLA, D. (1954) Action de la cystéamine et de la cystamine sur la fonction neuromusculaire. *Arch. internat. Physiol. Bioch.* **62**: 455–75.

GOFFART, M. and GRÉVISSE, J. (1960) Action de la cystéamine, de la cystamine et de l'éthanolamine sur l'utérus vierge isolé de la chatte. *C.R. Soc. Biol.* **154**: 2143–4.

GOFFART, M. and PATON, D. W. (1955) Action de la cystéamine et de la cystamine sur un ganglion sympathique. *Arch. internat. Physiol. Bioch.* **63**: 477–99.

GOFFART, M. and PIRET, J. (1955) Pouvoir anesthésique local de la cystéamine. *Arch. internat. Physiol. Bioch.* **63**: 534–5.

HALÁSZ, P., MECHLER, F., FEHÉR, O. and DAMJANOVICH, S. (1960) The effect of SH-inhibitors on ganglionic transmission in the superior cervical ganglion of the cat. *Acta Physiol. Acad. Sc. Hungar.* **18**: 47–55.

HULSE, E. V. (1963) The acute effects of cysteamine and their modification by X-irradiation. *Int. J. Rad. Biol.* **6**: 323–9.

JOUANY, J. M. and WEBER, B. (1961) Substances de réveil. Pharmacologie succincte et utilisations cliniques de l'AET (Aminoéthylisothiouronium). *Agressologie* **2**: 30–6.

LABORIT, H., BROUSOLLE, B., JOUANY, J. M., NIAUSSAT, P., REYNIER, M. and WEBER, B. (1959) Etude pharmacologique du bromhydrate de 2-aminoéthylisothiouronium (AET). *Thérapie* **14**: 1116–35.

LABORIT, H., WEBER, B. and BARON, C. (1967) Activité dite béta sympatholytique de certains réducteurs: aminoéthylisothiouronium (AET), cystéine et glutathion réduit. *Agressologie* **8**: 427–51.

LECOMTE, J. and BACQ, Z. M. (1965) Propriétés vasomotrices de la 2-mercaptoéthylguanidine (MEG) chez le rat. *Arch. int. Pharmacodyn.* **158**: 480–97.

LECOMTE, L., CESSION-FOSSION, A., LIBON, J. CL. and BACQ, Z. M. (1964) Sur quelques effets pharmacodynamiques généraux de la cystamine chez le rat. *Arch. int. Pharmacodyn.* **148**: 487–510.

LOCKER, A. and PANY, J. E. (1964) Die Wirkung von Cysteamin und AET auf den Sauerstoffverbrauch und die Körpertemperatur der Maus. *Z. ges. exptl. Med.* **138**: 331–7.

MEER, VAN DER, C., VALKENBURG, P. W., KUILE, C. A. TER, and NEYHOFF, J. A. (1960) Farmacologische onderzoekingen van cysteamine, cystamine, cysteine en AET, in verband met hun profilactische werking tegen bestraling. *Rapport du Medisch Biologisch Laboratorium RVO-TNO* **25**: 15–19.

MUNDY, R. L. and HEIFFER, M. H. (1960) The pharmacology of radioprotectant chemicals. General pharmacology of β-mercaptoethylamine. *Rad. Res.* **13**: 383–94.

NEWSOME, J. R., KNOTT, D. H. and OVERMAN, R. R. (1962) Radioprotective effects of β-aminoethylisothiuronium Br-HBr in the dog. *Rad. Res.* **17**: 847–54.

PERRY, W. L. M. (1953) Acetylcholine release in the cat's superior cervical ganglion. *J. Physiol.* **119**: 439–54.

ROBBERS, H. (1937) Die pharmakologische Wirkung des Cystamins, einer blutdruksenkenden Substanz. *Arch. exp. Path. Pharmakol.* **185**: 461–91.

SINHA, H. K. (1936) The local anesthetic actions of certain pyrazoline and quinoline compounds. *J. Pharmacol. exp. Therap.* **57**: 199–220.

SMITH, J. C. and WEISKOPF, R. D. (1967) Effect of cysteine on acetylcholine synthesis. *Nature* **215**: 1379–80.

STEPANOVIĆ, G., VARAGIĆ, V. and HAJDUKOVIĆ, S. (1963) The effect of cysteamine on the responses to biologically active substances of the isolated guinea-pig ileum taken from normal and gamma-irradiated animals. *Bull. Boris Kidrich. Inst. Nucl. Sci.* **14**: 163–74.

VAN DE BERG, L. and LECOMTE, J. (1953) β-Mercaptoéthylamine, acétylcholine et histamine chez le lapin. *Arch. internat. Physiol.* **61**: 240–2.

VARAGIĆ, V., DEBIJADJI, R. and ELČIĆ, S. (1963) An analysis of adrenergic blocking activity of cysteamine. *Arch. int. Pharmacodyn.* **142**: 207–15.

3.6

SMOOTH MUSCLES *IN VIVO* AND *IN VITRO*

J. Lecomte

Liège, Belgium

A DISTINCTION must be made between: (a) reactions of smooth muscle fibers caused by the action of sulfur-containing radioprotective agents on isolated organs and (b) reactions registered *in situ* which include the possibility of compensatory mechanisms (catecholamine secretion, histamine release, etc.). The behavior of vascular fibers is dealt with in Chapter 3.1; antihistaminic activities in Chapter 3.2.

Concentrations and dosage of the radioprotective agents will be quantified according to the type of expression used by the authors cited.

3.6.1. FROG

INNER EYE

Cysteamine (10^{-3} to 10^{-2} M) (MEA) relaxes the intrinsic muscles of the iris: as a mydriatic, MEA is 50,000 times weaker than epinephrine. Cystamine has a comparable effect (Grévisse and Goffart, 1960).

3.6.2. MOUSE

SMALL INTESTINE *in situ*

Cysteamine is inactive when up to 16 mg/kg is intravenously (i.v.) injected. When intraperitoneally injected (i.p.) (200 mg/kg), the intestinal mobility is only slightly increased.

Aminoethylisothiourea (AET) (4 mg/kg, i.v.) temporarily increases peristalsis. This increase is not subject to tachyphylaxis. In radioprotective doses (200 mg/kg, i.p.), hyperperistalsis persists throughout the phase of arterial hypertension.

Aminopropylisothiourea in similar doses is more active than AET. However, 200 mg/kg injected i.p. reduces intestinal activity.

When APMT is administered i.v., it has practically no effect on intestinal activity; at 300 mg/kg, i.p., it reduces peristalsis (DiStefano et al., 1962).

3.6.3. RAT

Cystamine (1/800 M) causes a decrease in tonus of the *isolated uterus* which is not followed by hypertonia. It may thus be distinguished from histamine (Robbers, 1937).

3.6.4. GUINEA-PIG

BRONCHI *in situ*

Cysteamine (200 mg/100 g, i.p.) does not alter air-flow resistances (Lecomte, 1955). Cystamine, administered subcutaneously, in a dose of 500 mg/kg, has no effect on the resistances of the bronchi and does not cause dyspnea. On autopsy, the lungs have a normal volume and readily collapse (Robbers, 1937). Typical histamine-induced pulmonary damage is not found in cases of poisoning by sulfur-containing derivatives (Robbers, 1937).

ISOLATED INTESTINE

Cysteamine (10^{-4} M) causes a slight increase in the tonus of the terminal ileum (Grévisse and Goffart, 1960). Cystamine (50–200 mcg/ml) has no effect on the ileal tonus (Lecomte, 1955).

3.6.5. RABBIT

ISOLATED BRONCHI

Cystamine (10^{-4} M) does not cause contraction of the tracheal rings.

At a concentration 10^{-2} M, it causes a rise in tonus and a decrease in frequency of spontaneous contraction.

ISOLATED UTERUS

Cysteamine (10^{-3} M) produces an increase in tonus and a decrease in frequency of spontaneous contractions. These effects are similar to those of epinephrine, but the ratio of the activity of MEA to that of epinephrine is of the order of 1/4000. In the same concentration, cystamine is weakly excitatory, or inactive (Grévisse and Goffart, 1960).

ISOLATED INTESTINE

Cysteamine (10^{-3} M) affects intestinal pendular movements. The effect is often triphasic: first a reduction in contraction amplitude, then an increase in their height during a period varying between 2 and 15 min and finally a progressive decrease in tonus and pendular movements. These effects no longer resemble those due to epinephrine. The excitatory phase is not due to the eventual action of MEA on the ganglionic cells of the enteric plexus, since it persists in the presence of pentamethonium or hexamethonium (2×10^{-5} M) (Grévisse and Goffart, 1960).

Cystamine (10^{-3} M) is almost inactive on the intestine; however, it sometimes produces weak inhibition (Robbers, 1937; Grévisse and Goffart, 1960).

Aminoethylisothiourea (10^{-8} to 10^{-3} M) considerably increases the pendular activity. This can persist after washing out the product (Laborit *et al.,* 1959).

INTESTINE *in situ*

Aminoethylisothiourea (12 mg/kg) brings about powerful contractions and intense peristaltic movements of the small intestine (Laborit *et al.,* 1959).

Cystamine forms a complex with lead acetate (10^{-4} M) which causes contraction of isolated strips of aorta and tracheal rings of the rabbit. This "activation" does not affect the contraction of all types of smooth muscles (Grévisse and Goffart, 1959).

3.6.6.   CAT

NICTITATING MEMBRANE *in situ*

Cysteamine (120 mg/kg) causes contraction of the acutely denervated nictitating membrane of the cat adrenalectomized in order to eliminate the nicotinic effects of MEA. The effect is therefore direct, but not of great significance and varies between individuals (Goffart and Paton, 1955; Grévisse and Goffart, 1960).

In the adrenalectomized animal, MEA causes strong contractions of the nictitating membrane. There is no contraction on the side from which the ganglion is removed: this provides evidence of an excitatory ganglionic effect of a nicotinic type (Goffart and Paton, 1955).

In the intact cat the contraction induced by these two mechanisms can, in certain individuals, be reinforced by epinephrine liberated from the adrenal medulla, either directly (Lecomte, 1954; Goffart, 1955), or by activating homeostatic mechanisms to correct an eventual systemic arterial hypotension (Lecomte *et al.*, 1964). Thus, the contraction of the membrane observed in the intact cat demonstrates a complex mechanism in which direct, nervous and humoral effects are associated.

Cystamine has a direct effect but is weaker than MEA; it has similar excitatory ganglionic effects. However, it releases into circulation a larger quantity of adrenal medullary catecholamines which may cause the membrane to contract (Lecomte *et al.*, 1964; Beaumariage *et al.*, 1966).

The tonus of the membrane is directly inhibited by AET and APT, both blocking transmission in the superior cervical ganglion. No effect on tonus is observed with ABT, whereas 2-AT increases it, possibly by the homeostatic liberation of epinephrine (DiStefano *et al.*, 1956, 1959).

INTESTINE *in situ*

An increase in the motor activity of the small intestine is produced by AET 2.5–12.5 mg/kg, i.v. This decreases with increasing doses and is suppressed by atropine (DiStefano *et al.*, 1956).

An increase in the motor activity of the intestine comparable to that caused by AET is also produced by APT 2.5 mg/kg, i.v. It is blocked by atropine. Aminopropylisothiourea acts in the same way, while ABT is inactive.

Biphasic effects are produced by 2-AT: first inhibition which is probably due to a liberation of epinephrine, then excitation which is suppressed by vagotomy; they are dependent on a central mechanism (DiStefano *et al.*, 1959).

SPLEEN

An increase in the volume of the spleen is produced by APMT (4.8–16 mg/kg). It also increases the constrictor effects of epinephrine (DiStefano *et al.*, 1961).

ISOLATED NON-PREGNANT UTERUS

Cysteamine in a final concentration of 10^{-3} to 4×10^{-4} M produces a lowering of tonus and also inhibits to a lesser extent the spontaneous contractions of the uterus. For an equivalent lowering of tonus, the action of MEA is of longer duration than that of epinephrine. The sensitivity of various preparations is very variable. Cysteamine is 125–5000 times less active than L-epinephrine. These effects of MEA are spontaneously reversible.

After return to normal tonus, with the continued presence of MEA, the drop in tonus produced again by epinephrine is generally 2–10 times greater in intensity and in duration.

The inhibiting action of MEA is sometimes subject to tachyphylaxis.

Tolazoline and phentolamine (1×10^{-5} M) cause a decrease of 30–80% in the inhibition due to MEA, but have no effect on the response of the isolated uterus to epinephrine.

933 F (5×10^{-6} M), which inhibits the action of epinephrine by 50–80%, inhibits the effect of MEA to a greater extent.

Cystamine (10^{-3} M) does not alter or slightly lowers the tonus of the uterus. In the presence of cystamine, the action of epinephrine is increased by 80–100% (Goffart and Grévisse, 1960).

3.6.7. DOG

DIGESTIVE TRACT *in situ*

Intravenous administration of MEA (100 mg/kg) to the waking dog produces immediate vomiting, followed after 1 or 2 hr by diarrhea containing blood. These symptoms are suppressed by general anesthesia (Mundy and Heiffer, 1960).

Infusion or i.v. injection of AET (25–150 mg/kg) produces vomiting, tenesmus and defecation. These effects give evidence of an increase in peristalsis of the digestive tract. They are suppressed by general anesthesia (Knott and Overman, 1961).

EYE *in situ*

Cysteamine (100 mg/kg) produces mydriasis (Mundy and Heiffer, 1960).

Aminoethylisothiourea, while being infused i.v. (25–150 mg/kg) or being injected i.v. in a rapid single dose of 150 mg/kg, produces a relaxation of the nictitating membrane and dilatation of the pupils (Knott and Overman, 1961).

3.6.8. MAN

DIGESTIVE TRACT *in situ*

Cysteamine and cystamine are well tolerated in normal clinical dosages (Bacq, 1965). Cystamine, in very high doses (200–400 mg, i.v.), produces vomiting in some volunteers (Lecomte, 1952).

Aminoethylisothiourea i.v. in doses of up to 25 mg/kg produces nausea and vomiting. Sometimes this is followed by diarrhea, which may be delayed (Condit *et al.,* 1958).

3.6.9. DISCUSSION AND CONCLUSION

As a whole, smooth muscle layers which are not part of the structure of blood vessels react only slightly to sulfur-containing radioprotective agents. These reactions are of minor importance in the development of the general intoxication.

Cysteamine as an aliphatic amine cannot be included among agents having a sympathomimetic action, as was established by the results of various comparative investigations carried out by Goffart and Grévisse (1959, 1960).

In whole animals, smooth muscle reactions are complex. In a general way, there is a mixture of direct action, stimulation or inhibition of central origin, disturbances of ganglionic transmission and interference with homeostatic processes.

Sulfur-containing radioprotective agents do not have any significant direct effects on the functions of non-vascular smooth muscle.

REFERENCES

BACQ, Z. M. (1965) *Chemical Protection against Ionizing Radiation.* Charles C. Thomas, Springfield, Illinois, 328 pages.

BEAUMARIAGE, M. L., VAN CANEGHEM, P. and BACQ, Z. M. (1966) Etude de certaines propriétés pharmacodynamiques de la cystamine et de la cystéamine chez diverses espèces animales. *Strahlentherapie* **131**: 342–51.

CONDIT, P. F., LEVY, A. H., VAN SCOTT, E. J. and ANDREWS, J. R. (1958) Some effects of β-aminoethylisothiouronium bromide (AET) in man. *J. Pharmacol. exp. Ther.* **122**: 13A.

DiSTEFANO, V. and LEARY, D. E. (1959) The pharmacological effects of D- and L-2-amino-butylisothiouronium bromide and 3-aminopropyl-*N*′-methylisothiouronium bromide hydrobromide in the cat. *J. Pharmacol.* **126**: 304–10.

DiSTEFANO, V., LEARY, D. E. and DOHERTY, D. G. (1956) The pharmacology of β-aminoethylisothiouronium bromide in the cat. *J. Pharmacol.* **117**: 425–33.

DiSTEFANO, V., LEARY, D. E. and LITTLE, K. D. (1959) The pharmacological effects of some congeners of 2-aminoethylisothiouronium bromide (AET). *J. Pharmacol.* **126**: 159–63.

DiSTEFANO, V., KORN, P. S. and LEARY, D. E. (1961) The blood pressure effects of 3-amino-propyl-*N*′-methylisothiouronium bromide hydrobromide in the cat. *J. Pharmacol.* **134**: 341–6.

DiSTEFANO, V., KLAHN, J. J. and LEARY, D. E. (1962) The pharmacological effects of some radioprotective agents in mice. *Rad. Res.* **17**: 792–800.

GOFFART, M. (1955) Mode d'action de la cystéamine et de la cystamine au niveau de la médullo-surrénale. *Arch. internat. Physiol. Bioch.* **63**: 500–12.

GOFFART, M. and GRÉVISSE, J. (1960) Action de la cystéamine, de la cystamine sur l'utérus vierge de la chatte. *C.R. Soc. Biol.* **154**: 2143.

GOFFART, M. and PATON, W. D. M. (1955) Action de la cystéamine et de la cystamine sur un ganglion sympathique. *Arch. internat. Physiol. Bioch.* **63**: 477–99.

GRÉVISSE, J. and GOFFART, M. (1959) "Activation" de l'ion plomb par la cystéamine, sur certains muscles lisses isolés du lapin. *J. de Physiol.* **51**: 471–2.

GRÉVISSE, J. and GOFFART, M. (1960) La cystéamine est-elle douée de propriétés sympathicomimétiques? *C.R. Soc. Biol.* **154**: 2401–3.

KNOTT, D. H. and OVERMAN, R. R. (1961) Cardiovascular effects of radioprotective compound beta-aminoethyl isothiouronium Br-HBr (AET). *Am. J. Physiol.* **201**: 677–81.

LABORIT, H., BROUSSOLLE, B., JOUANY, J. M., NIAUSSAT, P., REYNIER, M. and WEBER, B. (1959) Etude pharmacologique du bromhydrate de 2-aminoéthylisothiouronium (AET). *Thérapie* **14**: 1116–35.

LECOMTE, J. (1952) Sur la pathogénie du choc nitritoide bénin. *Arch. int. Pharmacodyn.* **92**: 241–51.

LECOMTE, J. (1954) Cystéamine et médullo-surrénale. *Arch. internat. Physiol.* **62**: 431–2.

LECOMTE, J. (1955) Propriétés antihistaminiques des dérivés décarboxylés de la cystéine (cystéamine et cystamine). *Arch. internat. Physiol. Bioch.* **63**: 291–304.

LECOMTE, J., CESSION-FOSSION, A., LIBON, J. C. and BACQ, Z. M. (1964) Sur quelques effets pharmacodynamiques généraux de la cystamine chez le rat. *Arch. int. Pharmacodyn.* **148**: 487–510.

MUNDY, R. L. and HEIFFER, M. H. (1960) The pharmacology of radioprotectant chemicals. General pharmacology of β-mercaptoethylamine. *Rad. Res.* **13**: 381–94.

ROBBERS, H. (1937) Die pharmakologische Wirkung des Cystamins, einer blutdrucksenkenden Substanz. *Arch. f. exper. Path. u. Pharmakol.* **185**: 461–91.

3.7

EFFECTS OF CYSTAMINE AND CYSTEAMINE ON THE SKIN

P. Van Caneghem

Liège, Belgium

3.7.1. LOCAL APPLICATION

The doses of cystamine and cysteamine (MEA) injected intradermally usually vary between 0.5 and 0.75 mg. They correspond to the doses of MEA used in the study of local radioprotection. These doses can be increased if the substances are applied on the skin.

3.7.1.1. ACTION ON PIGMENTATION

When applied locally MEA causes a depigmentation of guinea-pig skin (Frenk *et al.,* 1968), as well as of the hair of young mice (Beaumariage, 1968). This loss of pigment may be attributed to the inhibitory action of the —SH groups on tyrosinase and to the cytotoxic action of MEA, since destruction of the melanocytes has also been observed (Frenk *et al.,* 1968).

3.7.1.2. EFFECT ON HAIR GROWTH

Cystamine and to a lesser extent MEA have a dysplasing effect (i.e. they induce constriction in the hair shaft and decrease or disappearance of the pigment) when injected into the skin of young mice (Beaumariage and Van Caneghem, 1968; Beaumariage, 1968). The dysplasia probably results from the non-specific, tissue-irritating action of the substances, since the same effects are seen with quite unrelated substances (such as formol), or anoxiating agents such as epinephrine.

137

3.7.1.3. ACTION ON SKIN BLOOD VESSELS

Cystamine produces cutaneous vasodilatation and therefore causes a decrease in the vascular resistance of the isolated rabbit ear. This effect is weaker with MEA (Van Caneghem and Beaumariage, unpublished experiments).

3.7.1.4. IRRITATING ACTION

Cystamine and MEA cause irritation when injected locally under the skin of rats and mice (Franchimont *et al.*, 1962; Lecomte *et al.*, 1964; Beaumariage *et al.*, 1966) (see also Chapter 3.2). An increase in capillary permeability and edema formation may be observed. In the rat intradermal injection of cystamine results in the formation of a wheal, resembling the histamine wheal. In the mouse, edema does not seem to be due to the liberation of the histamine by these two substances, but it seems that 5-hydroxytryptamine may be involved, since methysergide partially reduces the inflammatory reaction resulting from cystamine. Similar observations were made by Lecomte *et al.* (1964) after administration of methysergide or an antihistaminic in rats.

Trasylol® [2000 UKI/kg intraperitoneally (i.p.)] similarly inhibits the cystamine inflammatory reaction in the young mouse, probably by inhibiting proteolytic enzyme action (Beaumariage *et al.*, 1966). Trihydroxyethylrutosid (Vit. P_4) reduces vascular permeability, but has no effect on edema formation after cystamine injection (Van Caneghem *et al.*, 1967).

3.7.1.5. ACTION ON SKIN DEHYDROGENASE

Perfusion of an isolated rabbit ear with sodium tellurite (Na_2TeO_3) according to a technique described by Wels (1963) followed by injection of a thiol compound results in rapid reduction of the tellurite by direct action of the —SH group on the salt. However, if cystamine (with —SS— groups) is injected, tellurite reduction is inhibited by comparison with normal skin, instead of being accelerated. A white spot appears at the injection site (Fig. 1).

These experiments show that skin, unlike liver, is incapable of reducing —SS— groups to —SH— (Van Caneghem, 1968, 1969). A rise in skin potential may be seen after local injection of redox indicators, followed by cystamine, into rabbit skin. These observations support the previous conclusion.

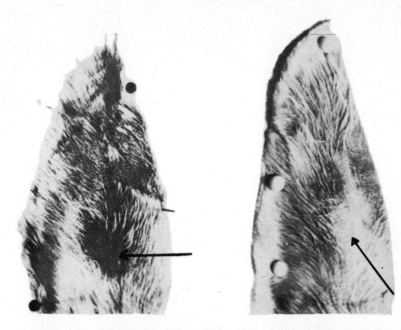

Fig. 1. Perfusion during 30 min of an isolated albino rabbit ear with Locke-Ringer solution containing 1 % sodium tellurite. On the left: black spot after intracutaneous injection of 0.1 ml MEA solution (10^{-1} M/l). On the right: white spot in grayish surroundings after injection of 0.1 ml cystamine solution (0.5×10^{-1} M/l) (Van Caneghem, 1969).

Cysteamine (MEA) has a weak local anesthetic effect (Goffart and Piret, 1955).

3.7.2. GENERAL ADMINISTRATION

The doses administered correspond with those used in radioprotection, that is 100–150 mg/kg, and are usually given by i.p. injection.

3.7.2.1. EFFECT ON SKIN TEMPERATURE

Cystamine causes a rapid fall in skin temperature, which is a symptom of a state of shock (see Chapter 3.3). A slower fall in temperature is observed with MEA (Fig. 2).

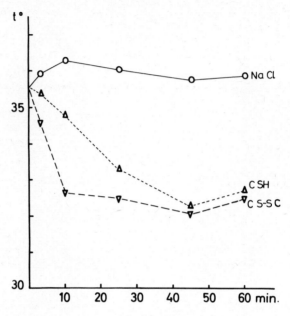

Fɪɢ. 2. Skin temperature measured in the hairless mouse after i.p. injection of cystamine or MEA (150 mg/kg) (Van Caneghem *et al.*, 1973). Abscissa: time in minutes after injection; ordinate: temperature in degrees Celsius;——: animals injected with NaCl; ......: animal injected with MEA (—SH); —— animals injected with cystamine (—SS—). Each point is the average of 30 measurements. After 3 min the difference between—SH and—SS—is significant ($P<0.05$), after 10 min and 25 min it is highly significant ($P < 0.01$).

3.7.2.2. EFFECT ON HISTAMINE AND 5-HYDROXYTRYPTAMINE (5-HT) CONTENT

Lecomte *et al.* (1964) have shown the weak histamine liberating action of cystamine in rats. Cystamine has no effect on the endogenous histamine content of the skin of the adult hairless mouse, but causes a reduction in the 5-HT content (Beaumariage *et al.,* 1968).

3.7.2.3. EFFECT ON THE PILOUS SYSTEM

Cystamine and MEA cause slight dysplasia after i.p. injection in young mice. In rare cases there is discoloration of the hair roots (Beaumariage, 1968).

3.7.2.4. EFFECT ON THE OXYGEN TENSION

In the young mouse, cystamine produces a significant and prolonged reduction of the partial oxygen tension in the subcutaneous cellular tissue. Only a small and irregular effect on the oxygen tension is observed with MEA (van der Meer and Beaumariage, 1962; Beaumariage, 1968; Van Caneghem and Beaumariage, 1973).

3.7.3. CONCLUSIONS

Cysteamine (MEA) causes depigmentation of the skin by the inhibitory action of its thiol group and its cytotoxic action. Cystamine and to a lesser degree MEA have a dysplasing effect on the hair of young mice. Cystamine inhibits the skin dehydrogenases. At the applied doses, the skin is unable to reduce the —SS— groups to —SH—; cystamine and MEA act as local irritants, liberating a negligible quantity of histamine, but causing an appreciable decrease in the 5-HT content in the skin.

After general administration, cystamine causes cutaneous hypothermia and a fall in partial oxygen tension. These effects may be attributed to the shock-producing action of cystamine; they are less significant with MEA.

From these observations, it may be concluded that the effects of cystamine and MEA on the skin are, in many ways, not identical. These differences may be explained at least partly in terms of the general pharmacological action of cystamine being stronger than that of MEA, the skin being very sensitive to this due to its homeostasic function; and secondly, reduction of cystamine to MEA does not occur to any significant extent in the skin. At the subcellular level (mitochondria and lysosomes), the action of thiols and their disulfides is not identical, as mentioned in Chapter 3.3.

REFERENCES

BEAUMARIAGE, M. L. (1968) Contribution à l'étude de la radioprotection du système pileux du souriceau contre le rayonnement X. *Thèse de Licence en Sciences Nucléaires.* Liège, pp. 173.

BEAUMARIAGE, M. L. and VAN CANEGHEM, P. (1968) Modification of hair dysplasia curve by radioprotectors containing sulfur as a function of the X-ray dose. *Rad. Res.* **33**: 74–8.

BEAUMARIAGE, M. L., VAN CANEGHEM, P. and BACQ, Z. M. (1966) Etude de certaines propriétés pharmacodynamiques de la cystamine et de la cystéamine chez diverses espèces animales. *Strahlentherapie* **131**: 342–51.

FRANCHIMONT, P., VAN CAUWENBERGE, H. and LECOMTE, J. (1962) Sur l'œdème local provoqué par la cystamine chez le rat. *C.R. Soc. Biol.* **156**: 549–52.

FRENK, E., PATHAK, M., SZABÓ, G. and FITZPATRICK, T. (1968) Selective action of mercaptoethylamines on melanocytes in mammalian skin. Experimental depigmentation. *Arch. Derm.* **97**: 465–77.

GOFFART, M. and PIRET, J. (1955) Pouvoir anesthésique local de la cystéamine. *Arch. internat. Physiol. Bioch.* **63**: 534–5.

LECOMTE, J., CESSION-FOSSION, A., LIBON, J. and BACQ, Z. M. (1964) Sur quelques effets pharmacologiques généraux de la cystamine chez le rat. *Arch. int. Pharmacodyn.* **148**: 487–510.

MEER, C. VAN DER and BEAUMARIAGE, M. L. (1962) Action des radioprotecteurs soufrés sur la pression partielle d'oxygène au niveau du revêtement cutané. Communication présentée à la 2ème réunion des Radiobiologistes de l'Euratom, Bruxelles.

VAN CANEGHEM, P. (1968) Radiobiologie cutanée, pp. 1069–70. In: *XIII Congrès Int. de Dermatologie.* JADASSOHN, W. and SCHIRREN, C. G. (eds.). Springer–Verlag, Berlin.

VAN CANEGHEM, P. (1969) Vergleich der Strahlenschutzwirkungen von Cystamin und Cysteamin auf die Haut. *Strahlentherapie* **137**: 231–7.

VAN CANEGHEM, P. and BEAUMARIAGE, M. L. (1973) pH und kutane Strahlenschutzwirkung von Cysteamin. *Strahlentherapie* **145**: 663–73.

VAN CANEGHEM, P., DUNJIC, A., STEIN, F. and PESESSE, M. P. (1967) Action du trihydroxyéthylrutoside sur les réactions inflammatoires. *Path. europ.* **2**: 118–23.

WELS, P. (1963) Reduktionen und Oxydationen bei biologischen Strahlenwirkungen. *Photochem. Photobiol.* **2**: 268–323.

ADDENDUM

It is possible that the pharmacological actions of cysteamine are mediated by cAMP, as was suggested by Langendorff. Nevertheless, the experiments made on the subject allow no precise distinction between the effects of cysteamine as such and the effects of anoxia and of the adrenaline discharge following its administration. It is not impossible that cysteamine is modifying completely or partly the cellular content of cAMP by way of the last two mechanisms.

LANGENDORFF, H. and LANGENDORFF, M. (1972) Experimentelle Untersuchungen zum Wirkungsmechanismus strahlenresistenzerhöhender Substanzen. *Strahlentherapie* **143**: 432–43.

LANGENDORFF, H. and LANGENDORFF, M. (1972) Adenosin-Nukleotide und Strahlenempfindlichkeit. *Strahlentherapie* **144**: 451–56.

LANGENDORFF, H. and LANGENDORFF, M. (1973) Weitere Untersuchungen über die Beziehungen der Strahlenempfindlichkeit eines höheren Organismus zum Adelynst-Cyclase-System seiner Zellen. *Strahlentherapie* **146**: 436–43.

MITZNEGG, P. (1973) On the mechanism of radioprotection by cysteamine. II. The significance of cyclic 3′,5′-AMP for the cysteamine induced radioprotective effects in white mice. *Int. J. Radiat. Biol.* **24**: 339–44.

CHAPTER 4

CELLULAR EFFECTS AS SEEN WITH THE ELECTRON MICROSCOPE

J. S. Hugon

Sherbrooke, Quebec, Canada

4.1. INTRODUCTION

Since the first radioprotective studies by Bacq and Herve (1949) and Patt *et al.* (1949) a great many studies on the pharmacological and biochemical aspects of these compounds have been published (see Bacq, 1965). These aspects are discussed in the other chapters in this volume. It would be logical to suppose that these protective compounds, especially the most powerful of them, should be able to induce changes in cellular structures detectable under the microscope.

Initially, optical microscopic studies were only concerned with the anatomical manifestations of the protective power of these agents in irradiated animals pretreated with them. Protection against tissue lesions caused by the presence of these compounds was, however, the only aspect studied. The control animals did not show any alterations attributable to the radioprotective agent itself.

Nevertheless, it soon became apparent that in mitotically active cells such as intestinal crypt cells (Maisin *et al.,* 1968) or chicken fibroblasts in culture (Chèvremont, 1961) aminoethylisothiourea (AET) and cysteamine (MEA) clearly have an antimitotic effect. Maisin and Lambiet (1967) have shown that a mixture of several radioprotective agents produces considerable depression in the mitotic activity in mouse intestinal crypts, apparently due to a lengthening of the mitotic cycle.

Optical microscopy cannot produce evidence of fine alterations in the intracellular organelles, and there have been no histochemical studies performed following the use of radioprotective agents. Some of these interfere with the oxidizing enzymes present in the mitochondria, so that histochemical alterations might be expected.

143

The application of electron microscopic techniques in morphological research has made it possible to investigate more precisely the intracellular effects of radioprotective agents. A small number of studies have been devoted to this subject but their results are in good agreement.

These optical and electron microscopic investigations will be reviewed, and compared with information available on the ultrastructural localization of labeled radioprotective agents. Finally the ultrastructural lesions in irradiated and protected tissues will be discussed.

4.2. CELLULAR ALTERATIONS OBSERVED UNDER THE OPTICAL MICROSCOPE

Among the numerous protective agents studied, we shall discuss the experiments carried out with the principal ones: these were administered alone or in combination: AET, MEA, 5-hydroxytryptamine (5-HT), and dimethylsulfoxide; they have all been studied *in vivo*, or in tissue culture.

When used in concentration from 10^{-5}M AET considerably inhibits growth in cultures of mice cells (Eker and Pihl 1964; Peters, 1963). *In vivo*, an injection of 10 mg AET in 25 g mice, causes a slight decrease in mitotic activity. However, no other cytological alterations have been observed (Maisin *et al.*, 1960, 1968). Goutier *et al.* (1966) were able to show clearly a decrease in mitotic activity in regenerating liver.

Many tissue culture studies have been performed using MEA. Chèvremont (1961) showed that it affected or inhibited cytodieresis in chicken fibroblasts. The nuclei show irregularities in form, and variations in their DNA content. Therkelsen (1958) showed that MEA causes pyknosis and blocked metaphases when it is added to the time culture for periods of 2–24 hr.

The histological investigations performed by Highman *et al.* (1967) on rats injected with dimethylsulfoxide in a dose of 4.5 g/kg did not show any lesion under the optical microscope. On the other hand, the growth of HeLa cells is strongly inhibited by a concentration of 2% MEA. In addition it causes a slight increase in the activity of ribonuclease and β-galactosidase (Chang and Simon, 1968).

Radioprotective mixtures have been investigated by Maisin *et al.* (1967, 1968). They showed that the administration of glutathione, AET, and 5-HT produced a lengthening of the mitotic cycle in the stem cells of the intestine of the Balb/c mouse, an increase in the period of migration along the villi, and a decrease in the number of cells synthesizing DNA.

The mixture also has very toxic effects on spermatogonia (Léonard, personal communication).

In summary, observations made after the administration of radio-protective compounds, using light microscopy, have produced very little precise cytological data; most of the compounds studied caused a slowing of mitotic activity.

4.3. INTRACELLULAR MODIFICATIONS OBSERVED UNDER THE ELECTRON MICROSCOPE

4.3.1. RADIOPROTECTIVE AGENTS INJECTED ALONE

The action of some radioprotective agents, injected alone or in combination, have been studied on the undifferentiated duodenal crypt cells of the Balb/c mouse (Hugon *et al.*, 1964, 1966a, b).

Fifteen minutes after the administration of an intraperitoneal (i.p.) dose of 300 mg/kg AET considerable swelling of the mitochondria is observed, accompanied by the disappearance of the mitochondrial cristae. The double peripheral membrane may eventually show ruptures in its outer layer. It is possible that this latter result is really a fixation artefact. These alterations are accompanied by a thinning of the mito-chondrial matrix, which becomes more permeable to electrons. At the same time, the cisternae of the rough endoplasmic reticulum become dilated and contain a less electron-dense substance. They also seem to be fragmented into vesicles. The nuclear envelope exhibits also some swelling between the pores.

These alterations persist for 90 min and progressively regress, without extensive damage to the intracellular organelles. However, between 90 min and 3 hr after the injection of the protective agents, the number of bodies with a dense or membranous content seem to increase slightly in the Golgi region. Their dimensions remain normal. All traces of lesions have disappeared 24 hr after the injection of AET. During this period, no morphological alterations have been observed in the absorbing cells of the villi.

Glutathione was administered orally in a large dose of 16 g/kg. The structural changes which occurred in the epithelial cells of the duodenum were particularly notable in the stem cells of the duodenal crypt. These changes are essentially transitory, and are only observed at the level of the mitochondria. The swelling of these organelles is very marked; the cristae are devaginated and stretched along the double membrane, leaving

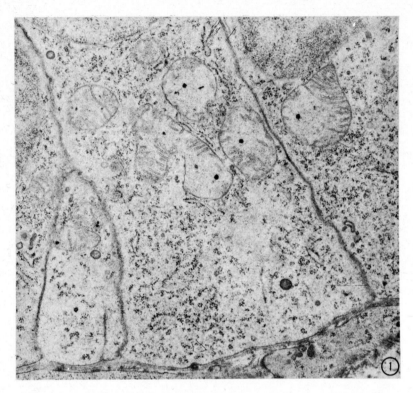

FIG. 1. Undifferentiated cells of the duodenal crypt of the mouse 10 min after glutathione given orally: considerable dilatation of the mitochondria, with obliteration of the cristae (× 28,000).

a very clear matrix (Fig. 1). No other structure showed any alterations. Thirty minutes after the administration of AET the mitochondria recovered their normal appearance. Ueno and Yamano (1960) did not, however, observe mitochondrial lesions in the hepatic cells of mice that had been injected with a large quantity of mixture of 10:1 oxidized glutathione and its reduced form. For comparison, 5-HT (a non-sulfur-containing radioprotective agent) was injected in a dose of 40 mg/kg i.p. The mitochondria of the undifferentiated cells had an abnormal appearance: after 15 min the organelles appeared longer compared with the controls, extending over several microns in the cytoplasm. The cristae remained very sharp, and multilobular constrictions were frequently observed. The intramitochondrial granules were dense and numerous.

TABLE 1. PERCENTAGE OF VARIOUS ASPECTS OF THE MITOCHONDRIA IN THE RED PULP OF
RAT SPLEEN AFTER INJECTION WITH CYSTAMINE (100 mg/kg, i.p.)
(Firket and Lelièvre, 1966)

Type of mitochondria observed	Controls	Minutes after injection					
		10	20	30	50	90	120
Normal appearance	71	54	45	57.5	43	61	62.5
Abnormal appearance	6.5	22	30.5	20.5	31	19.5	10
Non-classified	22.5	24	24.5	22	26	19.5	27.5

These alterations were also transitory and disappeared 90 min after the injection. This mitochondrial appearance can be explained in terms of a lowering of the activity of the mitochondria.

Firket and Lelièvre (1966) studied the effects of MEA in the spleen, liver, kidney, lymphatic ganglion, and thymus of the rat. The dose injected was 100 mg/kg i.p. In the liver there were no alterations. Systematic alterations were, however, observed in the spleen, particularly in the reticulated cells of the red marrow (Table 1). There is an enlargement of the intracristal space 10 min after the administration of the radio-protective agent, and other mitochondria show considerable disorganization of their structure, or clearing of their matrix. All these anomalies disappear about 2 hr after the injection. They are not found in the lymphoid cells of the white marrow, lymphatic ganglia, or thymus, and there are apparently no alterations in the cells of the renal tubule. Using MEA in organotypic cultures of embryonic chicken intestine at concentrations of 16–64 mM Kirrmann (1967) observed very considerable lesions in the mitochondria and ergastoplasm 2 hr after impregnation with the radioprotective agent. Some parts of the cytoplasm were observed to be vacuolar.

Braun and Koch (1968) studied the ultrastructural aspects of duodenal crypt cells of mice, 3–30 min after the i.p. injection of radioprotective and non-radioprotective sulfhydryl compounds. Cysteamine (MEA), isocysteine, 5-mercaptopyridoxine, 5-mercaptomethylpyridine, and 4-mercaptopyridoxine have been tested. The radioprotective MEA and 5-mercaptopyridoxine caused fairly large mitochondrial lesions manifested by the swelling of the organelles and the disappearance of the cristae. The non-radioprotective agents, such as 4-mercaptopyridoxine, did not provoke any detectable alterations. Injection of β-mercapto-ethanol, a non-protective compound, did not result in any mitochondrial ultrastructural alterations. In the series of sulfur-containing compounds there therefore seems to be an important correlation between the possible radioprotective properties and the presence of mitochondrial lesions.

To summarize, sulfhydryl radioprotective agents produce transient mitochondrial and ergastoplasmic alterations in many tissues, whereas other non-sulfur-containing protective agents such as 5-HT have only very slight effects on these structures. It is debatable whether the lesions observed are, in fact, due specifically to the accumulation of radio-protective agents in these structures. Masurovsky and Bunge (1969) have used radioautography to approach this problem. Using cultures

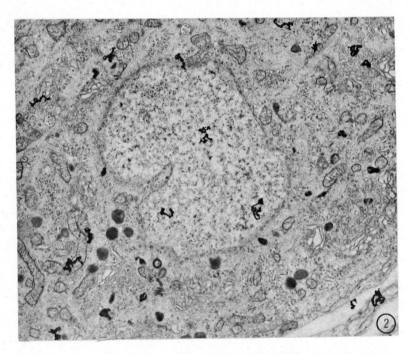

Fig. 2. Cultures of rat dorsal root ganglion neurons (with satellite cell investment) treated with 3 mmol ^{35}S AET solution, X-ray irradiated (40 Kr), and immediately fixed for electronmicroscopic autoradiography. Silver grains appear over the nucleus, near the nuclear envelope, over the mitochondria, Golgi complexes, ergastoplasm of the neuron, and near the plasma membrane of the satellite cell (× 14,000). (Courtesy of E.B. Masurovsky and R.P. Bunge, Department of Anatomy, Columbia University, New York, N.Y.)

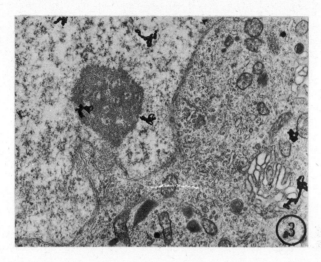

Fɪɢ. 3. Electronmicroscopic autoradiogram of ^{35}S AET-treated, X-ray irradiated rat dorsal root ganglion neuron, showing nucleolar, nuclear matrix, Golgi complex, and ergastoplasm labeling (× 10,000). (Courtesy of E. B. Masurovsky and R. P. Bunge.)

of rat fetus spinal ganglia, incubated for 20 min with 3 mmol ^{35}S-labeled AET, they followed the distribution of radioactivity. The nucleolus, nuclear membrane, nuclear matrix, mitochondria, ergastoplasm, and the Golgi complex were clearly labeled; less frequently, the lysosomes and a region adjacent to the plasma membrane (Figs. 2 and 3) were also found to be labeled. Counting the grains showed the mitochondria to be most heavily labeled with radioactive compounds, followed by the Golgi complex and ergastoplasm. There is a direct correlation between the intensity of lesions observed and the concentration of protective agents.

4.3.2. RADIOPROTECTIVE AGENTS INJECTED AS MIXTURES

Two mixtures have been studied because of their remarkable radio-protective effects: (1) Glutathione, AET, and 5-HT, in doses of 640, 300 and 40 mg respectively. (2) Glutathione, AET, 5-HT, MEA and cysteine in doses of 640, 300, 40, 100, and 600 mg/kg respectively.

(1) With the first combination the mitochondrial changes are less significant than with the injection of AET alone. However, the mito-chondria may be seen to swell with an enlargement of the cristae; the ergastoplasm is also dilated. After 3 hr there is a considerable increase

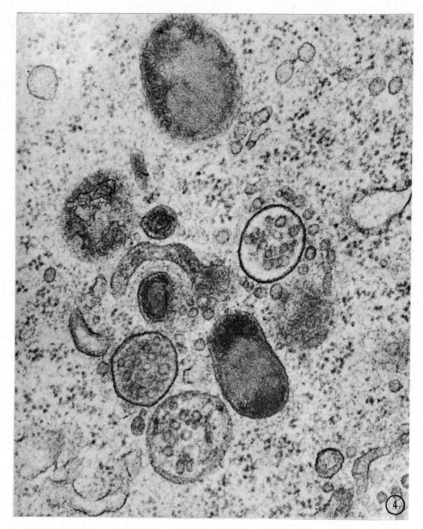

FIG. 4. Undifferentiated cells of the duodenal crypt of the mouse 90 min after injection of a radioprotective mixture of glutathione, AET, and 5-HT. Accumulation of dense bodies, multivesicular bodies, and small vesicles appears to indicate an increased lysosomal activity (× 90,000).

in the number of electron-dense bodies with fibrillar or vesicular content, which is a characteristic effect of this mixture (Fig. 4).

Some of these structures appear to merge, and the cisternae of the

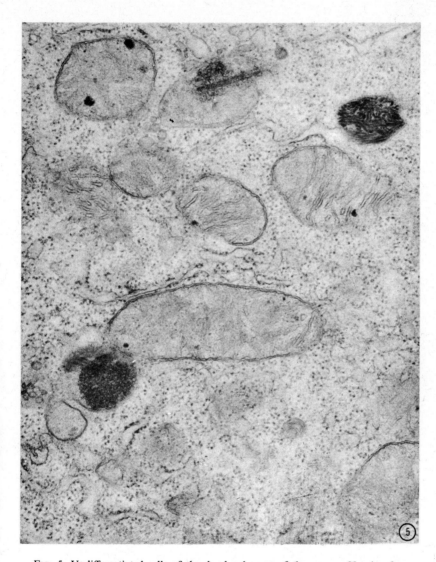

FIG. 5. Undifferentiated cells of the duodenal crypt of the mouse, 30 min after injection of a radioprotective mixture of glutathione, AET, 5-HT, cysteine, and mercaptoethylamine. Some mitochondria show a slight degree of obliteration of the cristae without dilatation of the matrix. One of them appears very close to a dense body having a myelin content ($\times$ 55,000).

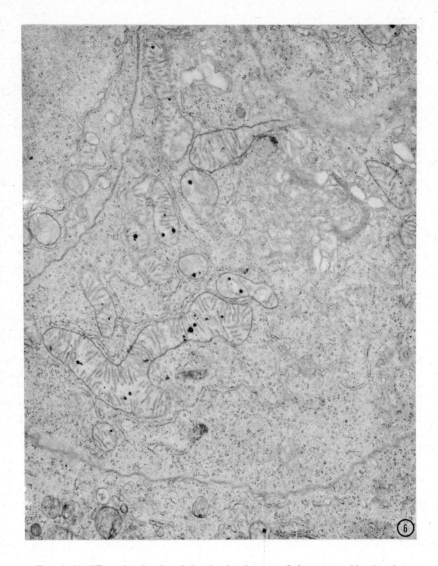

FIG. 6. Undifferentiated cells of the duodenal crypt of the mouse, 30 min after injection of a radioprotective mixture of glutathione, AET, 5-HT, cysteine, and mercaptoethylamine. In this cell, the mitochondria have relatively sharp cristae, but a somewhat cleared matrix. Certain mitochondria have twisted or drawn-out contours ($\times$ 25,000).

rough endoplasmic reticulum are found to be adjacent to their limiting membranes (Fig. 5). An ultrastructural, cytochemical study of these formations has given a positive result for the acid phosphatase test (Hugon and Borgers, 1966). It is therefore thought that they are secondary lysosomes. The nuclei, examined at various times after the injection of these mixtures, showed no clear lesions, although some stem cell nucleoli of the duodenal crypt showed slight dissociation comparable to that seen at the beginning of nuclear alterations following irradiation (Hugon and Borgers, 1968).

(2) The second mixture studied, whose considerable radioprotective power has been shown by Maisin *et al.* (1968), produced very similar alterations in the duodenal crypts, the mitochondria showing changes in the form of clear central plaques. The dilatation was very slight (Fig. 6). These lesions persisted for more than 3 hr but had totally disappeared 6 hr after administration of the mixture. The absorbing cells of the villus did not show any damage, although after 90 min the number of inclusions with dense fibrillar or granular content had also increased, frequently taking up an apical position in the cell. After 24 hr, the structures of the cells had completely returned to normal. Five months after the administration of the radioprotective mixture, no alterations in the cellular organelles of the duodenal epithelium could be seen.

From the collection of electron microscopic observations made on the intestine, spleen, kidney, and lymphatic glands of the mouse or rat, as well as those made on the tissue cultures after administration of radio-protective agents, it appears that (a) the only organelles regularly showing alterations are the mitochondria—these alterations are paralleled to the toxicity of the compound; and (b) an increased number of secondary lysosomes appear during the cell repair phase.

4.3.3. INTERACTION OF RADIOPROTECTIVE AGENTS AND IRRADIATION AT THE ULTRASTRUCTURAL LEVEL

Some cytological alterations produced by radioprotective agents resemble the changes caused by irradiation; therefore it was of interest to study the ultrastructural shape of the cells in protected and irradiated animals.

There have been few investigations on this subject. In the mouse duodenum, irradiated by 1350 r of X-rays and protected by a mixture of radioprotective compounds, the appearance of the lesions was delayed by up to 3–6 hr after the irradiation (Fig. 7). Mitochondrial and ergasto-

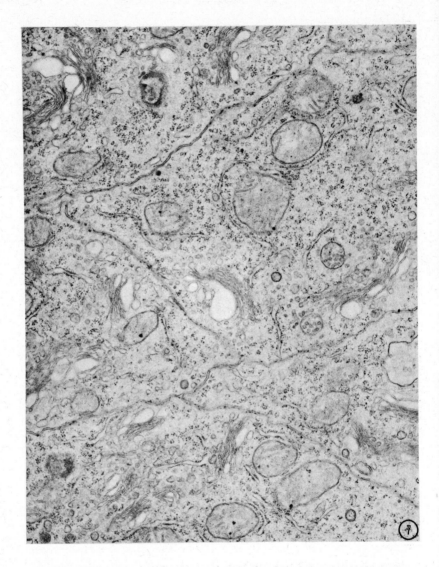

FIG. 7. Undifferentiated cells of the duodenal crypt of the mouse, 6 hr after injection of a radioprotective mixture of AET, 5-HT, and glutathione, and irradiation with 1350 r of X-rays. The cells show a very small number of lesions, slight swelling of the mitochondria with clearing of the matrix, and slight dilatation of the Golgi complex (× 25,000).

plasmic changes initially present in the first few minutes after administration of the single radioprotective agent were absent when the animal was irradiated. Also all the alterations observed in the organelles after irradiation without protection were absent immediately following irradiation. This fact seems important since it demonstrates the activity of the protective agent, which prevents or repairs the mitochondrial lesions due to irradiation. Paradoxically, irradiation lessens the morphological effect of the protective agent on the organelle. However, using organotypic cultures of chicken embryo intestine protected by MEA and irradiated Kirrmann and Cuminge (1965) found that the mitochondrial lesions produced by the protective agent alone were also observed in the irradiated and protected tissues. Masurovsky and Bunge (1969) using cultures irradiated after treatment with 3 mmol AET have verified that the mitochondria, the Golgi complex, and the ergastoplasm are morphologically normal in most of the neurons, even if the same structures are severely damaged in non-protected cell cultures.

Very blurred mitochondrial and cytoplasmic lesions have been observed in the intestinal cells 90 min–6 hr after the administration of the radioprotective agent and the irradiation. By this time, effects peculiar to the radioprotective agent have disappeared. The number of lysosomes, which is greatly increased in non-protected irradiated animals, is apparently unchanged in the protected intestine. Autophagic vacuoles are very rare and late in appearing. After 5 hr the number of ribosomes in the stem cells remain normal; the Golgi complex shows considerable vesicular activity, the vesicles containing a fairly opaque granular material. The content of the autophagic vacuoles may be clearly seen, with little lysis of the organelles they contain. The mitochondrial matrix is dense with intact transverse cristae; many nuclei have a normal structure; dilatations of the nuclear membrane are rare. The acid phosphatase enzyme reaction produces a lead phosphate precipitate, which is localized in the electron-dense bodies and in some smooth membrane profiles. The autophagic vacuoles are still localized in the cytoplasm of the cells, and are not extruded into the intestinal lumen 24 hr after irradiation with protection. Many cells are in mitosis, in spite of the presence of very large cytolysomes; this seems to demonstrate the integrity of their membrane and an absence of hydrolase diffusion into the cytoplasm.

To summarize, ultrastructural observations made on the irradiated intestine of mice, protected by a mixture of sulfhydryl compounds, confirm a delay in the appearance of lesions and their relative unimportance. Morphology and cytochemistry have provided evidence of greater lysosomal resistance to membrane rupture, with maintained localization of the hydrolases in the granules.

4.4.   DISCUSSION

From the electron microscopic observations made following the use of radioprotective compounds, it clearly appears that if these compounds can produce structural alterations at the level of certain cellular organelles, there is no strict correlation between the intensity of the lesion and the degree of radioprotection obtained. However, certain structures are visibly altered by the presence of sulfhydryl protective agents, the mitochondria among these being the most sensitive. Moreover, a review of the literature shows that mitochondrial dilatations can be obtained with a large number of toxic compounds, appearing 12–24 hr after their administration, except in the case of anoxia; in this condition they appear earlier (Green and Purdue, 1966). According to Amoore and Bartley (1958), and Malamed (1965), the mitochondria present a doubly compartmented structure. Their external and peripheral membranes are permeable to sucrose, while their cristae are not. Following osmotic shock, the dilatation would at first result from an unwinding of the cristae, followed by an eventual rupture of the peripheral membrane. The alterations that have been observed after AET or glutathione administration are similar to those observed after osmotic shock or pentachlorophenol.

Complete recovery is, however, seen within several minutes or hours. Weinbach *et al.* (1963) have shown that mitochondria greatly disorganized by immersion in a solution of pentachlorophenol, which inhibits oxidative phosphorylation, recover their normal structures after addition of serum albumin and ATP to the medium. However, the same authors (1967) could not obtain evidence of a correlation between any particular biochemical function and a mitochondrial structure. Nevertheless, the mitochondrial dilatations that have been observed under the electron microscope are very probably associated with changes in function. In fact, an important set of biochemical experiments has shown that cystamine considerably depresses oxygen consumption and oxidative phosphorylation in mitochondria (see Chapter 6).

In addition, Skrede and Bremer (1965) have demonstrated swelling of the mitochondria after incubation in a medium containing cystamine.

These facts support our morphological observations on early mitochondrial alterations following *in vivo* injection of radioprotective compounds. It has, on the other hand, been demonstrated that AET becomes localized in the mitochondria. The experiments of Maisin *et al.* (1963, 1965), after the injection of tritium-labeled AET, confirmed by the electron autoradiographs of Masurovsky and Bunge (1969) after ^{35}S-AET injection, have shown that radioactivity is found in the mitochondria.

Like cystamine, AET would interfere with the sulfhydryl enzyme systems and produce a transient inhibition of oxidative phosphorylation. This lowering of the metabolic activity of the cells can be demonstrated by reversible morphological modifications. The comparative biochemical and electronic studies by Firket and Lelièvre (1966) support this supposition.

Early mitochondrial dilatation is not observed in protected and irradiated individuals (Hugon *et al.*, 1966b). In this case one might think that the AET liberated from its protein linkages would leave the mitochondrial membranes intact. Sulfur-containing radioprotective agents also protect against the damage caused by some radiomimetics. It seems that in this case there is a neutralization of the toxic substance by the protective agent or competition for the same sites (see Chapter 8).

The alterations observed in the dense bodies or lysosomes appear to be of two types, according to whether the animals have or have not been irradiated after the administration of the radioprotective agents. In the latter case the lytic activity of the dense bodies appears to increase slightly with the disappearance of the protective activity. Their number increases and they appear to contain a considerable amount of membrane debris and osmiophilic substance apparently belonging to the phospholipid class. The acid phosphatase content is high and it could be postulated that they intervene in the detoxification of the protective product and participate in its elimination and degradation. This assumption is supported by the experiments of Masurovsky and Bunge (1969) who have observed the presence of labeled AET in the dense bodies during their study of cultured nerve cells.

In the former case, when irradiation follows administration of the protective agent, the lysosomic lability, characteristic of the intestinal cells of an irradiated unprotected animal, is very considerably diminished. The abrupt multiplication of vesicles rich in acid phosphatase followed by their rupture in the large autophagic vesicles is not observed. The absence of hydrolase dispersion after radioprotection must protect the cell against its own autolysis, and permit repair processes.

However, this effect could be due to a reinforcement of the lysosomal membrane or a decreased synthesis of hydrolytic enzymes. This decreased synthesis could be due to a lower metabolic rate induced by the radioprotective agent. Concurrent with the altered characteristics of the lysosomal granules, the number of cytolysosomes is very much decreased.

4.5. CONCLUSIONS

Radioprotective agents have an individual morphological action on cellular organelles and, in protective doses, drastically modify the structures of some of them. As biochemical tests have shown, these alterations are transitory, if the protective dose is given in a single injection. Electron microscopy has permitted the definition of the ultrastructures whose protection after irradiation is increased; these are mitochondria and lysosomes in the cytoplasm, and the nucleolus in the nucleus.

REFERENCES

AMOORE, J. and BARTLEY, W. (1958) The permeability of isolated rat liver mitochondria to sucrose, sodium chloride and potassium chloride at 0°C. *Biochem. J.* **69**: 223–38.

BACQ, Z. (1965) *Chemical Protection against Ionizing Radiation.* Charles C. Thomas, Springfield, U.S.A. 328 p.

BACQ, Z. and HERVE, A. (1949) Cyanure et rayons-X. *J. Physiol.* **41**: 124A-5A.

BRAUN, H. and KOCH, R. (1968) Untersuchungen über einen biologischen Strahlenschutz. 86. Mitteilung. Veränderungen der Mitochondrien nach strahlenschützenden Sulfhydrylkörpern bzw nicht schützenden Homologen. *Strahlentherapie* **135**: 628–31.

CHÈVREMONT, M. (1961) Le mécanisme de l'action antimitotique. *Path. Biol.* **9**: 973–1004.

CHANG, CHUNG-YI and SIMON, E. (1968) The effect of dimethyl sulfoxide (DMSO) on cellular system. *Proc. Soc. Exp. Biol. Med.* **128**: 60–6.

EKER, P. and PIHL, A. (1964) Studies on the growth-inhibiting and radioprotective effect of cystamine, cysteamine and AET on mammalian cells in tissue culture. *Rad. Res.* **21**: 65–79.

FIRKET, H. and LELIÈVRE, P. (1966) Effet de la cystamine sur la respiration, la phosphorylation oxydative et l'ultrastructure des mitochondries du rat. *Int. J. Rad. Biol.* **10**: 403–15.

GOUTIER, R., MAISIN, J. R., LÉONARD, A. and LAMBIET, M. (1966) Influence de la 2-β-aminoéthylisothiourée (AET) sur l'activité mitotique et sur la synthèse du DNA dans le foie de rat en régénération irradié. *Rev. Franç. Et. Clin. Biol.* **11**: 1001–6.

GREEN, D. and PURDUE, J. (1966) Correlation of mitochondrial structure and function. *Ann. N.Y. Acad. Sc.* **137**: 667–84.

HIGHMAN, D., HANSELL, J. and WHITE, D. (1967) Radioprotective effect of dimethylsulfoxide in rats. *Rad. Res.* **30**: 563–8.

HUGON, J. and BORGERS, M. (1966) Lysosomal modifications after administration of radioprotective drugs. *Experientia* **22**: 235–6.

HUGON, J. and BORGERS, M. (1968) Fine structure of the nuclei of the duodenal crypt cells after X-irradiation. *Am. J. Path.* **52**: 707–23.

HUGON, J., MAISIN, J. R. and BORGERS, M. (1964) Effet de l'aminoéthylisothiourée sur les ultrastructures des cryptes duodénales de la souris. *C.R. Soc. Biol.* **158**: 210–13.

HUGON, J., MAISIN, J. R. and BORGERS, M. (1966a) Ultrastructural aspects of duodenal crypts in X-irradiated mice after chemical protection. *Nature* **210**: 749–50.

HUGON, J., MAISIN, J. R. and BORGERS, M. (1966b) Modifications ultrastructurales après radioprotecteurs. *Int. J. Rad. Biol.* **11**: 105–16.

KIRRMANN, J. M. (1967) Protection chimique contre les effets précoces des rayons-X sur l'incorporation de thymidine tritiée ·dans l'intestin embryonnaire de poulet cultivé *in vivo. C.R. Acad. Sc. Paris* **265**: 1419–21.

KIRRMANN, J. M. and CUMINGE, D. (1965) Aspect ultrastructural de la protection exercée par la cystéamine contre les effets précoces des rayons-X sur un organe embryonnaire cultivé *in vivo. C.R. Acad. Sc. Paris* **261**: 567–9.

MAISIN, J. R. and LAMBIET, M. (1967) Influence of a mixture of chemical radioprotectors on the cellular renewal in the duodenum of mice. *Nature* **214**: 412–13.

MAISIN, J. R. and LÉONARD, A. (1963) Etude autoradiographique de la localisation de l'AET dans les tissus de la souris. *C.R. Soc. Biol.* **157**: 203–5.

MAISIN, J. R., NOVELLI, G. D., DOHERTY, D. G. and CONGDON, C. C. (1960) Chemical protection of the alimentary tract of whole-body X-irradiated mice. 1. Changes in weight, histology and cell division in relation to nucleic acid and protein synthesis. *Int. J. Rad. Biol.* **2**: 281–93.

MAISIN, J. R., LÉONARD, A. and HUGON, J. (1965) Tissue and cellular distribution of tritium-labeled AET in mice. *J. Nat. Concer Inst.* **35**: 103–12.

MAISIN, J. R., MATTELIN, G., FRIDMAN-MANDUZIO, A. and VAN DER PARREN, J. (1968) Reduction of short- and long-term radiation lethality by mixtures of chemical protectors. *Rad. Res.* **35**: 26–44.

MALAMED, S. (1965) Structural changes during swelling of isolated rat mitochondria. *Z. Zellforsch.* **65**: 10–15.

MASUROVSKY, E. B. and BUNGE, R. P. (1969) Radiation protection in mammalian spinal ganglion cultures treated with AET derivatives. Light and electron-microscopic auto-radiographic studies. *Acta Radiol. (Ther. Phys. Biol.)* **8**: 38–54.

PATT, H., TYREE, E., STRAUBE, R. and SMITH, D. (1949) Cysteine protection against X-irradiation. *Science* **110**: 213.

PETERS, K. (1963) Zur Frage der Wirksamkeit von Strahlenschutzsubstanzen in Gewebe Kulturen. *Strahlentherapie* **121**: 599–604.

SKREDE, S. and BREMER, J. (1965) The effect of disulphides on mitochondrial oxidations. *Biochem. J.* **95**: 838–46.

THERKELSEN, A. (1958) Studies in the cytotoxicity of cysteamine and related compounds in tissue culture. *Acta Path. Microbiol. Scand.* **92**: 201–15.

UENO, Y. and YAMANO, K. (1960) Electron microscopic studies on hepatic cells after the administration of glutathione mixtures. *Experientia* **25**: 60.

WEINBACH, E., SHEFFIELD, H. and GARBUS, J. (1963) Restoration of oxidative phosphoryla-tion and morphological integrity to swollen uncoupled rat liver mitochondria. *Proc. Nat. Acad. Sc.* **50**: 561–8.

WEINBACH, E., GARBUS, J. and SHEFFIELD, H. (1967) Morphology of the mitochondria in the coupled, uncoupled and recoupled states. *Exp. Cell. Res.* **46**: 129–43.

CHAPTER 5

DISTRIBUTION, METABOLISM, AND EXCRETION

P. Lelièvre (*Liège*), J. R. Maisin (*Mol*), and Z. M. Bacq (*Liège*)

Belgium

5.1. INTRODUCTION

It is outside the scope of this section of the *Encyclopedia* to discuss the metabolism, distribution, and excretion of such substances as cysteine or glutathione, which are normal constituents of all living organisms. But radiobiologists have used them at such high "pharmacological" doses (0.1% of the weight of rats or mice) that the normal mechanisms which regulate the fate of these substances in the body are completely saturated. Thus we must deal in this chapter with these high doses of normal substances. The metabolism, distribution, and excretion of large doses (generally the maximal tolerated dose) of the more powerful protective agents are much better known than those of small quantities. The reader should understand that the majority of the experimental studies discussed in this chapter have been undertaken essentially in order to discover the chemical nature, localization, and metabolites of the protective agents at the time of exposure to ionizing radiation. This knowledge is needed for an understanding of the mechanisms by which these substances decrease the effects of ionizing radiation (see Chapter 1) or radiomimetic chemicals (see Chapter 8).

A number of reactions common to all —SH or S—S containing protective compounds must be explained before presenting the data pertaining to each series.

5.2. GENERAL REACTIONS IN MODEL AND BIOLOGICAL SYSTEMS

5.2.1. "SPONTANEOUS" OXIDATION OF THIOLS

In vitro or *in vivo,* in biological fluids, the thiols are oxidized more or less rapidly to the disulfide in the presence of molecular oxygen. This reaction is accelerated by an alkaline pH and traces of metals like iron, copper, or manganese. At acid pH solutions of pure cysteine in pure water are quite stable. In order to prevent the oxidation of a thiol [for instance cysteamine (MEA)] the best technique is to add to the solution some thiolated Sephadex which will reduce the —SS— bridges as soon as they occur.

The reactivity of thiols increases with increasing pH, because for alkaline pH they exist as RS^- in aqueous solution which is the active form for many reactions, particularly alkylation. The chemical reactivity of SH substances also depends critically on the pK of the dissociation constant $R-SH \rightleftharpoons RS^- + H^+$. If it is high as in thioglycollic acid or mercaptoethanol, the thiols have low reactivity at physiological pH. The presence of a NH_2 group on the beta carbon atom (as in cysteine and MEA) lowers the pK (8.35 for MEA). The hydrogen of the thiol can be easily substituted, but a clear distinction must be made between the reactions in which it is the $R-SH$ form which reacts by hydrogen transfer* and those which are only concerned with the RS^- form, for instance alkylation by mustards or iodoacetate, because these agents are electrophilic; in alkylation the pK_a is important because it determines the fraction of the thiol which is in RS^- form under physiological conditions. The reaction of a thiol with a mustard [nitrogen or sulfur mustard, $R-N$ $(CH_2-CH_2Cl)_2$] to form $R-N (CH_2-CH_2-SR)_2$ is irreversible; the reaction product is catabolized and excreted in various forms. The —SH functions are not regenerated, as they may be after oxidation to disulfide, reaction with a metal, or an arsenoxide. Full detoxication occurs only when the organism has synthesized new —SH substances; restoration depends on the turnover of these substances.

The oxidation of $R-SH$ may be carried further than the disulfide, to the sulfoxide (SO), sulfone (SO_2), and finally the sulfate SO_4^{2-} which is

---

* This kind of reaction is the basis of the activity of CoA; there are other cases of physiological —SH substances functioning as specific coenzymes (for instance, reduced glutathione (GSH) for methylglyoxalase).

the final metabolite. As soon as the S—O stage is reached, the reaction in mammals is irreversible.

5.2.2. MIXED DISULFIDE FORMATION; REDUCTION OF SYMMETRICAL DISULFIDES

The property of certain thiols to form mixed disulfides when put in contact with reactive S—S groups (of proteins, peptides, or even the amino acid cystine), considered by Eldjarn and his associates as one of the reasons for their radioprotective effect, may now be regarded as fundamental,and of physiological significance. Similarly, certain disulfides form mixed disulfides by reaction with certain —SH groups of protides. If R represents a protide and X—SH or X—S—S—X the reduced or disulfide form of a chemical protective agent, the reactions may be expressed very simply in the following way:

$$R—S—S—R + X—SH \longrightarrow R—S—S—X + R—SH$$
$$R—SH + X—S—S—X \longrightarrow R—S—S—X + X—SH$$

(see also Fig. 1). Pihl and Eldjarn (1957) have shown, by using labeled

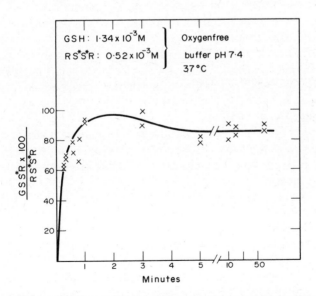

FIG. 1. Rate and extent of formation of the mixed disulfide GSS*R. Glutathione (GSH) and ³⁵S-cystamine (RS*S*R) were incubated for varying lengths of time in phosphate buffer and the mixed disulfide separated by paper electrophoresis. (Pihl and Eldjarn, 1957.)

substances, that the reaction proceeds (as, for example, in the case of cystamine and GSH) according to the equations:

$$GSH + XS^*S^*X \rightleftharpoons GSS^*X + XS^*H \tag{1}$$
$$GSS^*X + GSH \rightleftharpoons GSSG + XS^*H \tag{2}$$

Similarly in the case of a mixed disulfide exchange between protein S—S groups and MEA, the reaction proceeds in the following way:

$$\boxed{Prot}{-S \atop -S} + XS^*H \rightleftharpoons \boxed{Prot}{-SH \atop -SS^*X} \tag{3}$$

$$\boxed{Prot}{-SH \atop -SS^*X} + XS^*H \rightleftharpoons \boxed{Prot}{-SH \atop -SH} + XS^*S^*X \tag{4}$$

When these thiols or disulfides endowed with radioprotective activity are injected into a mammal, they come into contact with a great variety of —SH and S—S groups of proteins and peptides. The usual chemical techniques do not indicate the nature of the protein or the localization of the interested function in the binding molecule. It is usual only to speak of and titrate soluble —SH and S—S, or protein bound —SH or S—S. According to its position in a protein, an SH group or an S—S bridge may have very different chemical affinities and physiological significance. It is not known whether mixed disulfides normally exist in certain cells or what function they might have.

Not all thiols or disulfides are capable of forming mixed disulfides. After testing a large series of compounds, Eldjarn and Pihl (1956, 1960) concluded that only the radioprotective thiols or disulfides do form mixed disulfides (see Table 1). The importance of this fact is discussed in the last chapter of this section.

The rapid non-enzymic mixed disulfide formation is the first step in the reduction (and partial detoxication) of many disulfides and in particular those (cystamine, guanidoethyl disulfide) connected with radioprotective action.

Nesbakken (1963) has shown that in the presence of a large excess of GSH the S—S bridge of the mixed disulfide is broken, with formation of oxidized glutathione (GSSG) and MEA according to eqn. (2). In the presence of glutathione reductase and NADPH, the oxidized glutathione (GSSG) is reduced to GSH. There reactions are limited by the availability of NADPH; when the stock is exhausted, disulfides can no longer be reduced and disulfide poisoning occurs.

This mechanism of disulfide reduction postulates that the disulfide penetrates inside the cell; both GSH and glutathione reductase are intracellular. Cystine and GSSG cannot cross the membrane of erythro-

TABLE 1. Protective or Sensitizing Action *in vivo* of Various Thiols and Their Ability to Form Mixed Disulfides with Glutathione and Cystine (Eldjarn and Pihl, 1960)

Compound	Extent of mixed disulfide formation with CSSC and GSSG	Rate of mixed disulfide formation with CSSC and GSSG[a]
Protective thiols		
Cysteine	Extensive	Fast (2–3 min)
Homocysteine	Extensive	Fast (3–5 min)
Cysteamine (MEA)	Extensive	Fast (1–2 min)
Aminoethylisothiouronium bromide HBr (AET)	Extensive	Fast (2–3 min)
N-Methylcysteamine	Extensive	Fast (2–3 min)
N-Dimethylcysteamine	Extensive	Fast (2–3 min)
N-Diethylcysteamine	Extensive	Fast (2–3 min)
N-Morpholylcysteamine	Extensive	Fast (2–3 min)
N-Acetylcysteamine[b]	Extensive	Slow (10–15 min)
Glutathione	Extensive	Slow (10–15 min)
Aletheine[b]	Extensive	Slow (15–20 min)
Cysteine ethyl ester	Extensive	Fast (1–2 min)
2,3-Dimercaptopropanol[b]	Moderate	Slow (15–20 min)
Sensitizing thiols		
Thioethanol	Extensive	Slow (10–15 min)
Penicillamine	Extensive	Slow (12–17 min)
Inactive thiols		
Di-N-butylcysteamine[c]	Extensive	Fast (3–5 min)
Thioglycolic acid	Extensive	Slow (15–20 min)
Thiocholine	Slight	Fast ($\frac{1}{2}$–1 min)
N-Piperidylcysteamine[c]	Extensive	Moderate (4–6 min)
N-Benzylcysteamine[c]	Extensive	Moderate (4–6 min)
1-Amino-7-mercaptoheptane	Moderate	Slow (40–60 min)
Thioctic acid	Traces	Slow (15–30 min)
Dithiopentaerythrit	Traces	Slow (10–15 min)
o-Aminothiophenol	None	No interaction
Thiophenol	None	No interaction
2,4-Dinitrothiophenol	None	No interaction
4,6-Dimethyl-2-mercaptopyrimidine	None	No interaction
2-Mercaptothiazoline	None	No interaction
Thiolhistidine	None	No interaction
Ergothioneine	None	No interaction
Thioacetamide	None	No interaction
Thiocyanide	None	No interaction

[a] The figures in parentheses give the time needed to reach equilibrium.
[b] Doubtful protective effect.
[c] Protective action tested only with very low doses on account of the toxicity.

cytes and are not reduced by blood *in vitro* (Eldjarn *et al.*, 1962). This inability to penetrate the membrane is probably the reason why cystamine is not reduced *in vitro* by rabbit's blood (Fischer and Goutier-Pirotte. 1954) although it is reduced in the same conditions by the red cells of man and rat as well as by slices of kidney or brain (Pihl *et al.*, 1957). Mammalian cell cultures are not protected by cystamine which apparently does not cross the membrane. When injected either intravenously (i.v.) or into the peritoneal cavity (i.p.) of mammals (man, dog, rabbit, or rat) cystamine is rapidly converted to MEA (Bacq *et al.*, 1952; Fischer and Goutier-Pirotte, 1954; Mundy *et al.*, 1961; Heiffer *et al.*, 1962).

According to Eldjarn and Bremer (1963), isolated rat liver mitochondria reduce cystamine in the presence of an intermediate of the Krebs cycle (α-ketoglutarate for instance) in conditions where GSSG is not reduced. This reduction is not due to glutathione reductase because it does not occur in mitochondria. The electron donor in this system is thioctic acid. This acid in reduced form, at the aldehyde state of oxidation, is reoxidized by electron transfer to protein SS. The disulfides added to the medium are reduced by spontaneous exchange with the protein SH generated in this way (Fluharty and Sanadi, 1960).

Despite its rapid reduction, cystamine is not metabolized and excreted in exactly the same manner as MEA. For instance, the percentage of MEA oxidized to taurine is much greater than that of cystamine (Eldjarn, 1954). Cystamine (not MEA) is a substrate for diamine oxidase. Furthermore the injected doses of this disulfide are so great that a large fraction "overflows" and is excreted as such by the kidney, before the enzymatic processes in the body have had time to reduce the excess disulfide (Fischer and Goutier-Pirotte, 1954; Mundy *et al.*, 1961).

5.2.3. OTHER GENERAL REACTIONS

Mercaptoamines react with pyridoxal-5-phosphate (Vitamin B_6) which has been found to be highly radiosensitive (Nakken, 1960). Langendorff and his associates have published many facts in favor of the idea that the lack of pyridoxal-5-phosphate plays an important rôle in the biochemical aspects of radiation sickness.

Both MEA and cysteine react with the carbonyl group of, for instance, glyceraldehyde, methylglyoxal, dihydroxyacetone, or α-ketoglutaric acid (Pihl and Eldjarn, 1957). Cysteine reacts stoichiometrically with streptomycin, but not with dihydrostreptomycin which has no carbonyl group (Eldjarn *et al.*, 1957).

Thiols in radiochemistry are known as good "scavengers" of free OH radicals in dilute aqueous systems; they react with many organic radicals produced by either direct or indirect action. They can also act as energy transfer agents in systems where direct action of ionizing radiation predominates:

$$XSH + OH^\bullet \longrightarrow XS^\bullet + H_2O$$
$$R^\bullet + XSH \longrightarrow RH + X\dot{S}^\bullet$$

5.3. DISTRIBUTION AMONG ORGANS; CHANGES WITH TIME

5.3.1. CYSTEAMINE AND CYSTAMINE

5.3.1.1. *Non-isotopic Methods*

Lelièvre (1959) has elaborated a method which allows accurate estimation of MEA and cystamine* in complex biological systems (blood, homogenates) in the presence of —SH substances like cysteine or glutathione. With this method it is possible to determine the concentration of the protective agent in a given organ at any time after injection both in its protein-bound and free forms. The results obtained in the rat after i.p. injection of 100 mg/kg of cystamine are given in Table 2. It appears that in most tissues, with the exception of the testis, cystamine is massively bound to proteins a few minutes after injection; this confirms the importance *in vivo* of the mixed disulfide formation according to Eldjarn and Pihl. It is also perfectly logical and expected that the concentration of this bound form decreases regularly and rapidly following a course familiar to pharmacologists. But the striking feature is the slow increase in the free form which reaches a maximum in 30–45 min and clearly surpasses the concentration of the bound form. This fact is not clearly understood. The secondary liberation of the amine is logical, but the reason why it does not bind again to available S—S groups has not been explained.

Organs, like bone-marrow and spleen, which are particularly radiosensitive, concentrate more cystamine. The testis behaves differently; very little cystamine is combined with protein and it disappears rapidly.

5.3.1.2. *Isotopic Methods*
Biochemical techniques

Fundamental and well-conducted experiments have been performed by Verly and associates in 1954 and 1955. A pure (from radiological and chemical points of view) preparation of ^{35}S-MEA was injected i.p.

* The method does not allow separation of the reduced from the S—S form.

TABLE 2. DISTRIBUTION OF CYSTAMINE IN VARIOUS ORGANS OF THE RAT AT VARIOUS TIMES AFTER I.P. INJECTION OF 100 MG/KG OF CYSTAMINE. RESULTS ARE EXPRESSED IN MCG OF CYSTAMINE PER G OF FRESH TISSUE. B, BOUND FORM; F, FREE FORM; T, TOTAL (Lelièvre, 1961)

Time (min)	Blood			Spleen			Thymus			Bone-marrow			Testis		
	B	F	T	B	F	T	B	F	T	B	F	T	B	F	T
2	99	4	103	163	3	166	166	0	166	362	11	373	28	47	75
5	69	8	77	151	10	161	91	4	95	177	30	207	10	52	62
10	54	11	65	121	19	140	70	15	85	130	49	179	4	51	55
20	34	19	53	81	48	129	49	41	90	70	85	155	1	19	20
30	19	33	52	40	51	91	31	49	89	45	101	146	0	14	14
45	9	34	43	24	42	66	16	35	51	28	96	124	0	9	9

...

into mice with enough carrier to reach the usual radioprotective dose of 150 mg/kg. The radioactivity was measured in various organs and the whole carcass: (a) ^{35}S still attached to the original molecule (or to cystamine), (b) total ^{35}S after oxidation to SO_4^{2-}. Table 3 and Figs. 2 and 3 show that degradation and excretion are very rapid. Fifteen minutes after the injection, a large part of the radioactivity remains attached to the original molecule, but after $2\frac{1}{2}$ hr only 20 % of the administered dose is still in the form of MEA. Metabolites are retained longer and about

TABLE 3. TOTAL ^{35}S ACTIVITY IN DIFFERENT TISSUES AFTER I.P. INJECTION OF CYSTEAMINE (3.14 mg/20 g MOUSE (Verly *et al.*, 1954a)

	Radioactivity as counts/min/g of tissue $\times 10^{-5}$						
Time after injection	15 min		1 hr		6 hr	24 hr	
Mouse (No.)	1	2	3	4	5	6	7
Blood	1.14	1.11	0.69	0.69	0.18	0.14	0.15
Liver	5.10	4.55	4.38	4.34	5.60	2.86	3.54
Intestine + pancreas	3.78	2.98	2.22	3.04	2.55	3.24	3.46
Kidney	5.37	6.08	4.00	3.31	1.47	1.73	2.05
Brain	1.81	1.55	1.57	1.83	0.27	0.30	0.31
Remainder	1.94	1.63	1.44	1.63	0.80	0.80	0.63

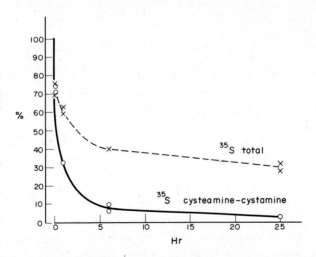

FIG. 2. Remaining radioactivity in the whole mouse at various times after i.p. injection of 150 mg/kg of ^{35}S-MEA (Verly *et al.*, 1954b).

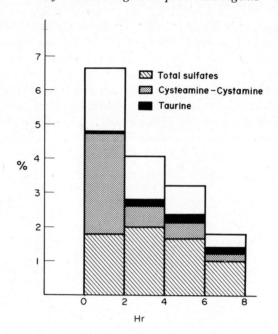

FIG. 3. Distribution of radioactivity in the urine of a dog after i.v. injection of 15 mg/kg of ^{35}S-MEA (Verly and Koch, 1954). The radioactivity is expressed in per cent of the injected radioactivity: the white space indicates unidentified tagged metabolites.

34% of ^{35}S is still present in the body after 24 hr, although radioactive MEA can no longer be detected in significant amounts (Verly *et al.*, 1954a). A large part of the MEA injected is excreted unaltered in the urine. Radioactivity is high in the kidney (on its way to excretion) and in the liver, where the amine is actively metabolized.

Labeled cystamine administered by gastric catheter to mice is not more concentrated in the liver at 15 or 60 min than after i.p. injection of an equal dose; in fact the concentration is smaller at 15 min because 20% of the amine is still in the stomach. Also the concentration of metabolites (taurine, SO_4^{2-}, total ^{35}S) in liver is not increased by oral administration (Verly, 1955). For studies on radiation protection, doses administered orally are about 5 times higher than by i.p. injection (see Chapter 2).

Eldjarn and Pihl (1956) showed that after i.p. injection of a radioprotective dose of labeled MEA or cystamine to mice a significant amount of radioactivity is bound to plasma proteins and hemoglobin as mixed

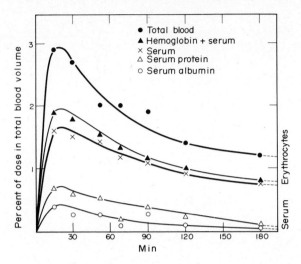

FIG. 4. The [35]SH distribution among certain blood fractions at various times after i.p. administration of 2.3 mg of ^{35}S-cystamine to a mouse weighing 28 mg. (Eldjarn and Pihl, 1956.)

disulfides (Fig. 4). During the period of maximal protection against irradiation very little free protective agent is found in the blood.

When a small non-protective dose (30 mg/kg) was injected subcutaneously into rats, the distribution of radioactivity in the tissues differed from that observed by Verly *et al.*, in particular the concentration in the liver was not as high (Eldjarn and Nygaard, 1954). Table 4 also shows that the thyroid is rather active and that radiosensitive tissues like the spleen and bone-marrow concentrate the amine. Gensicke *et al.* (1962) report that i.p. injected ^{35}S-cystamine is taken up to a large extent by the kidney, the liver, the skeleton (presumably including bone-marrow), and the intestinal tract within 15 min; the authors believe that the peritoneum itself may retain some of the i.p. injected substance. After 15 min the concentration of [35]S (mostly still attached to the original cystamine molecule) is highest in the kidney followed in decreasing order by pancreas > liver > lung > blood > testis > muscle. Arbusow *et al.* (1959) have followed the ^{35}S activity in the central nervous system, various organs, urine, and feces in the rat during 24 hr following injection of ^{35}S-MEA (100 mg/kg) in normal rats or rats irradiated 30 min after the injection. The ^{35}S activity is smaller for all organs (except for gastrointestinal tract) in irradiated animals at all times. Cysteamine penetrates easily to all

TABLE 4. RADIOACTIVITY IN SS ± SH AND TOTAL SULFUR FRACTIONS OF VARIOUS RAT ORGANS 30 MIN AFTER SUBCUTANEOUS INJECTION OF ^{35}S-CYSTAMINE OR ^{35}S-MEA. THE ACTIVITIES ARE EXPRESSED RELATIVE TO THAT OF SERUM SS ± SH AND PER G OF TISSUE (Eldjarn and Nygaard, 1954)

Compound administered	Cystamine				MEA			
Fraction analyzed for radioactivity	SS + SH		Total S		SS + SH		Total S	
Experiment No.	I	II	I	II	III	IV	III	IV
Thyroid	2.5	2.5	3.2	3.6	—	7.9	5.8	8.0
Kidneys	1.9	3.3	6.4	6.9	0.4	—	6.6	—
Bone-marrow	1.2	2.6	2.9	3.3	(5.2)	(3.9)	3.8	3.3
Adrenals	0.8	1.5	2.7	3.0	—	3.3	6.1	6.3
Spleen	1.6	1.2	4.3	3.2	0.8	—	5.0	—
Serum	1.0	1.0	1.4	1.8	1.0	1.0	1.6	1.1
Lungs	0.5	1.2	2.4	2.6	0.4	—	3.4	—
Colon	—	—	—	—	0.7	—	2.5	—
Small intestine	—	—	—	—	0.3	—	3.9	—
Heart	0.4	0.5	2.1	2.2	—	—	—	—
Brain	0.3	0.7	0.9	1.3	0.3	—	0.9	—
Skeletal muscle	0.2	0.3	0.7	0.7	—	—	—	—
Epididymis	0.1	0.2	0.7	0.7	—	—	—	—
Liver	0.2	0.7	8.8	4.8	0.1	0.2	3.4	3.1
Testes	0.02	0.2	0.4	0.6	0.06	—	0.6	—

parts of the central nervous system, if one considers the data for 30 min after injection, and may be five times more concentrated than in blood.

It is very difficult to interpret the data of Arbusow *et al.* (1959) giving ^{35}S activity from 1½ to 24 hr after injection because most of this activity is linked with metabolites (sulfate, taurine, etc.); nevertheless, it is certain that the ^{35}S activity does not change in the same way in irradiated and non-irradiated rats.

Figure 5 summarizes the observations of Lauber *et al.* (1958) concerning *total* radioactivity in various organs at various times, after injection in mice, of a moderate dose of ^{35}S-MEA. Concentration in liver, kidney and spleen is confirmed (see also Lauber *et al.*, 1960).

In vivo distribution and metabolism of MEA-*S*-phosphate (MEAP) has been studied in mice. The tissues contained mainly MEA–cystamine, some protein-bound MEA, and some MEAP at 20 min, the time of maximum protection. At 30 min when little MEAP was present in the

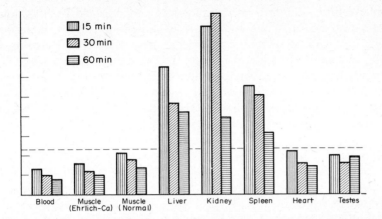

FIG. 5. Total ^{35}S activity in various organs after i.p. injection of a single dose of ^{35}S-cystamine (75 mg/kg) to mice with intramuscular inoculated Ehrlich ascites tumor. The dashed line indicates the theoretical average ^{35}S activity if the injected MEA had been evenly distributed throughout the body. The activity per gram of wet tissue is expressed in arbitrary units, the total ^{35}S activity of the blood after 30 min being taken as unity. (Lauber *et al.*, 1958.)

tissues the animals were still protected. These results indicate that protection is due to the dephosphorylation of MEAP and generation of MEA–cystamine in the tissues. Thus the advantages of MEAP are: (1) the temporary masking of the thiol group before the agent reaches the tissues, and (2) the generation of the protective form at the critical site (Shapiro *et al.*, 1970).

Autoradiography

1. Nelson and Ullberg (1960), using their technique of autoradiography of whole body slices, observed very high activity in the pituitary, salivary, and lacrimal glands, and eye and liver, when the mouse was killed 20 min after injection of 61 mg/kg of ^{35}S-MEA; the epididymis, spleen, thymus, lymph glands, gastric and intestinal mucosa as well as kidneys, adrenals, skin, arterial walls, and bone-marrow were also labeled. If the animal is killed after a delay of 1 hr (i.e. when most of the MEA is already metabolized) the activity in blood and salivary glands has decreased, but the liver, spleen, and gastrointestinal tract are still well labeled; in fetuses the bones and liver are particularly active.

2. Firket *et al.* (1963) estimated by autoradiography the density of silver grains in 21 tissues of the young adult rat from 5 to 60 min after i.p. injection of ^{35}S-cystamine or MEA (100 mg/kg). Their findings were

similar to those obtained with aminoethylisothiourea (AET). Maximum labeling is reached 10 min after i.p. injection, but apparently diminishes more slowly after cystamine injection than after AET. The testis contains little labeling. Organs like the lungs, the gastrointestinal tract, and the adrenals, however, are well labeled after the administration of cystamine. The skin, which is poorly protected against epilation, at least in young mice, contains a large amount of label after i.p. injection of MEA; it is poorly labeled after injection of cystamine which is a good protective agent. It is hazardous to draw conclusions from these observations on the skin because they show only the protein- (or structure-) bound amine; the free protective agent is lost during the preparation of the sections; as discussed in Chapter 9, the active form for protection against ionizing radiation is not necessarily the protein-bound form. ^{35}S-MEA accumulates to a significant extent in rabbit's spermatozoa (Nuzhdin and Nizhnik, 1965).

5.3.2. AMINOETHYLISOTHIOUREA AND RELATED SUBSTANCES

5.3.2.1. *Ingestion versus Injection*

Practically all the studies concerning the distribution of AET (or more correctly, of its transguanylation product mercaptoethylguanidine MEG) and its disulfide guanidoethyl disulfide (GED) have been carried with either ^{35}S or tritium labeled substances. Ingested MEG is absorbed more rapidly than GED, and gives higher tissue levels after 30 min. This explains the more effective radioprotective action from ingestion of MEG rather than GED. However, 30 min after oral administration of MEG or GED, a significant amount of protective agent still remains in the gastrointestinal tract. This accounts for certain differences between the oral and i.p. administration with respect to $LD_{50/30}$ values after an equal dose of protective agents (Maisin and Léonard, 1963).

Kollmann *et al.* (1963) found that the liver of animals acquires a concentration of three times more GED when given by stomach tube than that given by i.p. injection. On the other hand, bone-marrow and spleen contain twice the amount of protective agent in the latter case, although the degree of radioprotective action determined from $LD_{50/30}$ days after i.p. or stomach tube administration is the same. When ^{3}H-AET is given orally, maximal labeling is seen in the gastrointestinal tract during the initial 30 min.

5.3.2.2. Chemical Techniques

After i.p. injection of ^{35}S-AET Rusanov (1961) also found irregular distribution of radioactivity in the organs. Immediately after administration, the concentration of the substance was highest in the heart, kidneys, and small intestine and lowest in the lungs and liver. Very small amounts of AET were found in the spleen, brain and skin. Labeling decreased rapidly, 15–30 min after administration, in the heart and increased in the kidneys, liver and small intestine. Three hours after administration, all the organs examined showed a decrease in radioactivity.

Bradford *et al.* (1961) reported on the tissue distribution of ^{35}S activity in mice after injection of ^{35}S MEG; unfortunately the dose injected was low, much below the radioprotective dose, and the time between injection and killing was too long (45 min). It is not surprising to find small concentrations of ^{35}S in the liver and kidney, even smaller than in the bone-marrow, spleen, or intestinal mucosa; this happens when non-protective doses are injected; similar observations have been made with MEA. As far as the intracellular distribution is concerned, the same difficulty of interpretation as in the case of the experiments of Mondovi *et al.* (1962) can be raised: the technique of homogenization for subsequent separation of the various fractions requires dilution which shifts the equilibrium between free and bound —SH protective agents in favor of the free form. This dilution effect is well shown by the following fact: when 27 mg/kg of MEG is injected, the ratio of nuclei/soluble in mouse liver homogenate is about 1/4; when ten times more MEG is injected (a really protective dose) the ratio is about 1/1. Several types of bound ^{35}S activity could be separated by various techniques (dialysis with various solvents, denaturants, oxidizing and reducing agents, etc.) (Bradford *et al.*, 1961).

The technique used by Shapiro *et al.* (1962, 1963b, c) involves homogenization of the organs of mice with a very small amount of ice-cold water, in such a way that there is little dilution and consequently the equilibrium between free and bound forms will be almost undisturbed. Labeled MEG or GED is injected in radioprotective doses; the various forms containing ^{35}S activity are separated by paper chromatography and electrophoresis. The following species were identified and titrated: protein bound ^{35}S, GED, taurocyamine, guanidoethanesulfinic acid, S-acetyl-2-mercaptoethylguanidine and sulfate. Mercaptoethylguanidine is not found in the tissues, but constitutes the major excretory product, even when pure GED is injected; the disulfide GED is reduced in the body to the —SH compound MEG just as cystamine is converted to MEA. Twenty minutes after injection of MEG or GED, the radioactivity

TABLE 5. CONCENTRATION OF S-AET IN PROTEIN BOUND (P.B.) AND FREE GED FORM
CHROMATOGRAPHICALLY SEPARATED IN TISSUE HOMOGENATES OF MAMMARY
ADENOCARCINOMA-BEARING MICE 20 MIN AFTER 140 OR 280 MG/KG I.P.
INJECTION OF MEG AND 20 OR 120 MIN AFTER 140 MG/KG I.P. INJECTION OF GED
(Shapiro, Schwarz and Kollmann, 1963b)

Organ	Injected form	Dose (mg/kg)	Time (min)	P.B. dry weight (mcg/mg)	GED dry weight (mcg/mg)
Spleen	MEG	280	20	0.045	0.031
	MEG	140	20	0.023	0.016
	GED	140	20	0.047	0.029
	GED	140	120	0.024	—
Small intestine	MEG	280	20	0.090	0.072
	MEG	140	20	0.066	0.055
	GED	140	20	0.064	0.051
	GED	140	120	0.047	0.057
Liver	MEG	280	20	0.121	0.072
	MEG	140	20	0.074	0.052
	GED	140	20	0.048	0.032
	GED	140	120	0.016	0.022
Kidney	MEG	280	20	0.257	0.186
	MEG	140	20	0.102	0.086
	GED	140	20	0.141	0.092
	GED	140	120	0.046	0.044
Carcass	MEG	280	20	0.045	0.015
	MEG	140	20	0.031	0.006
	GED	140	20	0.032	0.016
	GED	140	120	0.018	0.005
Testes	MEG	280	20	0.035	0.012
	MEG	140	20	0.027	0.008
	GED	140	20	0.024	0.010
	GED	140	120	0.016	0.005
Tumor	MEG	280	20	0.026	0.010
	MEG	140	20	0.023	0.008
	GED	140	20	0.027	0.014
	GED	140	120	0.025	0.008
Serum[a]	MEG	280	20	13.97	4.65
	MEG	140	20	6.72	—
	GED	140	20	15.00	2.80
	GED	140	120	2.80	—

[a] Serum concentrations are given in mcg/ml.

TABLE 6. CONCENTRATION OF S-AET IN CHEMICAL FORMS CHROMATOGRAPHICALLY SEPARATED IN BONE-MARROW SUSPENSIONS (Shapiro *et al.*, 1963c)

Group[a]	P.B. (mcg/mg)	GED (mcg/mg)	RSO_2H (mcg/mg)	SO_4 (mcg/mg)	X (mcg/mg)
A	0.067	0.043	—	—	0.047
B	0.026	0.012	0.006	—	0.014
C	0.081	0.040	—	—	0.028
D	0.015	0.013	—	—	0.037
E	0.019	0.011	0.010	0.009	0.026

[a] The specimens were removed from groups of mice:
Group A : 20 min after 280 mg/kg of MEG.
Group B : 20 min after 140 mg/kg of MEG.
Group C : 20 min after 140 mg/kg of GED.
Group D : 60 min after 140 mg/kg of GED.
Group E : 120 min after 140 mg/kg of GED.

TABLE 7. CONCENTRATION OF S-AET IN THE CHEMICAL FORMS CHROMATOGRAPHICALLY SEPARATED IN SPLEEN HOMOGENATES (Shapiro *et al.*, 1963c)

Group[a]	P.B. (mcg/mg)	GED (mcg/mg)	RSO_2H (mcg/mg)	RSO_3H (mcg/mg)	X (mcg/mg)
A	0.100	0.057	0.028	0.012	0.056
B	0.056	0.024	0.008	—	0.028
C	0.055	0.021	0.006	0.007	0.022
D	0.037	0.012	0.009	—	0.052
E	0.015	—	0.010	—	0.031

[a] The specimens were removed from groups of mice:
Group A : 20 min after 280 mg/kg of MEG.
Group B : 20 min after 140 mg/kg of MEG.
Group C : 20 min after 140 mg/kg of GED.
Group D : 60 min after 140 mg/kg of GED.
Group E : 120 min after 140 mg/kg of GED.

(mainly protein-bound) is greater in the kidney > liver > intestine > spleen > bone-marrow > carcass than in serum; the proportion of protein-bound ^{35}S (which is nearly always the highest, even after 2 hr) to free GED and other radioactive metabolites varies with time, and from one organ to another (Tables 5, 6 and 7). The protective agent appears to be linked to proteins by a mixed disulfide, a thioester, and by a third, so far unidentified, bond which has no importance in protective action since it is present 2 hr after injection, at a time when protective action has faded away. The cautious conclusion of Shapiro *et al.* (1963b) is that the protective form of AET in the animal is either GED itself or protein-bound S-AET or both. Although radioprotective action is about the same in animals receiving 140 mg/kg of MEG or of GED, the concentration of protein-bound ^{35}S is greater after injection of MEG than after the equivalent amount of GED. This might be due to the fact that MEG crosses vascular and cell membranes more easily than GED.

According to Shigetoshi (1964), after injection of ^{35}S-MEG, in mice, peak activities are reached, within 5 min, in the blood, liver, and spleen; at 10 min in the kidney; at 20 min in the small intestine, lung, and thymus; and at 30 min in the bone-marrow. The gastrointestinal tract and the brain are more extensively labeled than the lymph nodes, bone-marrow, spleen, and testes. Free-^{35}S and bound-^{35}S activities in tissues correspond to the total ^{35}S.

Yarmonenko *et al.* (1965) reported maximal activities in the blood and liver $2\frac{1}{2}$ min after i.p. injection of AET in mice. Later (after 30 min), activity decreases in these organs whereas it still increases in the brain.

5.3.2.3.   *Autoradiographic Studies*

Five minutes after administration of 5.8 mg of AET (Cl, HCl) labeled with tritium on the methylene carbon, all tissues in the mouse are labeled as shown by autoradiography, but the intensity of labeling varies widely. Most radioactivity is found in the kidney, liver, heart, and digestive tract. The radioactivity is lower in the epididymis, the pancreas, brain, spleen, bone-marrow, lymph-glands, and in the lungs, and still lower in the testes, ovaries, striated muscle, and bone (Maisin and Léonard, 1963).

It is not surprising that the highest concentrations of radioactivity occur in the kidney and liver since AET is eliminated preferentially by the kidney and is metabolized by the liver. The administration of a non-toxic dose of AET (175 mg/kg) to normal laparatomized rats becomes highly toxic when a part of the liver is removed 10 min before or after administration of the compound (Maisin *et al.*, 1965). A detailed examination of the kidney demonstrates that after injection of labeled AET, labeling of the cortex and medulla of the kidney is about the same during the first 30 min. Later, the medulla is more strongly labeled than the cortex. In the liver, the bile ducts contain less activity than the blood vessels or the cells of the parenchyma. The gastric and small intestine mucosae are labeled more intensively than the mucosa of the colon. Throughout the intestinal tract, the mucus in goblet cells is less strongly labeled than the cytoplasm in other intestinal cells. The epididymis contains significantly more label than the testes. In the latter

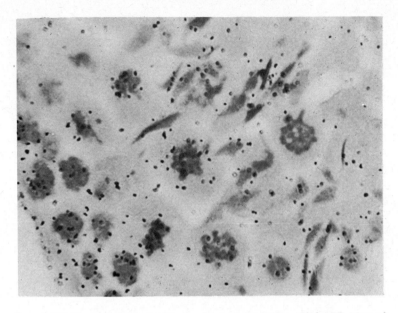

FIG. 6. Tubule of a mouse testes 30 min after an i.p. injection of ³H-AET. Most of the spermatogenic cells are labeled. (Maisin *et al.*, 1965.)

organs, there is an irregular distribution of activity, only a few spermatogenic cells being labeled in some tubules, whereas almost all cells are labeled in others (Fig. 6).

Although labeled, AET is found in the testes only in an irregular distribution, and at a low concentration it protects the spermatogenic cells against death and decreases the frequency of lethal mutants induced by irradiation (Léonard and Maisin, 1964).

The islets of Langerhans and the exocrine part of the pancreas are labeled about equally. Three days after treatment, certain tissues, including the liver and kidney, still contain radioactivity (Maisin and Léonard, 1963).

The advantages and the limitations of autoradiography studies are obvious. They allow interpretation of the data from chemical analysis and, for example, demonstrate whether any ubiquitous structure (vessels, connective tissues) take up a large percentage of protective agent. But classical autoradiography merely detects protective agents or metabolites fixed to insoluble macromolecules. This form may, however, be ineffective in protective action. A few studies on freeze-dried sections, where water

soluble compounds are retained, show, however, a similar localization of
AET labeled in the tissues, although with higher activities than those after
fixation in formalin.

5.3.3. CYSTEINE

Calcutt and Connors (1963) have titrated the total free —SH in the
spleen of rats after i.p. injection of various amounts of cysteine. The
increases shown in Fig. 7 must be attributed to cysteine itself, at least
for 90% (Ball, 1966).

Obviously, the highest concentration is not reached until about 30 min
after the injection. The same curve has been obtained by Ball and Connors
(1967) for the Yoshida sarcoma of the rat, and by Connors *et al.* (1965)
for a plasma cell tumor of the mouse, where the increase in acid soluble
—SH is about three times higher (and occurs somewhat later) than in
spleen or liver (Fig. 8).

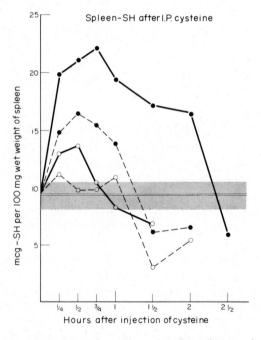

FIG. 7. Free SH levels in the spleen of rats at various times after i.p. injection of
various doses of cysteine HCl. (Calcutt and Connors, 1963.)

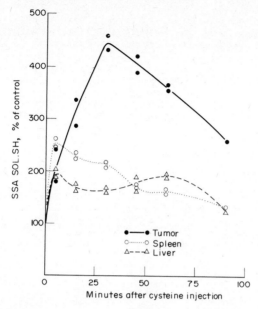

Fig. 8. Free SH levels in spleen, liver and tumor of rats after i.p. injection of 1 g/kg of cysteine. The tumor is a Yoshida sarcoma. (Ball and Connors, 1967.)

5.3.4. GLUTATHIONE

When large amounts of glutathione are injected in rats, a new fact appears besides the confirmation of the curve in the form of a dome with a maximum at about 30 min. The increase in —SH groups is not due only to glutathione itself; the majority of the —SH groups are attached to a new substance, an unidentified β-aminothiol, which does not exist normally and which might be a dipeptide (i.e. glutathione minus one amino acid) (Ball, 1966). This observation is important because it shows that, contrary to what is generally assumed, the —SH substance titrated after injection of large amounts of a thiol is not necessarily identical to the injected substance.

5.4. INTRACELLULAR LOCALIZATION

5.4.1. CHEMICAL STUDIES

Mondovi *et al.* (1962) have studied the distribution of ³⁵S radioactivity

TABLE 8. DISTRIBUTION OF RADIOACTIVITY IN THE SUB-CELLULAR FRACTIONS OF THE ORGANS OF RATS, 15 MIN FROM THE INJECTION OF 0.5 MC OF ^{35}S-CYSTAMINE PER 100 G BODY-WEIGHT (Mondovi *et al.*, 1962)

Tissue	Total homogenate activity in c.p.m. referred to 1 mg/N	Activity in per cent of total homogenate activity		
		Bound to structures; centrifuged at 10^5 g .	Bound to proteins in super-natant	Free in supernatant
Liver	2173	18.2	4.3	77.5
Spleen	3362	25.7	8.3	66
Kidneys	8085	12	5	83
Brain	2289	24.5	10	65.5
Testicles	1438	10.5	2	87.5
Mucosa of the small intestine	3732	14.5	3	82.5
Thymus	2016	29.5	3.5	67
Bone-marrow	1655	39	2.5	58.5
Psoas muscle	1073	17.5	4.5	78
Heart	1207	18	5	77
Lungs	3590	27	14.5	58.5
Adrenals	805	18.5	15.5	67
Pancreas	1750	23	4	73
Lenses	63	—	—	—
Salivary glands	7986	21.5	6	72.5
Lymph nodes	895	25.5	1.5	73

in various fractions (separated by classical ultracentrifugation) of homogenates of rat's organs, 15 min after injection of labeled cystamine. Radioactivity is bound not only to soluble proteins but also to subcellular particles (Table 8). The nuclei, microsomes, and mitochondria of the liver and spleen show ^{35}S activity. There seems to be a correlation between the degree of protection and the concentration in the subcellular structures. The lens and testicles, which are only weakly protected, show little localization of radioactivity. There are some discrepancies between the results of Lelièvre (1961) and those of Mondovi *et al.* (1962), but these are easily explained. Mondovi *et al.* have injected a smaller dose (58 mg/kg), and their technique of separating the free from the bound form is different. Lelièvre precipitates by acid alcohol without preliminary dilution so that the equilibrium between free and bound forms which exists at the moment when the organ is manipulated is "frozen". Mondovi *et al.* prepare a classical homogenate and dilute one part of tissue with 10 parts of 0.25M sucrose, then, after ultracentrifugation, they add trichloracetic acid to the supernatant. This dilution and rather brutal manipulation may displace the equilibrium in favor of the free form. This may be the reason why the free form represents 59–87% of the total activity, and from three to forty-four times the activity bound to the soluble proteins. The merit of the work of Mondovi *et al.* is to prove that, at a time when protection against irradiation is excellent, an important fraction (10–40%) of MEA–cystamine is bound to subcellular structures which, according to some radiobiologists, are the sites of primary damage during exposure to radiation.

Vladimirov (1967) investigated the labeling in the nuclei and mitochondria after injection of AET, cystamine (HCl), or 5-thiopentylamine disulfide, all labeled with ^{35}S, into mice at the maximal tolerable doses (125, 80 and 45 mg/kg, respectively). 5-Thiopentylamine is a cystamine analog which, however, does not protect against ionizing irradiation. After as little as 5 min following i.v. injection, AET and cystamine accumulate in significant amounts in the nuclear and mitochondrial fractions, isolated from liver and spleen cell homogenates by fractional centrifugation. Five to ten minutes after injection of cystamine, more radioactivity is found in the cytoplasm of liver cells than after injection of AET. An i.p. injection of 225 mg/kg of cystamine yields higher levels of activity in liver nuclei and cytoplasm, 10–30 min after administration, than does i.v. injection of 125 mg/kg. No such difference is observed with respect to liver mitochondria and spleen nuclei, mitochondria, or cytoplasm. From 10 min after administration, the radioactivity of cystamine decreases with time. 5-Thiopentylamine, a more toxic compound than AET or MEA, accumulates mainly in the mitochondria of the liver and spleen (Vladimirov, 1967).

5.4.2. AUTORADIOGRAPHIC STUDIES

Figure 9 shows the distribution of AET in the nuclei of the liver, the crypts of the small intestine, the kidney cortex and the white pulp of the spleen during the first hour after an i.p. administration of a protective dose of AET. These autoradiographic data demonstrate that maximal labeling is reached within 10 min after injection. At this time the activity in the liver, intestine, and spleen was 71, 48 and 35% respectively of that in the kidney. Twenty minutes after injection, the labeling decreased to about 20–40% of the maximal value, depending on the tissue.

Ten minutes after administration of AET, all the liver and kidney nuclei and most nuclei of the small intestine are labeled. Sixty minutes

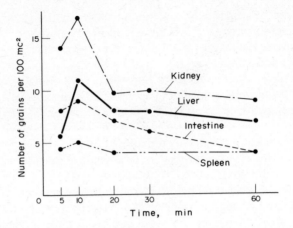

FIG. 9. Distribution of radioactive material in nuclei of the liver, parenchyma, intestinal crypts, convolute tubules of the kidney, and white pulp of the spleen cells at different times after injection of ^{3}H-AET into mice. (Maisin *et al.*, 1965.)

later, about the same percentage of nuclei is labeled but the number of grains in the nuclei has decreased markedly. On the other hand, in the spleen only 76% of the nuclei are labeled after 10 min, whereas 60% are still labeled 50 min later (Table 9). A detailed examination of the intestinal mucosa showed that the percentage of labeled nuclei and the degree of labeling is the same in the nuclei of the crypts and of the villi (Table 10).

TABLE 9. DISTRIBUTION OF RADIOACTIVE MATERIAL IN NUCLEI OF THE LIVER PARENCHYMA, INTESTINAL CRYPTS, CONVOLUTED TUBULES OF THE KIDNEY AND WHITE MARROW OF THE SPLEEN CELLS AT DIFFERENT TIMES AFTER INJECTION OF ^{3}H-LABELED AET INTO MICE (Maisin *et al.*, 1965)

Time after injection (min)	Liver		Intestinal crypts		Kidney		Spleen	
	Number of grains[a]	Percent of labeled nuclei	Number of grains[a]	Percent of labeled nuclei	Number of grains[a]	Percent of labeled nuclei	Number of grains[a]	Percent of labeled nuclei
5	5	100	8	54	14	100	4	73
10	11	100	9	98	17	100	5	76
20	8	100	7	96	10	100	4	61
30	7	100	6	95	10	100	4	61
60	7	100	4	89	9	100	6	70

[a] Number of grains per 100 mc^2.

TABLE 10. DISTRIBUTION OF RADIOACTIVE MATERIAL IN NUCLEI OF CRYPTS AND VILLI OF THE SMALL INTESTINE OF MICE AT DIFFERENT TIMES AFTER ADMINISTRATION OF ^{3}H-AET (Maisin *et al.*, 1965)

Time after injection (min)	Crypts		Villi	
	Number of grains[a]	Percent of labeled nuclei	Number of grains[a]	Percent of labeled nuclei
10	9	98	12	100
10	7	96	7	92
30	6	95	7	92
60	4	89	4	83

[a] Number of grains per 100 mc^2.

TABLE 11. DISTRIBUTION OF RADIOACTIVE MATERIAL IN NUCLEI AND IN CYTOPLASM OF LIVER CELLS OF MICE AT DIFFERENT TIMES AFTER AN INJECTION OF ^{3}H-AET (Maisin *et al.*, 1965)

Time after injection (min)	Nuclei		Cytoplasm	
	Number of grains[a]	Percent of labeled nuclei	Number of grains[a]	Percent of labeled cytoplasm
10	11	100	15	100
20	8	100	9	100
30	7	100	9	100
60	7	100	7	100

[a] Number of grains per 100 mc^2.

Nuclei in mitosis are labeled to the same degree as those at rest, and the membrane of the villi contains large amounts of activity.

The nuclei and cytoplasm of liver cells are labeled to the same extent (Table 11). The label seems evenly spread over the whole nucleus, but careful examination reveals that activity is concentrated near the nuclear membrane. Nuclei of other tissues behave similarly. Erythrocytes are not labeled except at the membrane (Fig. 10). In the bone-marrow, labeling of the cells is irregular. Some were faintly labeled, others, like megakaryocytes, were highly radioactive (Fig. 11). The serum also showed a certain amount of activity.

An electronmicroscopic–autoradiographic technique was employed to determine whether a correlation exists between the ultrastructural binding sites of AET and its derivatives and the degree of radiation pro-

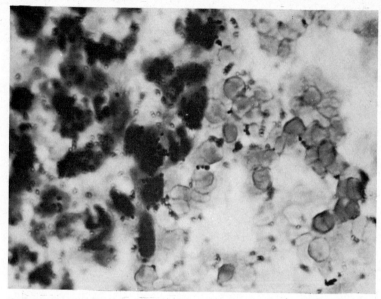

FIG. 10. Autoradiography of transversal section of blood vessel (to the right) which shows labeling near the membrane of red blood cells. (Maisin *et al.*, 1965.)

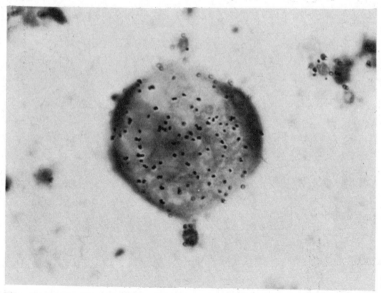

FIG. 11. Autoradiography of a megakaryocyte which shows the grains evenly spread over the cells. (Maisin *et al.*, 1965.)

tection given to the cellular structure. Cultures of rat dorsal root ganglion cells were treated with 3×10^{-3}M ^{35}A-AET (pH 7.4) for 20 min prior to irradiation and subsequently exposed to 20–40 Kr of 184 kV X-rays. Labeling, marking the binding sites, is observed over the nucleolus, nuclear matrix and near the nuclear membrane of control and irradiated cultures. Within the cytoplasm, grains appear mainly over the Golgi complex, the mitochondria, the cytoplasmic reticulum, and near the plasma membrane (Masurovsky and Bunge, 1969).

According to Pliess and Herbert (1963) ^{35}S-AET is homogeneously distributed in the base of the rat tooth but only the young odontoblasts are protected after head irradiation with 100, 500, or 1000 r. They concluded, from these data, that the effect of radioprotective agents does not depend only on their quantitative distribution in the tissues, but also on specific biological interactions with certain tissue components.

5.5. METABOLISM AND EXCRETION

5.5.1. CYSTEINE

Cysteine, ingested or synthesized by the mammalian organism from methionine, in normal amounts, is catabolized mainly to taurine and sulfate.

Cysteine is oxidized to cysteine sulfinic acid which is destroyed in two ways: (1) Degradation to SO_2 and alanine by a desulfinase; SO_2 is further oxidized to SO_4^{2-}. (2) Decarboxylation to hypotaurine which is further oxidized to taurine.

Cysteine may also be decomposed into alanine and H_2S which is oxidized to sulfate.

Mammals vary in their ability to dispose of an excess of cysteine. The taurine excretion of the guinea-pig is less than 10% that of the rat after injection of equivalent amounts of cysteine; as a consequence of this slow metabolism, cysteine is much more toxic in the guinea-pig than in the rat (Hewitt, 1963).

The marked increase in taurine excretion observed in rats soon after exposure to ionizing radiation is not due to an accelerated catabolism of cysteine, but to an increased mobilization and excretion of the taurine stores within the cells (Boquet and Fromageot, 1967).

When very large doses (1 g/kg) are injected, much of the amino acid is excreted as such in the urine; the rest is metabolized in the normal way.

5.5.2. CYSTEAMINE AND CYSTAMINE

5.5.2.1. *Metabolism*

Mercaptoethylamine does not exist free in living systems; it constitutes a fragment of coenzyme A. Cysteine, not MEA, is incorporated during the synthesis of this universal coenzyme; N-pantothenyl cysteine is decarboxylated to N-pantothenyl MEA, which after phosphorylation and binding to adenylic acid constitutes CoA. Cysteine is not decarboxylated when free in cells or fluids. As a corollary to this situation, the cells have to metabolize only the minute amounts of MEA resulting from the unavoidable turnover of CoA. The quantities of MEA and cystamine utilized in radioprotective action are thus in the pharmacological range, and it is no surprise if one of the conclusions, on which all authors agree, is that the capacity of the organisms to dispose of this large excess is completely overwhelmed. One speaks of "inundation" by —SH or S—S substances which "overflow" into the urine. Cysteamine or cystamine is not incorporated in polypeptides or proteins except in minute quantities; the incorporation of amines is only conceivable at the end of a polypeptide chain, like the incorporation of NH_3. Several complete studies and reviews have been published by Eldjarn (1954a), Verly (1955), Bacq (1965) about the metabolism of MEA and cystamine. All authors agree that the main metabolites are taurine and sulfate in all mammals (mouse, rat, dog, or man).

The following data illustrate these conclusions. MEA, a small molecule soluble in both water and lipid solvents, crosses all barriers easily and is rapidly metabolized. The metabolites, taurine and SO_4^{2-}, normal constituents of the body, share their fate and are logically excreted much more slowly than the original molecules which "overflow". This is well demonstrated by the results of Verly *et al.* (1954) in mice (Fig. 2). After 24 hr practically all the radioactivity remaining in the organism after i.p. injection of a radioprotective dose of MEA is linked to metabolites.

The catabolism of MEA to taurine may follow the same pathway as that of cysteine (with the exception of the decarboxylation), through aminoethane sulfinic acid ($SO_2H—CH_2—CH_2—NH_2$). Eldjarn (1954), using paper chromatography of the incubation products of cystamine in the presence of rat liver slices, has found a spot with an R_f value corresponding to this acid. Another possible pathway is that suggested by Cavallini and his associates (1957, 1960a, b, 1962), starting not from MEA but from cystamine, which, being a diamine, is a substrate for diamine oxidase.* The sequence of events proposed by Cavallini *et al.* (1960b) is given in Fig. 12. Hypotaurine is converted to taurine. The presence of ^{35}S-thiotaurine in the liver and kidney of a rat 15 min after injection of ^{35}S-cystamine has been established by Mondovi and Tentori (1961). By two-dimensional paper chromatography and subsequent autoradiography Gensicke *et al.* (1962) have separated the following compounds in the urine of rats injected i.p. with a large radioprotective dose of ^{35}S-cystamine: cystamine, MEA, cystine, cystine disulfoxide, cysteine, cysteinic acid, taurine, hypotaurine, sulfoconjugates of phenol and indoxyl, probably methionine and many unidentified substances.

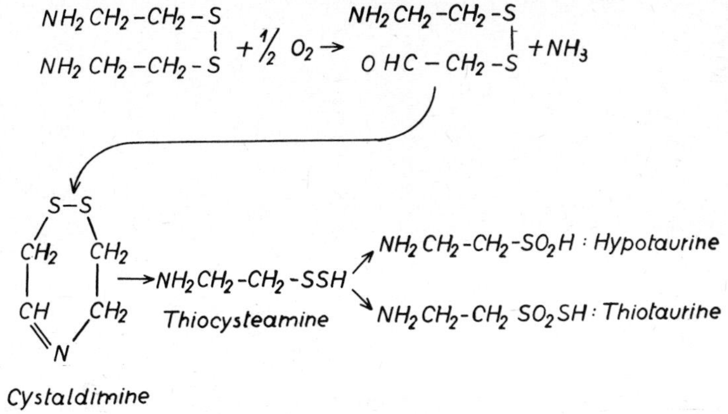

Fig. 12. Sequence of events proposed for the oxidative metabolism of cystamine by diamino oxidase. (Cavallini *et al.*, 1957)

---

* Monoaminoxidase from rat liver mitochondria does not oxidize cystamine.

The fact that labeled amino acids appear in the urine needs confirmation and quantitative evaluation, because it conflicts with the generally accepted rule that MEA or cystamine cannot be carboxylated in amino acids. After prolonged administration of ^{35}S-MEA or cystamine to growing rats, a very small radioactivity could be found in the cystine isolated from the hair (Eldjarn, 1954a).

Lauber *et al.* (1960) found that 10 days after injecting ^{35}S-MEA into rats, 75–90% of the remaining activity was in taurine; in skin and hair, a large proportion (22–30%) of the very small activity was bound to proteins, largely in the form of mixed disulfide, but also as cystine and sulfate.

5.5.2.2. *Urinary and Fecal Excretion*

The rapid disappearance of MEA or cystamine from the blood after

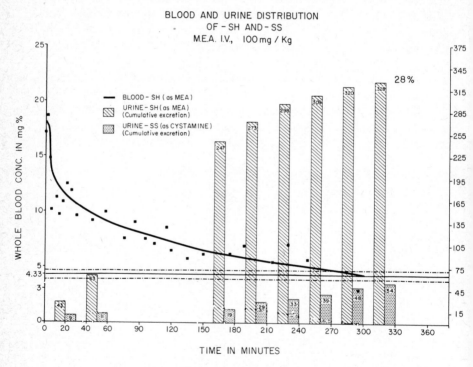

FIG. 13. Blood and urine —SH and S—S levels in dogs after i.v. injection of MEA (100 mg/kg). Zero time represents + 6 min from beginning of MEA administration. Solid line at 4.33 mg/ml of blood represents control values for —SH reactant material in normal dogs. (Mundy *et al.,* 1961.)

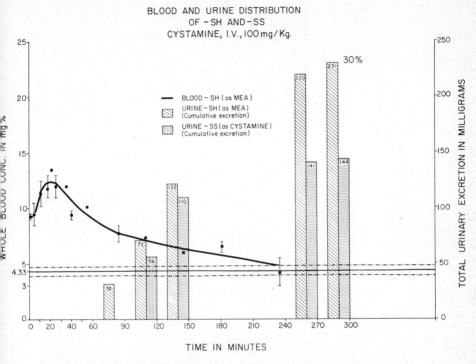

FIG. 14. Blood and urine —SH and S—S levels in dogs after cystamine (100 mg/kg i.v.). Compare with Fig. 13. (Mundy *et al.*, 1961.)

i.v. injection in rabbits (Bacq *et al.*, 1952; Fischer and Goutier-Pirotte, 1954) or dogs (Mundy *et al.*, 1961; Heiffer *et al.*, 1962) is due to three factors: (a) excretion as such by the urine, (b) binding to proteins, (c) rapid catabolism to taurine and SO_4^{2-}. The state of shock induced by a large dose of the amine may stop the secretion of urine and alter the pattern of elimination (see Figs. 13 and 14).*

In 4 hr, 30–35% of MEA injected into rabbits is recovered as such, or as cystamine, in the urine. In this animal, cystamine as such or reduced to MEA is also recovered in large quantities in the urine after i.v. injection of radioprotective doses of cystamine (Fischer and Goutier-Pirotte, 1954). In the dog, the same phenomena have been described (Figs. 13 and 14) but excretion is slower than in rabbits. More disulfide appears in the

* In rabbit's blood, there also appear, after i.v. injection of MEA, large quantities of reducing substances (ascorbic acid and others) which interfere with some titration techniques.

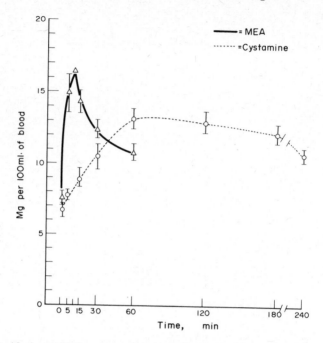

F I G. 15. A graphical representation of blood sulfhydryl levels of rats after the i.p. administration of 125 mg of mercaptoethylamine per kilogram or 100 mg/kg of cystamine. Bars indicate ± one standard error of the mean. (Heiffer *et al.,* 1962.)

urine when cystamine has been injected than after administration of MEA. Figure 15 is a good illustration of the ability of the mammalian organism to detoxicate disulfides; 70 min after i.v. injection of a large amount of cystamine, only traces of disulfides are found in the plasma.

Verly *et al.* (1954) found that injection of labeled MEA in mouse (150 mg/kg) or dog (22 mg/kg) is quickly followed by urinary excretion of MEA, cystamine, taurine and SO_4^{2-}. During the first 2 hours, excretion of the unaltered amines predominates, but later, usually after 8 hr, metabolites form the bulk of the excreted radioactivity.

When small doses (0.5 mg/kg) of labeled cystamine are injected into the rat, sulfate is the main metabolite; in man (0.35 mg/kg) or rabbit (3 mg/kg) taurine and sulfate. ^{35}S-Taurine is, as expected, found in the bile of man and rabbit after injection of small amounts of ^{35}S-cystamine (Eldjarn, 1954b). In man, subcutaneously injected MEA is oxidized more rapidly to SO_4^{2-} than cystamine (Eldjarn, 1954a), probably as a result of its easier penetration within the cells.

A number of authors have compared the metabolism and excretion of MEA and cystamine in normal and irradiated animals. According to Salvador *et al.* (1957) irradiated rats excrete into the urine, in 8 hr, only 70% of the radioactivity eliminated by the controls after i.p. injection of 150 mg/kg of labeled cystamine. The substances identified are taurine, cysteic acid, hypotaurine, cystamine disulfoxide, MEA, cystamine and sulfate.

The radioactivity in all organs (except for the gastrointestinal tract) is smaller after injection of ^{35}S-MEA into irradiated rats than in controls; this may be due to a decreased urine output in irradiated rats (Arbusow *et al.,* 1959). The peculiar behavior of the gastrointestinal tract is secondary to the physiological effect of the ionizing radiation—marked delay in emptying of the stomach. The contents of stomach and intestine should be carefully studied; we have no data to clarify this point. A larger proportion of ^{35}S, in form of thioesters, is also found in the urine of irradiated rats, as compared with controls, during the first day after injection of ^{35}S-MEA; this fact is considered by the Soviet authors as an indication of increased detoxication in irradiated animals.

Aebi *et al.* (1957) have observed differences in the metabolism and excretion of labeled MEA if it is injected 5 min before, or 60 min after, exposure to X-rays. Cysteamine injected before irradiation is a substrate for taurine synthesis but also, by its radioprotective action, decreases the wave of taurine excretion induced by irradiation. In 10 days, the rats injected before exposure eliminate about 66% of the radioactivity; those injected 1 hr after eliminate 72%. The very small radioactivity which remains after 10 days is firmly bound, not extractable by trichloracetic acid, acetone, or MEA. This observation confirms the possibility of a very small incorporation in the macromolecules of the skin and hair proteins or as $^{35}SO_4^{2-}$ in mucopolysaccharides.

Lauber *et al.* (1960) have also observed a smaller retention of radioactivity from ^{35}S-MEA in irradiated rats (500r of X-rays). If MEA is injected before irradiation, the retention is less than in control animals, but also less than if administration occurred after exposure to radiation.

Little attention has been paid to fecal excretion. A large fraction of the taurine of the bile is probably reabsorbed. Arbusow *et al.* (1959) maintain that after the first day following i.p. injection of ^{35}S labeled MEA, fecal excretion of ^{35}S predominates over urinary elimination.

5.5.3.   AET AND RELATED COMPOUNDS

As mentioned earlier, when separating the radioactive species from homogenates of organs of mice injected with radioactive (MEG (SH active form of AET) or GED (disulfide of MEG), Shapiro *et al.* (1962, 1963b, c) identified various metabolites which are also found in the urine: taurocyamine, guanidoethanesulfinic acid, *S*-acetyl-2-mercaptoethylguanidine and sulfate. Thus, as in the case of MEA, oxidation of the sulfur occurs progressively. An *S*-acetyl derivative of MEA has never been found; however, no attempts have been made to find it. Many metabolites of MEA (see Verly *et al.,* 1954) and AET (Shapiro *et al.,* 1963a; Tables 6 and 7) remain unidentified. For some unknown reason, MEG is not found in tissues after injection of either MEG or GED, but constitutes the major excretory product in the urine even after administration of pure GED. In the tissues of mice 20 min after i.p. injection of ^{35}S-AET, about 50% of ^{35}S is bound to proteins, 20% is free as GED; the rest of the radioactivity is attached to various metabolites. Two hours after injection of the protective agent both bound and free forms have decreased, the concentration of the metabolites is unchanged or increased. These changes are seen in all organs except the intestine; the behavior of this particular organ may be correlated with the observation of Maisin (1966) that AET has a marked protective effect on the intestinal cells. The *S*-acetylated MEG is recovered in the spleen, testis and bone-marrow in significant amounts, sometimes exceeding the protein bound form, 1 or 2 hr after injection, i.e. at a time when the protection against ionizing radiation has practically disappeared.

In the urine, the majority of radioactivity is found as MEG, even after administration of the S—S form GED; the quantities of tagged taurocyamine and $^{35}SO_4^{2-}$ are relatively small because the ability of the organism to metabolize the radioprotective agent is limited. What is true for MEA or cystamine (Eldjarn and Nygaard, 1954; Eldjarn, 1954) is also true for AET: when a small (non-protective dose) is injected in animals or man, the proportion of the final metabolite SO_4^{2-} found in the urine is much greater. The smaller the dose, the smaller the proportion of unchanged molecules recovered in the urine. If 1 g of AET is ingested by a 70 kg man, no MEG or GED is found in urine; sulfate is by far the main metabolite.

Twenty minutes after i.p. injection of 140 mg/kg of labeled MEG to mice, only 9% of the ^{35}S activity is recovered in the urine. Fifteen minutes after an injection of 150 mg/kg MEA i.p. into mice, about 25% of the activity is eliminated in the urine (Verly *et al.,* 1954), but one should not forget that 150 mg of MEA corresponds in molecular weight (hence in ^{35}S) to 550 mg of AET, nearly four times as much. The more rapid urinary excretion of MEA may be explained by this consideration; the fact that the changes in the intensity of radioprotective action with time after injection are not the same for MEA and AET becomes easily understandable.

The earlier increase of $^{35}SO_4^{2-}$ in animals injected with MEG as compared with GED injected mice may be accounted for by the fact that MEG penetrates more rapidly inside the cells to get in contact with the intracellular oxidizing enzymes.

Orally administered MEG and GED (400 mg/kg) are metabolized and excreted by mice in the same fashion as the injected compounds, but 30 min after intragastric administration, 40% are still present in the gastrointestinal tract. Absorption of GED from the intestine is slower (Kollmann *et al.,* 1963; Shapiro *et al.,* 1964).

Exposure to 1000 r of X-rays 10 min after injection of the radioprotective dose of 140 mg/kg only slightly alters the distribution and metabolism of labeled GED. The stomach, 20 min after injection, contains a good deal of radioactivity because irradiation slows down its emptying; 2 hr after, gastric concentrations are comparable, but excretion is still smaller than in non-irradiated controls (Shapiro *et al.,* 1963a). In mice grafted with a mammary tumor (BW 10232 of the Jackson Memorial Laboratory), 20 min after i.p. injection of MED or GED certain differences are found with respect to non-cancerous controls (Shapiro *et al.,* 1963a; Kollmann *et al.,* 1963). The urine and feces of cancerous mice contain about 30% only of the radioactivity found in the excreta of the controls; the kidneys of cancerous animals have about twice as much radioactivity as the controls. At 2 hr, most of the organs of the grafted mice show greater radioactivity than in the corresponding organs of the controls; this is due to a higher level of protein-bound ^{35}S activity, as well as to free GED. The tumor itself seems to concentrate less of the protective agent and to produce more of the *S*-acetylated MEG and of SO_4^{2-} than the other tissues of the mice. Grafted mice excrete MEG and GED less rapidly than do controls. But the radioactivity of the plasma is the same in cancerous and non-cancerous mice. Thus the renal clearance remains good and the higher radioactivity of the kidneys of grafted mice is not a sign of impairment.

Similar results were obtained with leukemic mice (myeloid leukemia C 1498 of the Jackson Memorial Laboratory) with MEG or GED by oral (400 mg/kg) or i.p. (140 mg/kg) route. Twenty minutes after injection or 30 min after ingestion, the radioactivity in the tumors is smaller than in the principal organs. Slices of cancerous tissue incubated *in vitro* with labeled GED absorb the protective agent as well as slices of liver or spleen. The most plausible interpretation is that the less efficient circulatory system of the tumor brings less of the substance to these cells than to the normal cells of other organs (Urbach, 1962). In cancerous tissue, the proportion of labeled protective agent, forming thioester links, is much smaller than that found in intestine, liver, or kidneys.

Among the numerous substances synthesized in the series of *S*-alkyl-thioureas, the butyl derivative merits special attention because (after the usual intramolecular transguanylation) this compound is very active as a protective agent against irradiation (see Khym *et al.*, 1958). The metabolism and distribution of this mercaptobutylguanidine (MBG) in rats and mice do not differ significantly from those of MEG. However, there is a more significant concentration of D or L MBG (and metabolites) in the radiosensitive and metabolically active tissues (Bradford *et al.*, 1961). Radioactivity is high on microsomes. It is loosely bound; a simple dialysis breaks the bond. It is suggested that MBG is adsorbed on microsomes in a manner resembling the enzyme–substrate complex. The L-isomers of MBG and MEG, which are less protective against ionizing radiation than the corresponding D-isomers, have also a smaller affinity for microsomes. Part of MBG is linked to proteins in the form of mixed disulfides and cannot be detached by dialysis. An excess of —SH (thioglycollate, for instance) succeeds in breaking the bond, just as in the case of mixed disulfides of MEG or GED. The proportion of MBG forming mixed disulfide with proteins is definitely smaller than in the case of MEG. Finally a third type of bonding seems to exist, because drastic chemical treatments (powerful oxidizing or reducing agents), capable of breaking very resistant disulfide bridges, do not liberate all the protein-linked ^{35}S; the nature of these bonds has not been established.

5.5.4. *N*-DIETHYLDITHIOCARBAMATE (DEDTC)

This compound, well known for its chelating properties, is a good protective agent against ionizing radiation (Bacq *et al.*, 1953b); the whole family of dithiocarbamates has been studied by van Bekkum (1956) with respect to their radioprotective action. The disulfide form of DEDTC is the famous Antabuse® or disulfiram, which is the subject of an important monograph in the *International Encyclopedia*.

TABLE 12. ^{35}S Metabolites in Urine of Rats after the Administration of Labeled Disulfiram (ASSA) or N-Diethyldithiocarbamate (ASH) (Strömme, 1965b)

Expt. no.	Compound	Dose (mc moles S)	Time after dose (hr)	^{35}S metabolites in urine			
				Total (mc moles S)	ASH (%)	S-glucur. (%)	Sulfate (%)
1	ASSA	138	1	10.11	0.00	91.5	8.5
2	ASSA	138	2	15.90	0.26	77.5	22.2
3	ASSA	138	4	26.45	0.10	57.4	42.5
8	ASH	222	1	46.15	0.03	96.1	3.9
10	ASH	222	2	78.90	0.06	80.6	19.3
10	ASH	222	4	95.31	0.06	76.3	23.6

We will deal here mainly with the facts established in connection with radioprotective action.

Disulfiram is a very insoluble substance; when injected in suspension it is slowly reduced to the soluble SH form* which is rapidly excreted and never reaches a sufficient concentration in the body to exert any protective action against radiation. This fact is the logical reason why disulfiram completely lacks radioprotective effects. The rate of excretion of labeled DEDTC is much more rapid than that of disulfiram. The S-glucuronoconjugate is the main constituent of the excretion products. Only traces of free thiol appear. Labeled mineral sulfate becomes abundant after 2 hr (Table 12, Strömme, 1965a). A significant fraction of radioactivity is recuperated in the expired air as CS_2. Again the elimination of CS_2 is much faster and more important ($\pm 10\%$ of the radioactivity) after injection of the reduced DEDTC than after disulfiram (only 2%) (Strömme, 1965b).

In deproteinized blood plasma and liver extracts, one finds only $^{35}SO_4^{2-}$ and labeled S-glucuronoconjugate after injection in rats of 10 mg of ^{35}S-disulfiram; a very small amount of labeled free thiol is found only after injection of a large dose (40 mg). On the other hand, 15 min after injection of the reduced form (25 mg), a significant fraction of the unaltered thiol is found free in the plasma, together with a high level of S-glucuronoconjugate (Table 13). After 1 hr, only traces of the free thiol are recovered while the ^{35}S-conjugate and SO_4^{2-} are still predominant. On the other

* In exactly the same way as cystamine.

TABLE 13. NON-PROTEIN-BOUND ^{35}S METABOLITES IN PLASMA FROM RATS GIVEN LABELED DISULFIRAM (ASSA) 10 MG OR N-DIETHYLDITHIOCARBAMATE (ASH) 25 MG (Strömme, 1965b)[a]

Expt. no.	Compound	Time after dose (hr)	Total	ASH	S-glucur.	Sulfate	%[b] identified
1	ASSA	1	169	0	37	132	100
2	ASSA	2	93	0	15	68	89
3	ASSA	4	64	0	7	54	95
4–6[c]	ASH	1/4	1561	567	772	142	95
7	ASH	1/2	672	72	377	124	86
8	ASH	1	305	2	106	128	77
9	ASH	2	148	0	13	127	95
10	ASH	4	65	0	10	52	95

[a] All amounts are expressed as nmoles sulfur per g liver (wet weight).
[b] Per cent of total non-protein-bound ^{35}S metabolites.
[c] Means of three experiments.

hand, in the liver, 15 min after injection of labeled DEDTC, a very small fraction (0.5%) of the radioactivity is linked to the free thiol. Thus the synthesis of the S-glucuronoconjugate of DEDTC is very active in the liver of the rat.

As might be expected, part of the radioactivity of injected ^{35}S-disulfiram or DEDTC is bound to plasma proteins and to the soluble liver proteins (Table 14). The highest proportion is found 15 min after injection; it decreases slowly with time, but this fall is not as rapid as the decrease in total radioactivity. *In vitro,* disulfiram forms mixed disulfides with SH proteins which are easily broken, in the case of plasma proteins, by addition of GSH and liberation of DEDTC. *In vitro,* DEDTC in presence of proteins does not readily form mixed disulfides. Thus it may be assumed that the mixed disulfides found *in vivo,* after injection of DEDTC, are formed after preliminary oxidation of DEDTC to disulfiram. Cytochrome *C* and methemoglobin easily oxidize DEDTC *in vitro* (Strömme, 1963).

Disulfiram is never found free in plasma, liver, or urine, probably because its affinity for the thiols and —SH groups of proteins is very great (Johnston, 1953; Strömme, 1963, 1965).

The metabolic pathway which produces SO_4^{2-} from DEDTC or disulfiram is not known. This SO_4^{2-} might be derived from the oxidation

TABLE 14. ^{35}S Bound to the Soluble Proteins of Liver and to the Proteins of Plasma from Rats Given Labeled Disulfiram (ASSA) 10 mg or N-Diethyldithiocarbamate (ASH) 25 mg (Strömme, 1965b)[a]

Expt. no.	Compound	Time after dose (hr)	^{35}S in supernt. of liver homogenate	^{35}S in plasma	^{35}S released from plasma prot.-^{35}S by GSH (%)[b]	
					Total	Identified as ASH
1	ASSA	1	18	36	92	86
2	ASSA	2	17	29	92	87
3	ASSA	4	10	11	94	77
4–6[c]	ASH	1/4	53	45	83	74
7	ASH	1/2	42	32	81	63
8	ASH	1	35	30	56	—
9	ASH	2	34	22	45	32
10	ASH	4	18	15	75	—

[a] The amounts are expressed as nmoles sulfur per g liver (wet weight).
[b] Per cent of total radioactive sulfur bound to the proteins.
[c] Means of three experiments.

of CS_2, since in mice and guinea-pigs about 30% of the radioactivity is found in the urine as sulfate after administration of $C^{35}S_2$.

The metabolites found in rats have also been observed in men and mice, but in different proportions. Forty-five per cent of a small dose of disulfiram (500 mg) ingested by man is metabolized in 80 hr to carbon disulfide (Merlevelde and Casier, 1961); 80% of ingested DEDTC is converted to CS_2 in 7 hr. The acidity of the gastric secretion may be responsible for this difference; disulfiram is more resistant to acid. The smell of CS_2 in expired air is most marked between 10 and 30 min after ingestion of DEDTC.

The yield of S-glucuronoconjugate is much smaller in man than in rat (Kaslander, 1963).

In mice, generally speaking, the metabolism of disulfiram and DEDTC and the formation of mixed disulfides with proteins are about the same as in rat (Strömme and Eldjarn, 1966). The same metabolites are found: S-glucuronoconjugate, sulfate and carbon disulfide, besides free DEDTC. Again the reduction of disulfide is a prominent feature; no disulfiram may be found even after injection of the very high toxic dose of 60 mg. The well-tolerated radioprotective dose of DEDTC is 15 mg/mouse;

during the period of protective action, a large proportion of the thiol is found unaltered in the plasma. In the liver, the free thiol is less concentrated than in the plasma, and the proportion of S-glucuronoconjugate increases more rapidly than in plasma.

The distribution of radioactivity in the various organs is the same after injection of the non-protective labeled disulfiram as after administration of the protective reduced compound. The radioactivity of radiosensitive organs (bone-marrow, spleen, intestinal mucosa) is not particularly high. The concentration of ^{35}S at the time of protective action is 10 to 20 times higher after injection of DEDTC than after an equal amount of disulfiram, and this again explains why disulfiram is not radioprotective. No free thiols are found in plasma after injection of disulfiram suspensions. The resorption of disulfiram is so slow that the thiol is metabolized as soon as it is formed and therefore thiol cannot accumulate in the tissues.

REFERENCES

AEBI, H., LAUBER, K., SCHMIDLI, B. and ZUPPINGER, A. (1957) Die Wirkung ionisirender Strahlen auf die Taurinausscheidung der Ratte. *Biochem. Zeit.* **328:** 391–404.

ARBUSOW, S. J., BASANOW, V. A., NEKATSCHALOWA, I. Y., PATALOWA, W. N., PETELINA, W. W. and SCHAMOWA, E. K. (1959) Über die Verteilung des ^{35}S Merkaptoethylamins in den Organen und Geweben bestrahlter und nicht bestrahlter Ratten. *Acta Biol. Med. Germ.* **3:** 417–32.

BACQ, Z. M. (1965) *Chemical Protection against Ionizing Radiation.* Charles C. Thomas, Springfield, Ill., U.S.A., 330 pages.

BACQ, Z. M., FISCHER, P. and PIROTTE, M. (1952) Métabolisme de la cystéamine et de la cystamine chez le lapin. *Arch. Int. Physiol.* **60:** 535–43.

BACQ, Z. M., HERVE, A. and FISCHER, P. (1953b) Rayons X et agents de chelation. *Bull. Acad. Roy. Méd. Belg.* **18:** 266–74.

BALL, C. R. (1966) Estimation and identification of thiols in rat spleen after cysteine or glutathione treatment. Relevance to protection against nitrogen mustards. *Biochem. Pharmacol.* **15:** 809–16.

BALL, C. R. and CONNORS, T. A. (1967) Reduction of the toxicity of "radiomimetic" alkylating agents by thiol pretreatment—VI. The mechanism of protection by cysteine. *Biochem. Pharmacol.* **16:** 509–19.

BEKKUM, D. W. VAN (1956) The protective action of *N*-diethyldithiocarbamate against lethal effect of X-irradiation in mice. *Acta Physiol. Pharmacol. Neurol.* **4:** 508–20.

BOQUET, P. L. and FROMAGEOT, P. (1967) Sur l'origine de la taurine urinaire excrétée par le rat soumis à une irradiation par les rayons gamma du ^{60}Co. *Int. J. Rad. Biol.* **13:** 343–53.

BRADFORD, R. H., SHAPIRA, R. and DOHERTY, D. G. (1961) The intracellular distribution and binding of radiation protective mercaptoalkylguanidines. *Int. J. Rad. Biol.* **3:** 595–608.

CALCUTT, G. and CONNORS, T. A. (1963) Tumour sulfhydryl levels and sensitivity to nitrogen mustard Merophan. *Biochem. Pharmacol.* **12:** 839–45.

CAVALLINI, B. and TENTORI, L. (1960) Inability of thiotaurine to protect mice against ionizing radiation. *Nature* **186:** 254–8.

CAVALLINI, D., DE MARCO, C. and MONDOVI, B. (1957) Cystaldimine: the product of oxidation of cystamine by diaminooxidase. *Biochem. Biophys. Acta* **24:** 353–8.

CAVALLINI, D., DE MARCO, C. and MONDOVI, B. (1960a) Conversione enzimatica della cistamine in tiotaurina. *Boll. Soc. Ital. Biol. Sper.* **36:** 1915–18.

CAVALLINI, D., DE MARCO, C. and MONDOVI, B. (1960b) A non-enzymic conversion of thiocysteine into cysteine sulfinic acid and alaninthiosulfonate. *Arch. Biochem. Biophys.* **87:** 281–9.

CAVALLINI, B., DE MARCO, C. and SCANDURRA, R. (1962) Ossidazione enzimatica della cisteamina a ipotaurina in presenza di donatori di zolfo. *Giorn. di Biochim.* **11:** 201–7.

CICCARONE, P. and BACQ, Z. M. (1966) Inhibition of oxygen consumption of liver homogenates from mice injected with radioprotectors in the presence of pyruvate. *Nature* **210:** 648–9.

CONNORS, T. A., JENEY, A. J. and WHISSON, M. E. (1965) Reduction of the toxicity of radiomimetic alkylating agents in rat by thiol pretreatment—V. The effect of thiol pretreatment on the anti-tumor action of Merophan. *Biochem. Pharmacol.* **14:** 1681–3.

DICKENS, E. A. and SHAPIRO, B. (1961) The mechanism of action of AET—II. The interaction between proteins and 2 MEG and bis(2 guanidoethyl) disulfide in aqueous buffered solution. *Radiation Res.* **14:** 308–22.

DOHERTY, D. J. and BURNETT, W. T. JR. (1955) Protective effect of *S*-aminoethylisothiouronium bromide bromhydrate and related compounds against X radiation death in mice. *Proc. Soc. Exp. Biol. Med.* **89:** 312–21.

ELDJARN, L. (1954a) The conversion of cysteamine to taurine in rat, rabbit and man. *J.B.C.* **206:** 483–90.

ELDJARN, L. (1954b) The metabolism of cysteamine and cystamine studies on the formation of taurine in mammals. *Scand. J. Clin. Lab. Invest.* **6:** Suppl. **13:** 1–11.

ELDJARN, L. and BREMER, J. (1963) The disulfide reducing capacity of liver mitochondria. *Acta Chem. Scand.* **17:** 59–66.

ELDJARN, L. and NYGAARD, O. (1954) Cysteamine–cystamine. Intestinal absorption, distribution among various organs and excretion. *Arch. Int. Physiol.* **52:** 476–84.

ELDJARN, L. and PIHL, A. (1956) On the mode of action of X-ray protective against. I. The fixation *in vivo* of cystamine and cysteamine to proteins. *J.B.C.* **223:** 41–52.

ELDJARN, L. and PIHL, A. (1960) Mechanisms of protective and sensitizing action. In: *Mechanisms in Radiobiology,* vol. 2, ERRERA, M. and FORSSBERG, A. (Eds.). Academic Press, New York, p. 231.

ELDJARN, L., NAKKEN, K. F. and PIHL, A. (1957) The interaction of cysteamine and cysteine with various carbonyl compounds. *Acta Chem. Scand.* **11:** 1085.

ELDJARN, L., BREMER, J. and BØRRESEN, H. C. (1962) The reduction of disulfide by human erythrocyte. *Biochem. J.* **82:** 192–9.

FIRKET, H., LELIÈVRE, P. and SMOLIAR, V. (1963) Distribution précoce de la radioactivité dans les organes du rat après injection de cystéamine-^{35}S et de cystamine-[35]S. Introduction et résultats autoradiographiques. *C.R. Soc. Biol.* **157:** 677–80.

FISCHER, P. and GOUTIER-PIROTTE, M. (1954) Métabolisme de la cystéamine et de la cystamine chez le lapin et le chien. *Arch. Int. Physiol.* **62:** 76–100.

FLUHARTY, A. and SANADI, D. R. (1960) The oxidation of the thioctic acid. *Proc. Natl. Acad. Sci. U.S.* **46:** 608–14.

GENSICKE, F., SPODE, E. and VENKER, P. (1962) Die [35]S Verteilung und Ausscheidung nach Injektion ^{35}S markierten Cystamin bei der Maus. *Strahlentherapie* **118:** 561–9.

HEIFFER, M. H., MUNDY, R. L. and MEHLMAN, B. (1962) The pharmacology of radioprotective chemicals. *Radiation Res.* **16:** 165–73.

HEWITT, R. R. (1963) *Metabolism of Protectant Dose of L-cysteine by Rats and Guinea-pigs with Reference to Post-irradiation Taurinuria.* Thesis, University of Rochester, Rochester.

JOHNSTON, C. D. (1953) The *in vivo* reaction between tetraethylthiuram disulfide (Antabuse) and glutathione. *Arch. Biochem. Biophys.* **44**: 249–52.

KASLANDER, J. (1963) Formation of *S*-glycuronide from tetraethylthiuram disulfide (Antabuse) in man. *Biochem. Biophys. Acta* **71**: 730–4.

KHYM, J. X., DOHERTY, D. G. and SHAPIRA, R. (1958) Ion exchange studies of transguanylation reactions.—2. Rearrangement of *S*-2 aminopropylisothiouronium and *N*-substituted aminoethyl and aminopropylisothioureas to mercaptoalkylguanidine and 2-aminothiazoline or penthiazoline. *J. Am. Chem. Soc.* **80**: 3342–9.

KOLLMANN, G., SHAPIRO, B. and SCHWARZ, E. E. (1963) The mechanism of action of AET. V. The distribution and the chemical forms of 2-mercaptoethylguanidine and bis (2-guanidoethyl) disulfide given orally in protective doses to mice. *Radiation Res.* **20**: 17–23.

LAUBER, K., ZUPPINGER, A. and AEBI, H. (1958) Distribution pattern and retention of cysteinamine-^{35}S in mammals. *U.N. 2nd Intern. Conf. Peaceful Uses Atomic Energy, Geneva* **25**: 97–9.

LAUBER, K., AEBI, H. and ZUPPINGER, A. (1960) Untersuchungen über die [35]S Retention nach Belastung mit [35]S Cysteamin bei der Ratte. *Biochem. Zeitschr.* **332**: 434–48.

LELIÈVRE, P. (1959) Une méthode de dosage chimique de la cystéamine dans les milieux biologiques. *Bull. Soc. Chim. Biol.* **41**: 1207–21.

LELIÈVRE, P. (1961) *Contribution à l'étude de l'interaction cystamine-protéines sulfhydrylées. Quelques conséquences sur le plan biologique.* Thèse de Doctorat, Université de Liège.

LÉONARD, A. and MAISIN, J. R. (1964) Effect of 2-β-aminoethylisothiourea (AET) against genetic damages induced by X-irradiation of male mice. *Radiation Res.* **23**: 53.

MAISIN, J. R. (1966) *Radiations ionisantes, radioprotecteurs et syndrome gastro-intestinal.* Masson et Cie, Paris, p. 193.

MAISIN, J. R. and LÉONARD, A. (1963) Etude autoradiographique de la localisation de l'AET dans les tissus de la souris. *C.R. Soc. Biol.* **157**: 203–6.

MAISIN, J. R., LÉONARD, A. and HUGON, J. (1965) Tissue and cellular distribution of tritium-labeled AET in mice. *J. Natl. Cancer Inst.* **35**: 103–12.

MASUROVSKY, E. B. and BUNGF, R. P. (1969) Radiation protection in mammalian spinal ganglion cultures treated with AET derivatives. *Acta Radiologica; Therapy Physics Biology* **8**: 38–54.

MERLEVELDE, E. and CASIER, H. (1961) Teneur en sulfure de carbone de l'air expiré chez des personnes normales ou sous l'influence de l'éthanol au cours du traitement par antabuse (disulfiram) et *N*-diéthyldithiocarbamate de soude. *Arch. Int. Pharmacodyn.* **132**: 427–44.

MONDOVI, B. and TENTORI, L. (1961) Metabolite della cistamina ^{35}S nel ratto. *Giorn. Biochim.* **10**: 444–52.

MONDOVI, B., TENTORI, L., DE MARCO, C. and CAVALLINI, D. (1962) Distribution of cystamine ^{35}S in the subcellular particles of the organs of the rats. *Int. J. Rad. Biol.* **4**: 371–8.

MUNDY, R. L., HEIFFER, M. H. and LEIFHEIT, H. C. (1961) Blood and urine sulfhydryl and disulfide levels after large doses of mercaptoethylamine or cystamine. *Radiation Res.* **14**: 421–5.

NAKKEN, K. F. (1960) The interreaction of mercaptoamines with pyridoxal-5-phosphate. *Acta Physiol. Scand.* **50** suppl. 175, 109.

NELSON, A. and ULLBERG, S. (1960) Distribution of ^{35}S in mice after injection of ^{35}S-cysteamine. *Acta Radiol.* **53**: 305–13.

NESBAKKEN, R. and ELDJARN, L. (1963) The inhibition of hexokinase by disulfide. *Biochem. J.* **87**: 526–32.

NUZHDIN, N. I. and NIZHNIK, G. V. (1965) Protection of spermatozoa of rabbits against genetic damage caused by irradiation *in vitro*. *Tr. Inst. Genet. Akad. Nauk SSR* **32**: 229–37.

PIHL, A. and ELDJARN, L. (1957) Studies on the mechanism of protection against ionizing radiation by compounds of the cysteamine–cysteine group. *Advances in Radiobiology,* Oliver & Boyd, Edinburgh, pp. 147–59.

PIHL, A., ELDJARN, L. and BREMER, J. (1957) On the mode of action of X-ray protective agents. *J.B.C.* **227**: 339–45.

PLIESS, G. and HERBERT, F. (1963) Autoradiographic studies with a radiation protection material. *Strahlenther.* Sonderbände **52**: 295–301.

RUSANOV, A. M. (1961) Pharmacological characteristics of certain mercaptoamines and their effectiveness in the prophylaxis of radiation sickness. In: *Diagnosis and Treatment of Acute Radiation Injury.* W.H.O., Geneva, pp. 347–60.

SALVADOR, R. A., DAVISON, C. and SMITH, P. K. (1957) Metabolism of cysteamine. *J. Pharmacol. Exptl. Therap.* **121**: 258–65.

SHAPIRO, B., SCHWARZ, E. E. and KOLLMANN, G. (1962) Further studies on the distribution and metabolism of 2-mercapto-ethyl guanidine and bis(2-guanidoethyl) disulfide in mice. *School of Aerospace Medicine, Brooks A.F. Base, Tex. SAM TDR,* 62–8.

SHAPIRO, B., KOLLMANN, G. and SCHWARZ, E. E. (1963a) The distribution and chemical forms of AET administered as bis(2-guanidoethyl) disulfide in irradiated mice. *Radiation Res.* **19**: 230.

SHAPIRO, B., SCHWARZ, E. E. and KOLLMANN, G. (1963b) The distribution and the chemical forms of the radiation protective agents AET in mammary tumour bearing mice. *Cancer Res.* **23**: 223–8.

SHAPIRO, B., SCHWARZ, E. E. and KOLLMANN, G. (1963c) The mechanism of action of AET. IV. Distribution and chemical forms of 2-mercaptoethylguanidine and bis(2-guanido-ethyl) disulfide in protected mice. *Radiation Res.* **18**: 17–30.

SHAPIRO, B., KOLLMANN, G. and SCHWARZ, E. E. (1964) The distribution and metabolism of orally administered 2-mercaptoethylguanidine and bis(2-guanidoethyl) disulfide in protected mice. *Ann. N.Y. Acad. Sci.* **114**: 597–601.

SHAPIRO, B., KOLLMANN, G. and MARTIN, D. (1970) Mechanism of action of radiation protective agents: *In vivo* distribution and metabolism of cysteamine-*S*-phosphate (MEAP). *Radiation Res.* **44**: 421–33.

SHIGETOSHI, A. (1964) The mechanism of chemical protection against ionizing radiation. II. Distribution of ^{35}S-MEG in various tissues in mice injected with ^{35}S-MEG. III. Sulfhydryl contents in various tissues of mice injected with mercaptoethylguanidine. *Proc. Res. Inst. Nucl. Med. Biol. (Japan)* **5**: 64–5 and 76–9.

STRÖMME, J. H. (1963a) Methemoglobine formation induced by thiols. *Biochem. Pharmacol.* **12**: 937–46.

STRÖMME, J. H. (1963b) Inhibition of hexokinase by disulfiram and *N*-diethyldithio-carbamate. *Biochem. Pharmacol.* **12**: 705–15.

STRÖMME, J. H. (1965a) Interactions of disulfiram and *N*-diethyldithiocarbamate with serum proteins studied by means of a gel filtration technique. *Biochem. Pharmacol.* **14**: 380–91.

STRÖMME, J. H. (1965b) Metabolism of disulfiram and *N*-diethyldithiocarbamate in rats with demonstration of an *in vivo* ethanol induced inhibition of the glycuronic acid conjugation of the thiol. *Biochem. Pharmacol.* **14**: 393–410.

STRÖMME, J. H. and ELDJARN, L. (1966) Distribution and chemical forms of *N*-diethyl-dithiocarbamate and tetraethylthiuram disulfide (disulfiram) in mice in relation to radioprotection. *Biochem. Pharmacol.* **15**: 287–97.

URBACH, F. (1962) Anatomy and pathophysiology of skin tumor capillaries. *Nat. Cancer. Inst. Monogr.* 10. Conf. on Biol. of Cutaneous Cancer, pp. 539–59.

VERLY, W. G. (1955) Le métabolisme de la cystéamine. *Bull. Acad. Méd. Belg.* VIth series, **20**: 447–64.

VERLY, W. G. and KOCH, G. (1954) Metabolism of β-mercaptoethylamine. II. In the dog. *Biochem. J.* **58**: 663–5.

VERLY, W. G., BACQ, Z. M., RAYET, P. and URBAIN, M. (1954a) Distribution du soufre radioactif après injection intrapéritonéale à la souris de benzoate de ^{35}S mercapto-éthylamine. *Biochim. Biophys. Acta* 1: 233–5.

VERLY, W. G., GREGOIRE, S., RAYET, P. and URBAIN, M. F. (1954b) Metabolism of β-mercaptoethylamine. I. In mice. *Biochem. J.* 58: 660–2.

VLADIMIROV, V. G. (1967) Intracellular distribution of ^{35}S in the liver and spleen of white mice after injection of ^{35}S-labeled $S,β$-aminoethylisothiouronium, cystamine and 5-thiopentylamine disulfide. *Radiobiologyia* 7: 71–5.

YARMONENKO, S. P., OVAKIMOV, V. G., PALYGA, G. F., FEDOSEEV, V. M. and TARASENKO, A. G. (1965) Action of chemical radioprotectors during fractionated irradiation. I. AET distribution in the animal organism as a function of protector dose, means of administration and irradiation conditions. *Radiobiologyia* 5: 423–7.

CHAPTER 6

METABOLIC EFFECTS OF SULFUR-CONTAINING RADIOPROTECTIVE AGENTS*

P. Lelièvre and C. Liébecq

Liège, Belgium

6.1. RESPIRATION AND RESPIRATORY QUOTIENT IN LIVING ANIMALS

In higher organisms and particularly in mammals, the central nervous system has an important place among the functional control systems and enables the organism, through nervous reflexes, to react very rapidly to stimuli coming from outside or inside the organism. These stimuli, such as a variation in temperature, are accompanied by a transient variation of the activity of a certain number of enzyme systems. Pospíšil and Novak (1957) and Novak (1958) measured the adaptative respiratory exchange to estimate the variations in the activities of the central nervous system and its enzyme systems.

6.1.1. EFFECTS OF RADIOPROTECTIVE AGENTS IN MICE

Novak and Vacek (1959) observed that intraperitoneal (i.p.) administration of cysteine in mice (1 g/kg) decreases the O_2 consumption and

---

Thiols and disulfides. AET, S-(aminoethyl)isothiourea; MEG, mercaptoethylguanidine; GED, *bis*(guanidinoethyl) disulfide; GSH, glutathione; GSSG, oxidized glutathione.

Pyridine nucleotides. NAD and NADP, nicotinamide adenine dinucleotide and its phosphate (NAD^+ and $NADP^+$ for the oxidized forms; NADH and NADPH for the reduced forms).

Others. ATP and ADP, adenosine tri- and diphosphates; EDTA, ethylenediamine tetraacetate.

Code numbers of enzymes [EC]:

Aconitase, or aconitate hydratase, or citrate (isocitrate) hydro-lyase [4.2.1.3]; adenosinetriphosphatase, or ATPase, or ATP phosphohydrolase [3.6.1.3]; aldolase, or fructose-1,

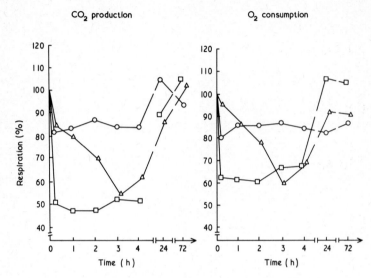

FIG. 1. CO_2 production and O_2 consumption in mice injected with cysteine. o, controls receiving no injection; △, controls receiving physiological saline; □, mice receiving 0.3–1.5 g L-cysteine/kg. (Novak, 1966.)

6-*bis*-phosphate D-glyceraldehyde-3-phosphate-lyase [4.1.2.13]; *S*-aryl transferase [no EC number]; catalase, or hydrogen-peroxide: hydrogen-peroxide oxidoreductase [1.11.1.6]; citrate synthase, or condensing enzyme, or citrate-oxaloacetate-lyase (CoA-acetylating) [4.1.3.7]; cytochrome oxidase, or ferrocytochrome c: oxygen oxidoreductase [1.9.3.1]; diamine oxidase, or diamine: oxygen oxidoreductase (deaminating) [1.4.3.6]; *S*-epoxide transferase [no EC number]; glucose-6-phosphate dehydrogenase, or D-glucose-6-phosphate: $NADP^+$ oxidoreductase [1.1.1.49]; glutamate dehydrogenase, or L-glutamate: NAD^+ oxidoreductase (deaminating) [1.4.1.2]; glutathione-homocystine transhydrogenase, or glutathione: homocystine oxidoreductase [1.8.4.1]; glutathione-insulin-transhydrogenase, in fact a protein disulfide reductase, or glutathione: protein-disulfide oxidoreductase [1.8.4.2]; glutathione peroxidase, or glutathione: hydrogen peroxide oxidoreductase [1.11.1.9]; glutathione reductase, or NAD(P)H: oxidized-glutathione oxidoreductase [1.6.4.2]; glyceraldehydephosphate dehydrogenase, or triosephosphate dehydrogenase, or D-glyceraldehyde-3-phosphate: NAD^+ oxidoreductase (phosphorylating) [1.2.1.12]; hexokinase, or ATP-hexose-6-phosphotransferase [2.7.1.1]; β-hydroxybutyrate dehydrogenase, or D-3-hydroxybutyrate: NAD^+ oxidoreductase [1.1.1.30]; 2-oxoglutarate dehydrogenase, or 2-oxoglutarate: lipoate oxidoreductase (decarboxylating and acceptor succinylating) [1.2.4.2]; lactate dehydrogenase, or L-lactate: NAD^+ oxidoreductase [1.1.1.27]; lipoyl dehydrogenase, or lipoamide dehydrogenase, or reduced NAD: lipoamide oxidoreductase [1.6.4.3]; malate dehydrogenase, or L-malate: NAD^+ oxidoreductase [1.1.1.37]; nitroglycerol reductase [no EC number]; phosphofructokinase, or ATP: D-fructose-6-phosphate 1-phosphotransferase [2.7.1.11]; pyruvate dehydrogenase, or pyruvate: lipoate oxidoreductase (acceptor acetylating) [1.2.4.1]; succinate dehydrogenase, or succinate: (acceptor) oxidoreductase [1.3.99.1]; triosephosphate isomerase, or D-glyceraldehyde-3-phosphate ketol-isomerase [5.3.1.1].

CO_2 elimination within 15 min. This effect is still present 4 hr later. Twenty-four hours later, when there is no longer any radioprotective action, values slightly higher than normal are observed, and after 72 hr O_2 consumption and CO_2 production return to normal (Fig. 1). Lowering of the O_2 absorption and CO_2 elimination do not develop in a parallel manner, so that the respiratory quotient varies. A few minutes after the injection of cysteine, it drops to 0.7, and 4 hr later it reaches 0.64. This alteration of the metabolism, induced by the radioprotective agent, is quite considerable, since 24 hr after the start of the experiment, the respiratory quotient is still lowered if compared to that of control animals and returns to normal only about 72 hr later.

The extent of the metabolic disturbance caused by the injection of radioprotective agents varies according to the quantity of the compound injected. Using non-toxic doses of cysteine (up to 1.5 g/kg), the O_2 consumption and elimination of CO_2 decrease in parallel with the dose injected. With larger doses (3 g/kg), respiration again increases. However, if the dose of cysteine is increased to 6 g/kg, one again sees a lowering of O_2 consumption and of CO_2 elimination (Fig. 2). It is probable that toxic doses which cause the more or less rapid death of the animal bring in other mechanisms to disturb the metabolism.

The respiratory quotient also varies according to the dose of cysteine administered to the animal, but its change does not parallel the change in O_2 consumption and CO_2 elimination. With increasing non-toxic doses (0.5 g/kg), a lowering of the respiratory quotient is observed. On the

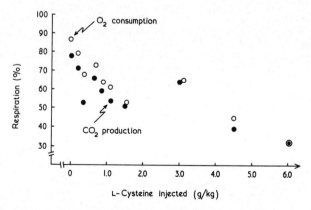

FIG. 2. O_2 consumption (o) and CO_2 production (●) in mice injected with L-cysteine. Mean values of measurements taken after 15, 60, and 120 min. (Novak, 1966.)

other hand, toxic doses (4 g/kg) of cysteine bring the respiratory quotient back to levels similar to those of control animals.

Other sulfur-containing radioprotective agents, especially cystamine succinate and aminoethylisothiourea (AET), in radioprotective doses, bring about a lowering of the respiratory quotient in mice; there appears to be some correlation between the fall of the respiratory quotient and the radioprotective efficiency of the compound used (Novak and Vacek, 1959). These results were confirmed by Locker and Pany (1964), who also observed in mice, after the i.p. injection of a radioprotective dose of cysteamine (MEA) or of mercaptoethylguanidine (MEG), a lowering of O_2 consumption that reaches a maximum about 15 min after injection. After 90 min, the O_2 consumption is brought to a level comparable with, or slightly higher than, that of the control animals.

They also stated that higher doses of MEA which cause severe poisoning, also after a phase of depression, cause an increase in O_2 consumption, which they attribute to the animals' abnormal motor activity at that time (Fig. 3).

Novak *et al.* (1967) compare certain sulfur-containing radioprotective agents (MEA and cysteine) with the non-sulfur-containing radioprotective

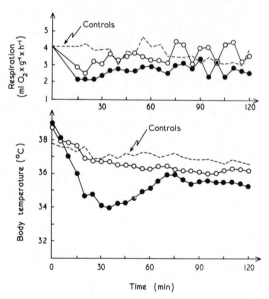

Fig. 3. Effect of MEA injection on the O_2 consumption and body temperature of mice. ----, controls; o, 100 mg/kg MEA; •, 250 mg MEA/kg. (Locker and Pany, 1964.)

agent, fluoroacetate, from the point of view of their effect on the O_2 consumption and respiratory quotient.

They stated that the respiratory quotient of mice treated with a radioprotective dose of fluoroacetate (5 mg/kg) is lowered during the period of radioprotective action. These variations are comparable to those caused by the administration of cysteine or MEA.

These authors also stated that a lowering of body temperature occurs in mice during the period of radioprotection, after treatment with fluoroacetate, as already noted by Bacq *et al.* (1960).

6.1.2. EFFECT OF RADIOPROTECTIVE AGENTS IN RATS

Novak and Vacek (1959) obtained similar results in rats, but less marked than those in mice (Fig. 4). A radioprotective injection of MEA (100 mg/kg) also causes a lowering of O_2 consumption and CO_2 elimination: these variations are less significant than those in mice. Initially the respiratory quotient of the rat is less than that of the mouse (about 0.7) and it alters relatively little after injection of MEA. Later, an increase of up to 0.8 in the respiratory quotient is observed. Romantsev and Savitch (1958) also observed that a dose of 150 mg/kg of MEA administered to a rat reduces its oxygen consumption, the maximum depression being

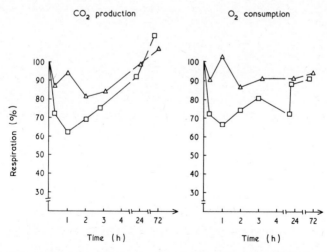

FIG. 4. CO_2 production and O_2 consumption in rats injected with MEA. $\triangle$, controls receiving physiological saline; $\square$, 100 mg MEA/kg (Novak, 1966.)

reached 20–50 min after injection. Eighteen hours after the MEA is injected, the oxygen consumption becomes normal again.

Betz *et al.* (1967), studying the possible relation between the living animal's O_2 consumption and the radioprotective efficacy of certain sulfur-containing protective agents, observed that MEA and cystamine in a dose of 100 mg/kg rapidly and considerably reduced the rat O_2 consumption. The maximum effect is obtained 10–20 min after injection, and is followed by progressive recovery (Table 1).

Under similar conditions, cysteine (1 g/kg) also produces a lower consumption of O_2, but this is less pronounced than that caused by the two radioprotective agents mentioned above. 2-Mercaptoethanol, or its oxidation product in equimolecular doses, does not affect O_2 consumption. There is some correlation between the lowering of the O_2 consumption and the radioprotective action. Actually, 10 min after the compound is injected, radioprotective action reaches a high level, coincident with a severe lessening of the O_2 consumption. The radioprotection then remains stationary, or decreases slightly with time, and then

TABLE 1. INHIBITION OF THE RESPIRATION OF THE RAT AFTER ADMINISTRATION OF VARIOUS RADIOPROTECTIVE AGENTS (Modified from Lelièvre, 1965c and Betz *et al.*, 1967)

Compound tested[a]	Respiration (%) after					
	10 min	20 min	30 min	45 min	60 min	90 min
Cystamine	57	60	62	64	69	86
MEA	54	66	73	75	83	93
Cysteine	66	74	78	80	94	100
GSH	69	61	62	64	70	86
MEG	64	64	62	64	73	92
GED	64	65	64	61	67	87
Diethyldithio-carbamate	71	75	67	64	63	76
Histamine	47	67	81	94	103	109
5-HT	47	60	73	83	89	92
Epinephrine	55	64	70	80	85	93
Cyanide	31	65	85	95	98	100
Thiourea	59	66	65	71	74	92
EDTA	65	66	66	67	77	93
2-Mercaptoethanol	103	102	99	100	99	99

[a] Doses injected: cystamine. $(HCl)_2$ and MEA.HCl, 100 mg/kg; cysteine.HCl.H_2O and GSH, 1 g/kg; MEG.HBr and GED.$(HBr)_2$, 175 mg/kg; sodium diethyldithiocarbamate, 700 mg/kg; histamine.HCl, 150 mg/kg; 5-HT (5-HT–creatinine-sulfate complex), 160 mg/kg; epinephrine.HCl, 1.25 mg/kg; sodium cyanide, 3 mg/kg; thiourea, 2.5 g/kg; Na_2H_2–EDTA, 250 mg/kg; 2-mercaptoethanol, 100 mg/kg.

TABLE 2. THIRTY-DAY SURVIVAL IN GROUPS OF RATS EXPOSED TO A WHOLE-BODY IRRADIATION OF 900 R AT VARIOUS INTERVALS AFTER ADMINISTRATION OF SULFUR-CONTAINING COMPOUNDS (From Betz *et al.*, 1967)

Interval after administration of the compound (min)	Survival[a] ($\% \pm$ S.D.) after administration of			
	MEA	Cystamine	Cysteine	Mercapto-ethanol
2	0	8 ± 5	0	0
10	33 ± 7	60 ± 7	23 ± 7	0
20	28 ± 8	47 ± 8	30 ± 8	
30	21 ± 8	40 ± 10		0
45	47 ± 7	73 ± 6	22 ± 6	0
60	19 ± 7	47 ± 13	20 ± 7	0
90	19 ± 7	16 ± 7	25 ± 10	

[a] No survival in the non-injected control groups.

noticeably increases about 45 min after injection (Table 2). At this time a partial recovery of O_2 consumption is already observed. The 2-mercapto-ethanol provides no protection against X-rays and in no way affects the O_2 consumption.

Injecting cystamine (100 mg/kg) causes the rat respiratory quotient to increase 10 min after the injection, and the increase is maintained until 60 min, and then disappears (Lelièvre *et al.*, 1969) (Table 3).

Cysteamine has a similar effect, although less marked, and the differences, taken singly, are not statistically significant, but from 10 min to 45 min, all respiratory quotients are subject to an increase. The effect of cysteine is less, and is not statistically significant.

Animals fasted for 72 hr show, as would be expected, a lower respiratory quotient than that of fed animals. After injection with sulfur-containing protective agents, the respiratory quotient varies in the same way as that of normally fed animals but to a less marked degree (Table 3).

Other sulfur-containing and non-sulfur-containing radioprotective agents were also tested for their possible action on the O_2 consumption of the rat *in vivo*. The results are shown in Table 1 (Lelièvre, 1965c): all the sulfur-containing radioprotective agents tested (*N*-diethyldithio-carbamate (DEDTC), reduced glutathione (GSH), thiourea, MEG and GED) reduce the consumption of O_2. The extent of this lowering and its development with time vary according to the nature of the compound tested. Finally, other non-sulfur-containing radioprotective substances,

TABLE 3. RESPIRATORY QUOTIENTS OF RATS INJECTED WITH SULFUR-CONTAINING
RADIOPROTECTIVE AGENTS (From Lelièvre *et al.*, 1969)

Time after injection (min)	Respiratory quotients after injection[a] of		
	Cystamine	MEA	Cysteine
Fed			
0	0.80	0.80	0.79
10	0.91	0.85	0.84
20	0.96	0.84	0.79
30	0.95	0.88	0.79
45	0.92	0.83	0.80
60	0.89	0.79	0.79
90	0.85	0.79	0.79
Fasted			
0	0.71	0.73	0.73
10	0.71	0.84	0.75
20	0.79	0.85	0.75
30	0.81	0.83	0.75
45	0.80	0.76	0.71
60	0.76	0.75	0.72
90	0.72	0.71	0.70

[a]Doses injected: cystamine.$(HCl)_2$ and MEA.HCl, 100 mg/kg; cysteine.HCl.H_2O, 1 g/kg.

potassium cyanide, ethylenediamine tetraacetate (EDTA), serotonin (5-HT), histamine, and epinephrine, also have the effect of reducing the quantity of O_2 consumed by the animal.

It should also be noted that MEG or MEA administered to the rat in a radioprotective dose before irradiation impedes the increase in O_2 consumption that is observed during the irradiation of non-protected animals. Belokonskii (1959) observes that in rats whose radioresistance has increased by becoming accustomed to hypoxia, or reduced by the opposite treatment (hyperoxia), there is, just as in normal rats, an increase of O_2 consumption during irradiation of the order of 30 %. The differences of radiosensitivity in no way affect this "O_2 effect" during irradiation.

6.1.3. ACTION OF RADIOPROTECTIVE AGENTS IN MAN

In man, the oral ingestion of a dose of cystamine of the order of 0.2–0.6 g (apparently insufficient to protect against a lethal dose of X-rays) increases the O_2 consumption and the metabolic rate. Mercaptoethylguanidine, however, in the same doses, causes a fall in metabolic rate, and lowers the O_2 consumption (Kuznetsov and Kushakovskii, 1963).

6.1.4. HYPOTHERMIA

Parallel with the changes in O_2 consumption, Locker and Pany (1964) measured the variations in body temperature in animals after the administration of radioprotective agents. They showed that MEA and MEG cause a drop in the body temperature of the mouse, which becomes more marked as the injected dose is increased (Fig. 3).

This action of cystamine on the body temperature has already been mentioned. Betz *et al.* (1962) showed that, in rats, after the administration of a radioprotective dose of cystamine (100 mg/kg) a body temperature drop occurs, which reaches a minimum value after about $2\frac{1}{2}$ hr. At that time there is no longer any radioprotective action. The body temperature drop observed by Locker and Pany (1964) in mice after treatment with cystamine is less than that observed in rats under the same conditions. It should be noted that the temperature of the rat or mouse after treatment with cystamine continues to decrease, and it remains at a level below normal when the O_2 consumption has returned to normal. The relation between hypothermia and radioprotective action has been studied in detail by Bacq *et al.* (1965a).

6.1.5. DISCUSSION

Novak (1966) considers that the lowering of the respiratory quotient in mice after the administration of a sulfur-containing radioprotective agent indicates a slowing down of the carbohydrate metabolism which could be due to an effect of the radioprotective agent on enzyme systems or on cellular structures. The following observations argue in favor of such a hypothesis:

(a) The rapid distribution of the sulfur-containing radioprotective agents (cysteine or cystamine) in the organism immediately after injection (Patt *et al.*, 1950; Verly, 1955; Lelièvre, 1959; Lelièvre *et al.*, 1963) and particularly the appearance of a high but transitory content of the cerebral tissue in the radioprotective agent.

(b) The observations of Betz *et al.* (1962) and Smoliar and Betz (1962) show the best period of radioprotective action in rats to be 10–45 min after the injection of MEA or cystamine.

(c) The disturbances in the metabolism of the carbohydrates in the presence of cystamine, which can be summarized as follows: inhibition of the anaerobic glycolysis and of hexokinase, inhibition of oxygen consumption by homogenates or mitochondria of tissues or suspensions of cells *in vitro*, and disturbances of oxidative phosphorylation (Lelièvre, 1959; Lelièvre, 1960; Lelièvre and Betz, 1963; Lelièvre 1965a; Ciccarone and Milani, 1964; Nesbakken and Eldjarn, 1963). Ciccarone (1965) and Ciccarone and Bacq (1966) show that the injection of a radioprotective dose of cystamine (170 mg/kg) or of 5-HT (80 mg/kg) inhibits, in the presence of pyruvate, the oxygen consumption of liver slices from animals injected 10–20 min before.

(d) Numerous observations indicate that the integrity of cellular structures is attacked (Emmelot *et al.*, 1962; Hugon *et al.*, 1964; Maisin *et al.*, 1964; Firket and Lelièvre, 1966) by the action of cystamine, AET, or MEA. It is certain that the deep structural changes of mitochondria lead to considerable disturbances of oxidative metabolism.

In rats, in contrast to mice, an increase of the respiratory quotient after treatment with MEA or cystamine is observed (Lelièvre *et al.*, 1969). Novak (1966) points out that the administration of MEA in radio-protective doses for rats only slightly modifies the respiratory quotient in the first few minutes after injection, but that there is a clear increase in the respiratory quotient later on.

The hypothesis of a change in the energy-producing metabolism toward an increased use of carbohydrates cannot be excluded, although it is not supported by observations showing that cystamine inhibits cellular oxidation. Also the increase in respiratory quotient persists when the rats are fasted and their reserves of glycogen are exhausted. This fact also argues against an increased consumption of carbohydrates. One may well ask whether the increase in the respiratory quotient observed is not related to tissue anoxia and acidosis, which liberates a certain quantity of carbon dioxide from the bicarbonate pools. In support of this hypothesis, there is a close correlation between tissue hypoxia and changes in the respiratory quotient.

The mechanisms by which radioprotective agents lower the O_2 consumption certainly differ according to the nature of the compound used. Sulfur-containing radioprotective agents may directly interfere with essential reactions, e.g. inhibition of an enzyme system.

Fluoroacetate must be metabolized first and then be incorporated in a molecule of fluorocitrate before it is able to inhibit aconitase (Peters, 1952). The biological amines, histamine and tryptamine, seem to intervene through their pharmacological activities (van der Meer and van Bekkum, 1959, 1961). In normal animals, cyanide produces hypoxia in the spleen and bone-marrow, caused by vasoconstriction following vaso-motor stimulation (van der Meer *et al.*, 1962).

All things considered, as far as sulfur-containing radioprotective agents are concerned, their effect on O_2 consumption is not directly linked to the addition of a certain quantity of thiol or disulfide groups. Indeed, 2-mercaptoethanol, reduced or oxidized and administered in equimolar doses to those of cystamine or MEA, adds to the organism the same amounts of thiols or disulfides. However, the 2-mercaptoethanol produces no radioprotection in rats or mice, and does not affect either the O_2 consumption or the respiratory quotient.

6.2. OXYGEN TENSION IN LIVING TISSUES

It is well known that O_2 plays an important role in the action of X-rays. Oxygen at normal partial pressure (about 150 mmHg) multiplies the intensity of X-ray action by a factor of 2 or 3 in a large majority of biological systems (Gray and Scott, 1964). Total or partial anoxia has an opposite effect, and diminishes considerably the action of ionizing radiation (Bacq and Alexander, 1955, 1961). The hypothesis has been expressed that the radioprotective activity of certain compounds could be due to anoxia induced at radiosensitive sites.

Salerno and Friedell (1954) and Salerno et al. (1955) have shown that cysteine administered to a rat or to a dog in a radioprotective dose causes a lowering of the O_2 content of the blood in the femoral vein, although the O_2 pressure in the blood of the femoral artery remains normal. This deoxygenation of the venous blood develops in a manner similar to the radioprotection. Cysteamine, injected under similar conditions in a radioprotective dose, does not alter the O_2 content of the venous or arterial blood (Salerno and Friedell, 1954). Cystamine behaves like cysteine and distinctly lowers the O_2 content of the venous blood in rats.

These results were confirmed by Bacq et al. (1955) who observed that blood taken from the inferior vena cava of the rat 10 min after injection of nembutal and cystamine (the latter in a dose of 150 mg/kg) is much more deoxygenated than that of the control animals who have not received cystamine.

This deoxygenation of the venous blood is not due to an increased consumption of O_2, because the same authors have shown that the administration of cystamine causes a slight lowering of the O_2 consumption. Bacq et al. (1955) attribute this pronounced deoxygenation of venous blood to a decreased rate of blood flow.

Implanting electrodes in tissues made it possible to measure the O_2

content at properly selected places. The results obtained with this method provide information on the O_2 pressure in the interstitial fluid in contact with the cells, but give no precise information on the intracellular O_2 pressure. The sulfur-containing radioprotective agents (cysteine, MEA, cystamine, AET) do not systematically cause intra-tissue anoxia.

6.2.1. EFFECT OF CYSTEINE

Cater (1960) observed that the administration of cysteine in rats does not cause variations in the partial pressure of O_2 in the mammary gland during lactation, but the doses injected were small and gave no radio-protection. An analogous observation was made by Grayevsky *et al.* (1962), who showed that the administration of a radioprotective dose of cysteine to a mouse does not change the partial pressure of O_2 in the spleen and liver. The experiments of van der Meer *et al.* (1961) partly confirm Grayevsky's observations. These authors find that injection of a radioprotective dose of cysteine in a mouse may alter the O_2 content of the spleen in different ways. In certain cases, the extracellular O_2 pressure remains unchanged. Against this, other tests provide results indicating a positive or negative variation in the O_2 content of the tissue. It is only with very high, just sub-lethal doses of cysteine that a considerable lowering of the tissue O_2 content is observed. The same variations in partial pressure of O_2 are observed in the femoral bone-marrow (Table 4).

In rats (van der Meer *et al.*, 1961), a radioprotective dose of cysteine causes variations of the oxygen content of the bone-marrow similar to those observed in mice. There is either a decrease, an increase, or no change in the partial pressure of O_2. In the spleen, however, it seems that a strong dose of cysteine causes a constant drop in the dissolved O_2 content, reproducible from animal to animal (van der Meer *et al.*, 1961) (Table 5).

These observations on the partial pressure of O_2 in the spleen after treatment with cysteine were confirmed subsequently (Lelièvre *et al.*, 1969). After injecting the rat with a radioprotective dose of cysteine (1 g/kg), a slight but not significant hypoxia in the spleen is observed after 10 min; after that, the O_2 partial pressure rapidly returns to normal.

6.2.2. EFFECT OF AET

Aminoethylisothiourea, administered in mice in the form of MEG in a radioprotective dose, has an irregular action on the O_2 pressure in the spleen, but always in the direction of increasing it (van der Meer *et al.*,

TABLE 4. CHANGES IN THE O_2 PARTIAL PRESSURE IN VARIOUS ORGANS AFTER INJECTION OF RADIOPROTECTIVE AGENTS (From Bacq, 1965)

Compound	Animal	Organ	Result	Reference
Cysteine	Rat	Lactating mammary gland	0	Cater (1960)
	Mouse	Spleen and liver	0	Grayevsky et al. (1961)
	Rat	Spleen	↑, 0, or ↓→	van der Meer et al. (1961)
		Bone-marrow	↑	van der Meer et al. (1961)
		Spleen	↑ to ↓↓	van der Meer et al. (1961)
		Bone-marrow	↑ to →	van der Meer et al. (1961)
Cysteamine	Mouse	Spleen and liver	0	Grayevsky et al. (1961)
		Spleen and bone-marrow	↑ to →	van der Meer et al. (1961)
	Rat	Spleen	↑ or 0	van der Meer et al. (1961)
Cystamine	Mouse	Spleen	↓↓ or 0	van der Meer et al. (1961)
		Spleen and liver	0	Grayevsky et al. (1961)
AET	Mouse	Spleen	↑↑	Zeitounian et al. (1962)
		Liver	↑	Zeitounian et al. (1962)
		Spleen and liver	0	Grayevsky et al. (1961)
		Spleen	↑	van der Meer et al. (1961)
Thiourea	Mouse	Spleen	±	Zeitounian et al. (1962)
		Liver	↓→	Zeitounian et al. (1962)
KCN	Mouse	Spleen	↓↓↓	van der Meer et al. (1962)
		Spleen and liver	0	Grayevsky et al. (1960)

TABLE 5. CHANGES IN THE O_2 TENSION IN THE SPLEEN AND BONE-MARROW AFTER INJECTION OF RADIOPROTECTIVE AGENTS
(Modified from van der Meer *et al.* 1961)

Animal	Compound tested (g/kg)	Organ	Number of animals	Number of animals showing changes of		
				more than −10%	from −10 to +10%	more than +10%
Mouse	Cysteamine (0.15)	Spleen	18	6	2	10
		Femur	4	2	—	2
	Cystamine (0.25)	Spleen	10	10	—	—
	Cysteine (1.3)	Spleen	6	2	1	3
	AET (0.15)	Spleen	5	1	—	4
Rat	Cysteamine (0.1)	Spleen	11	1	1	9
	Cysteine (1.0)	Spleen	6	1	—	5
	(1.5)	Femur	3	1	—	2
	(2.0)	Spleen	6	5	—	1

1961). These results are not confirmed by Grayevsky *et al.* (1961) who find no change in the partial pressure of O_2 in the liver and spleen after injecting mice with MEG. Against this, Zeïtounian *et al.* (1962) confirm the results of van der Meer *et al.* (1961), and observe, after treatment with MEG, a distinct increase in the O_2 pressure in the spleen, and to a lesser degree in the liver (Table 4).

6.2.3. EFFECT OF MEA AND CYSTAMINE

Grayevsky *et al.* (1961) observed no variations of O_2 pressure in the spleen and liver of mice treated with a radioprotective dose of MEA. Against this, van der Meer *et al.* (1961) find that similar treatment causes positive or negative variations of the partial pressure of O_2 in the bone-marrow of mice (Table 4).

After treatment with cystamine, Grayevsky *et al.* (1961) found no change at all in the partial pressure of O_2 in the liver or spleen of mice. On the contrary, van der Meer *et al.* (1961) observed a very distinct drop in the spleen (Table 5).

In rats, after a MEA injection, van der Meer *et al.* (1961) observed that the partial pressure of O_2 in the spleen may remain unchanged, or may increase. However, Lelièvre *et al.* (1969) showed that MEA causes a definite drop in partial pressure of O_2 in the spleen (Table 6). Cystamine behaves in a similar way, and seems to cause more marked and premature hypoxia than does MEA. The timing is different. Hypoxia due to MEA is more gradual than that caused by cystamine; the maximum is attained

TABLE 6. PARTIAL PRESSURE OF O_2 IN THE SPLEEN OF THE RAT AFTER ADMINISTRATION OF SOME SULFUR-CONTAINING RADIOPROTECTIVE AGENTS (Modified from Lelièvre *et al.*, 1969)

Time after injection (min)	Partial oxygen pressure (% of initial values) after injection[a] of		
	Cystamine	MEA	Cysteine
10	59	82	79
20	59	75	88
30	63	74	94
45	67	77	98
60	74	87	99
90	88	97	100

[a] Doses injected: cystamine.$(HCl)_2$ and MEA.HCl, 100 mg/kg; cysteine.HCl, 1 g/kg.

only after about 20 min. Against this, an equimolar dose of cystamine causes rapid serious hypoxia. These results have been compared with those obtained after treatment of animals with 2-mercaptoethanol, a sulfur-containing substance of structure very similar to that of MEA, but devoid of radioprotective activity. It is shown that 2-mercaptoethanol in no way affects the intra-tissue partial pressure of O_2.

It seems that hypoxia caused by administration of sulfur-containing radioprotective agents cannot be attributed to just one mechanism.

It is known that the —SH group of the sulfur-containing radioprotective agents (MEA, cysteine, MEG, or GSH) can be easily oxidized *in vitro* in a neutral or slightly alkaline solution, producing disulfide. This oxidation is accompanied by a consumption of dissolved O_2. This oxido-reduction may cause hypoxia in certain cases, such as a suspension of cells (Gray, 1956). *In vitro* cysteine may cause sufficient anoxia to protect a suspension of thymocytes against the action of X-rays (van Bekkum and Zaalberg, 1960). In bacterial cultures, according to the experimental conditions, sulfur-containing compounds can drain the O_2 present (Hollaender and Stapleton, 1953; Kohn and Gunter, 1959, 1960).

If one considers the case of an animal injected with a radioprotective dose of cysteine, MEA, or MEG, it is seen that the quantity of O_2 necessary to transform the thiols into disulfides is insignificant in relation to the quantity of O_2 consumed by the animal. Injecting a 20 g mouse with 2 mg MEA base (that is about 0.04 mmol) must involve the consumption of about 0.2 ml of O_2 (at 0°C and 760 mmHg pressure). The O_2 consumption of a 20 g resting mouse can be estimated, according to the authors, at 0.3–0.6 ml/min. As the MEA is not oxidized instantaneously, it cannot reduce the partial pressure of oxygen to a level likely to modify the radio-sensitivity of the tissues. Further, cysteine which at equivalent dose in —SH function is about 5 times less active than MEA as a radioprotective agent, consumes exactly the same quantity of O_2. Finally, it should be noted that the oxidation of MEA in the animal is far from complete, and that a considerable part of the radioprotective agent is eliminated in a reduced form. Cystamine, which is an excellent radioprotective agent, is partly reduced in the organism by the glutathione-reductase system, and excreted in the form of MEA. These arguments suggest that the anoxia cannot be attributed to the oxidation of the radioprotective agent.

The anoxia could be the consequence of a pharmacological effect, for example a slowing down of the blood circulation or prolonged hypotension. In fact, cystamine causes a considerable drop in the arterial pressure in animals (Lecomte, 1952) and also causes a lowering of the

O_2 content of venous blood (Bacq *et al.*, 1955; Heiffer *et al.*, 1961, 1962). Against this, MEA, which is at most only slightly hypotensive in rats (Heiffer *et al.*, 1962), does not affect the O_2 content of the venous blood (Bacq *et al.*, 1955; Salerno and Friedell, 1954).

6.3. CHANGES IN REDOX POTENTIAL

6.3.1. OXYGEN TENSION AND TISSUE RESPIRATION

As already mentioned, the administration of radioprotective agents to animals brings about variable changes in the O_2 tension measured by an electrode, and these essentially relate to extracellular O_2 tension.

6.3.1.1. *Heterogeneity of O_2 Tension*

The absolute measurements made under these conditions have really no physiological significance, because the O_2 tension of the cells in a tissue is extremely variable (this does not apply to the variations in O_2 tension measured with an electrode).

The O_2 tension of the blood diminishes from the arterial extremity of a capillary (where it is of the order of 80 mmHg) toward its venous end (where it is about 40 mmHg). The O_2 tension of the tissue also falls farther away from the capillaries (see Opitz and Schneider, 1950; Diemer, 1963, 1965a, b; Lübbers, 1968). Intracellular O_2 tension is necessarily lower than the surrounding extracellular liquid, and thus varies from one cell to another.

6.3.1.2. *Affinity of Cytochrome Oxidase for O_2*

It should be noted that the affinity of cytochrome oxidase for O_2 is very high; the Michaelis constant, $K_m = 0.5–2 \mu M$, corresponds to an oxygen tension of 0.25–1 mmHg for liver cytochrome oxidase (Chance, 1957). Therefore, the O_2 tension must fall to this level to bring about a reduction of 50 % of the catalytic activity. There is an excess of this enzyme in the respiratory chain.

The measurements by Kessler and Lübbers (1964), and those of Kessler (1968), have shown that the critical tension below which the respiration of isolated liver mitochondria is reduced may range from 1 to 7 mmHg; it seems to depend not on the properties of the mitochondrial catalysts, but rather on the properties of the measuring devices (Starlinger and Lübbers, 1973).

It is not therefore *a priori* that the reduction in O_2 tension already mentioned necessarily causes decreased respiration. So it would seem justified to investigate the possible effects of reduced respiration that might occur as the consequence of lower O_2 content.

6.3.1.3. *Interactions with the Respiratory Chain*

It seems likely that inhibition of respiration by direct action of thiols and disulfides on the respiratory chain may be excluded. Thus, oxidation of succinate and of NADH is not sensitive to cystamine, and the respiration of the intact mitochondria is insensitive to MEA (Skrede *et al.*, 1966). Also, the redox state of the cytochromes a_3, *b* and *c* in the mitochondria is not affected by the presence of MEA (Klingenberg and Liébecq, 1963).

Although it is known that cysteine, glutathione, and MEA can reduce the oxidized cytochromes, and that their corresponding disulfides can reoxidize the reduced cytochromes (Thors and Jackson, 1959), it would appear that these reactions are too slow, as compared with the normal turnover rate of the respiratory catalysts, to affect their steady-state redox potential (Liébecq, 1964). High concentrations of thiols are required to produce only moderate inhibition of cytochrome oxidase (Cooperstein, 1963a, b), a phenomenon partly reversed by adding disulfides.

6.3.2. CELLULAR REDOX POTENTIAL

If the lowered O_2 tension results *per se* in a reduction of activity in the respiratory chain, the NADH formed in the cells will not be normally oxidized and the relative proportions of nucleotides NAD^+ and NADH will be altered, the ratio $NADH/NAD^+$ increasing.

The determination of the ratio [total NADH]/[total NAD^+] is of no value because it does not differentiate between the free and bound nucleotides and it gives no indication whatever of their distribution across the different cellular compartments, which is known to be unequal. The usual method for fractionation of the cellular constituents cannot resolve this problem, because the reduced state of the NAD^+–NADH pair would be affected during the fractionation process.

6.3.2.1. *Cellular Equilibria*

These difficulties can be avoided by measuring the ratio of concentrations of reduced and oxidized metabolites coupled with NAD by the dehydrogenases located in the different cellular compartments. Because of the very high activity of the enzymes catalyzing these reactions, these metabolites are practically in thermodynamic equilibrium with the NAD^+–NADH system according to eqn. (1):

$$\frac{\text{[oxidized substrate] [NADH]}}{\text{[reduced substrate] [NAD}^+\text{]}} = K' = \frac{[K]}{[\text{H}^+]} \tag{1}$$

where K is the equilibrium constant of the reaction. Knowing K' and the pH, the ratio $[\text{NADH}]/[\text{NAD}^+]$ can be calculated from the concentrations of the substrates.

The redox potential can be calculated from eqn. (2):

$$E'_h = E'_o - \frac{RT}{nF} \ln \frac{\text{[reduced substrate]}}{\text{[oxidized substrate]}} \tag{2}$$

where E'_o represents the potential of the half-reduced system at pH 7 and at a temperature equal to the internal temperature of the animal.

6.3.2.2. *Redox Potential of the Cytoplasm*

The ratio $[\text{NADH}]/[\text{NAD}^+]$ of the cytoplasm was measured by Bücher and Klingenberg (1958), and by Hohorst *et al.* (1959), by means of the three ratios: [lactate]/[pyruvate], [α-glycerophosphate]/[dihydroxyacetone phosphate] and [malate]/[oxaloacetate] (see Klingenberg and Bücher, 1960).

The three dehydrogenases establish an equilibrium between their substrate and the free nucleotides that are in the cellular compartment where the dehydrogenases are located. The redox potentials measured by these three systems are identical (Hohorst *et al.*, 1959).

The [lactate]/[pyruvate] ratio of the blood is the one most often measured, because of its convenience. This ratio is the same as in the tissues (Bücher and Klingenberg, 1958), because lactate and pyruvate diffuse quite rapidly, do not become linked with the blood constituents, and because the ratio of their concentrations is not altered by oxidation of lactate into pyruvate, the red cells containing no cytochrome oxidase.

It has been verified that ischemia (Hohorst *et al.*, 1961) and anoxia (Gudbjarnason and Bing, 1962) cause significant changes in the [lactate]/[pyruvate] ratio.

6.3.2.3. *Effect of Sulfur-containing Radioprotective Agents*

Duyckaerts *et al.* (1969), and Duyckaerts and Liébecq (1970), studied the influence of an injection of cystamine on the redox potential of rat or mouse blood. The doses injected correspond to those used by Betz *et al.* (1967), and by Bacq (1966): 68 mg/kg of cystamine or of MEA (base) for rats and 150 mg/kg of cystamine (base) for mice.

They observed that the [lactate]/[pyruvate] ratio in rat blood increases progressively, until it reaches a maximum after 45 min (Fig. 5 and Table 7),

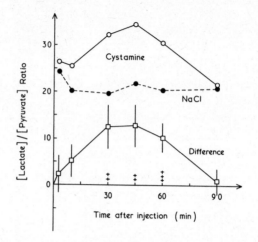

FIG. 5. [Lactate]/[pyruvate] ratio in the blood of rats injected with 68 mg cystamine/ kg. Difference (mean and standard error) statistically significant at the 1% (+ + +) or at the 2% (+ +) level. (Duyckaerts and Liébecq, unpublished graph; cf. Duyckaerts and Liébecq, 1970; Duyckaerts *et al.*, 1969.)

that is to say at the moment when the radioprotection curve as a function of time presents a second maximum (Table 3).

This change in the [lactate]/[pyruvate] ratio corresponds, after correction for changes in the rat's internal temperature, to a drop in the redox potential of 4.7 mV, and a significant increase of the $[NADH]/[NAD^+]$ ratio provided that the pH has not changed (Table 7).

Hyperglycemia is also observed, with a maximum 90 min after cystamine injection. Hypothermia is moderate and maximum between 100 and 300 min after injection.

TABLE 7. REDOX POTENTIAL OF RAT BLOOD 45 MIN AFTER I.P. INJECTION OF A SOLUTION OF 0.2 M CYSTAMINE (68 mg/kg) (From Duyckaerts and Liébecq, 1970)

	Controls	Cystamine	Difference
Lactate (μmol/g)	2.301	4.642	+ 2.341[a]
Pyruvate (μmol/g)	0.113	0.139	+ 0.026
[Lactate]/[Pyruvate]	21.8	34.5	+12.7[a]
Body temperature (°C)	37.54	36.78	− 0.76[a]
E_h (mV)	−245.8	−250.5	− 4.7[a]
$10^3 \times [NaDH]/[NAD^+]$	2.42	3.58	+ 1.16[a]
Glucose (μmol/g)	8.370	9.986	+ 1.615[a]

[a] Statistically significant at the 5% level.

TABLE 8. EFFECT OF SUBCUTANEOUS INJECTION OF 10 MG/KG OF DICHLOROISOPROTERENOL
(DCI) 30 MIN BEFORE INJECTION OF A SOLUTION OF ISOTONIC NaCL OR 0.2 M
CYSTAMINE (68 mg/kg) IN RATS (From Duyckaerts and Liébecq, 1970)

	Effects of cystamine after 45 min		
	Without DCI	With DCI	Difference
Lactate (μmol/g)	$+1.917^a$	-0.178	-2.094^a
Pyruvate (μmol/g)	$+0.043^a$	-0.014	-0.056^a
[Lactate]/[Pyruvate]	$+8.5^a$	$+1.9$	-6.5^a
Body temperature (°C)	-1.01^a	-0.51	$+0.50$
E'_h (mV)	-2.1^b	$+0.4$	$+2.5^b$
$10^{3-} \times$ [NADH]/[NAD$^+$]	$+0.61^a$	$+0.07$	-0.54^b
Glucose (μmol/g)	$+3.830^a$	$+1.027^a$	-2.803^a

[a] Statistically significant at the 5 % level.
[b] Statistically significant at the 10 % level only.

It seems likely that these changes may be the result of the release of
catecholamines, in connection with the fall of blood pressure. Dichloroisoproterenol, a well-known antagonist of the β-effects of the catecholamines, injected in a 10 mg/kg dose 30 min before the cystamine inhibits
the increase of both the [lactate]/[pyruvate] ratio and of the glycemia
(Table 8).

In mice, an increase is also observed in the [lactate]/[pyruvate] ratio
after cystamine injection. Hypothermia is doubtless partly responsible
for this phenomenon, because after appropriate correction the reduction
of the redox potential is slight and statistically insignificant.

Neither MEA nor cysteine causes equivalent changes of the redox
potential in rats.

6.3.2.4. *Redox Potential of Mitochondria*

According to Williamson *et al.* (1967), the redox state of the system
NAD$^+$–NADH of the mitochondria can be measured (a) in the mitochondrial cristae from the [3-hydroxybutyrate]/[acetoacetate] ratio, (b) in
the mitochondrial matrix from the [glutamate]/[2-oxoglutarate].[NH$_3$]
ratio. The 3-hydroxybutyrate and glutamate dehydrogenases, although
located in different places within the mitochondria, have a common
NAD$^+$—NADH pool.

Up to the present time, the influence of sulfur-containing radioprotective agents on the redox state of the free nucleotides of the
mitochondria has not been studied.

6.3.2.5. *Direct Electrode Potential Measurements*

The direct measurement of the redox potential by means of electrodes has been carried out by some authors. They have shown that sulfur-containing radioprotective agents such as cystamine, cysteine, and AET cause a significant reduction of the redox potential (Sumarukov and Kudryashov, 1963; Konopolyanikov *et al.,* 1966) the extent of which is linked to the degree of hypoxia (Dobrovolskii, 1967).

As in the case of potentiometric measurement of the O_2 tension by means of electrodes, the measurements must correspond essentially to the redox potential of the extracellular fluid with which the electrodes are in contact.

6.3.2.6. *Redox Potential of Bound Nucleotides*

Whereas the measurement of the [lactate]/[pyruvate] ratio makes possible the determination of the redox potential of the pyridine nucleotides of the extramitochondrial cytoplasmic compartment, the spectrofluorimetric method (Chance *et al.,* 1962a, b, 1964, 1965) is used to measure the reduction state of these nucleotides bound to the enzymes. An increase of fluorescence due to a greater reduction of these coenzymes occurs when the intracellular O_2 falls to levels in the range of 0–1 mmHg.

These measurements are made *in vivo,* not distinguishing between the NADPH and the NADH, but they reflect more particularly the mitochondrial compartment where these nucleotides are most abundant.

Jamieson and van den Brenk (1966) applied these techniques to measuring the pyridine nucleotides in the ileum of a rat, anesthetized and injected with several radioprotective agents. These experiments have shown that, whereas *para*-aminophenol and chlorpromazine cause a significant reduction of the pyridine coenzymes, this is not so with AET (300 mg/kg), dimethylsulfoxide (5 g/kg), cystamine (90 mg/kg), MEA (165 mg/kg), nor with 5-HT (15 mg/kg). These observations do not seem to have been repeated at different time intervals after injection, except in the case of MEA where the measurement was taken after 5–10 and 40 min.

Galeotti *et al.* (1969) took separate measurements of the state of reduction of the free nucleotides (fluorescence at 443 nm), and the bound nucleotides (fluorescence at 464 nm). Working on samples of liver, they report that anoxia above all causes a reduction of the mitochondrial NAD(P).

6.4. GLYCOLYSIS AND GLYCOGENOLYSIS

6.4.1. EFFECTS OF MEA AND CYSTAMINE

6.4.1.1. In vivo *Effects*

Cysteamine causes a rapid and considerable drop in liver glycogen in the mouse (Bacq and Fischer, 1953). Half an hour after a MEA(HCl) injection (115 mg/kg), liver glycogen falls from 28.6 to 9.3 mg/g of fresh tissue; 1 hr after injection, there remains only 2.1 mg/g; and 3 hr later, only 1.6 mg/g: about 80% of the hepatic glycogen disappears in 1 hr. Later on, progressive reconstitution of the glycogen content of the liver may be observed. Cysteine and GSH have no effect on the glycogen content of the rat's liver.

The rapid disappearance of glycogen from the liver does not seem to have any grave consequence for the animal. If, for several consecutive days, a radioprotective dose of MEA is administered, one finds that 24 hr after the last injection the hepatic glycogen level is higher than that of the control animals (Bacq and Fischer, 1953). This observation is confirmed by Sokal *et al.* (1959) who observed, in addition, a fall in the muscular glycogen content both in rats and mice. In adrenalectomized pancreatectomized animals, MEA remains glycogenolytic, which would seem to indicate a direct effect on the liver independent of a possible liberation of epinephrine.*

Hietbrink *et al.* (1959) observed slight hyperglycemia in rats 30 min after treatment with up to 200 mg/kg MEA. The increase of blood glucose reaches its maximum 2 or 3 hr after administration of the radioprotective agent, and then returns to normal.

Duyckaerts *et al.* (1969) and Duyckaerts and Liébecq (1970) observed hyperglycemia in rats and mice after the administration of a radioprotective dose of cystamine; hyperglycemia is less pronounced after the administration of MEA.

In rabbits, Fischer (1956) observed the depletion of hepatic glycogen under the action of MEA and cystamine, but without hyperglycemia. He found that 30 min after injection with these radioprotective agents there was a significant increase in blood lactic acid, but less in pyruvic acid.

In the urine, Fischer found an abnormally high level of lactic, pyruvic, citric, and 2-oxoglutaric acid, which are all intermediates either of

---

*Duyckaerts *et al.* (1971) have recently observed an activation of liver and muscle phosphorylase kinase by 1 to 10 mM cystamine *in vitro*; the level of phosphorylase *a* is higher in the liver of rats injected with cystamine (68 mg/kg) even if the animals have been depleted of their catecholamines by repeated injections of reserpine (4 times 1 mg/kg).

glycolysis or of the tricarboxylic acid cycle (Fischer, 1956).

One should compare the effects of MEA and cystamine with those of another excellent radioprotective agent, sodium cyanide, which also causes, in radioprotective doses (5 mg/kg) in mice, the rapid disappearance of hepatic glycogen. In rabbits, sodium cyanide in doses of 2.5 mg/kg greatly increases the lactic acid content of the blood even more rapidly than MEA does under the same conditions. The lactic acid appears in the urine as early as 10 min after injection with cyanide. Fischer (1956) suggests that this rapid disappearance of organic acids derived from glycogen could be due to anoxia caused by the radioprotective agent.

Subsequent observations (Lelièvre and Betz, 1959) agree with this hypothesis: the administration of MEA or cystamine decreases the total O_2 consumption of the living animal: sodium cyanide behaves in the same manner, but a clearly more significant hypoxia is observed, which may be correlated with the length of radioprotective action, the rapid increase in the level of lactic acid in the blood, and the early excretion in urine.

It should also be noted that MEA injected into rats before irradiation has another effect during an aerobic glycolysis: it is known that irradiation causes an increase in hepatic glycogen in the fasting rat (McKee, 1952; Ross and Ely, 1951); the irradiated animal previously treated with MEA has, after irradiation, a level of liver glycogen comparable to that of non-irradiated animals (Fischer, 1954).

Fumigalli and Malaspina (1958), through histochemical observations, confirm Fischer's results, but observe further that, during the first hour following irradiation in the presence of MEA, glycogenolysis is followed by gluconeogenesis, bringing the glycogen content of the liver back to normal.

TABLE 9. EFFECT OF MEA AND CYSTAMINE ON THE ANAEROBIC GLYCOLYSIS OF HOMOGENATES OF RAT ORGANS (From Lelièvre and Betz, 1960)

Addition	Lactic acid production (mmol/g dry weight per 20 min) by homogenates of					
	Liver	Kidney	Brain	Spleen	Testes	Thymus
None	0.29	0.30	0.62	0.39	0.37	0.37
MEA (0.88 mequiv. S/l)	0.28	0.29	0.62	0.39	0.34	0.39
MEA (4.44 mequiv. S/l)	0.30	0.29	0.60	0.39	0.34	0.37
Cystamine (0.88 mequiv. S/l)	0.23	0.25	0.52	0.32	0.28	0.29
Cystamine (4.44 mequiv. S/l)	0.13	0.19	0.44	0.23	0.27	0.25

6.4.1.2. In vitro *Effects*

In vitro, cystamine inhibits the glycolytic activity of rat tissue homo-genates (Lelièvre and Betz, 1960) (Table 9). In contrast, MEA is inactive under the same conditions. The principal effect of the disulfide is on the enzymes whose metabolic activity is conditioned by the presence of the free —SH groups, and particularly the hexokinase, phosphoglycer-aldehyde dehydrogenase, and phosphofructokinase.

6.4.1.2.1. **Hexokinase**

The hexokinase activity of these liver and brain homogenates is inhibited by cystamine. In contrast, MEA seems to exercise slight activa-tion (Lelièvre, 1961). Eldjarn and Bremer (1962) show that inhibition by cystamine of glucose utilization by human erythrocytes *in vitro* is due to inhibition of the hexokinase. This could be reversed by the addition of thiol or under the action of glutathione reductase, which provides GSH at the expense of NADPH. This mechanism explains why the addition of adenosine can reverse the inhibition of hexokinase caused by cystamine

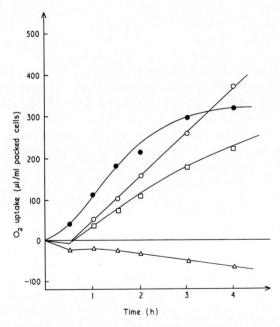

FIG. 6. Effect of cystamine on O_2 uptake by erythrocytes in the presence of methylene blue. o, glucose; △, glucose + cystamine; □, adenosine; •, adenosine + cystamine. (Eldjarn and Bremer, 1962.)

(Fig. 6). The degradation of adenosine leads to pentose phosphates, which are metabolized by the enzyme systems of the red blood cells with the production of NADPH, which enables the glutathione reductase system to continue its reducing effect.

Nesbakken and Eldjarn (1963) show that tetramethylcystamine, incubated anaerobically, decreases glucose uptake in certain tissues in the rat (diaphragm, brain, testes), whereas an increase in consumption of glucose appears in kidney slices. In anaerobiosis, one observes a much more significant production of lactic acid than that which could be accounted for by the tissue glucose consumption. These authors show that this lactic acid must be derived from an endogenous substrate which is glycogen. They consider that the utilization of glycogen is due to poisoning by the disulfide at the hexokinase level and that this phenomenon is quite general and common to all mammalian tissues.

The different degrees of inhibition obtained according to the nature of the tissue studied would depend on the capacity of that tissue to reduce the disulfides. It is known that the glutathione reductase varies considerably in different tissues in the same animal (Rall and Lehninger, 1952): the relative proportions of glutathione reductase in the muscle, brain and kidney of the rat are 22, 60 and 400 respectively. Therefore glutathione reductase provides the cells with a protective mechanism against intoxication by the disulfides; thus, the toxic effect will be high if the glutathione reductase content is low. This is in agreement with the observations of Nesbakken and Eldjarn (1963), who show that, with equal concentrations of tetramethylcystamine, the brain preparations display a more significant inhibition of hexokinase than that observed under the same conditions with kidney preparations. It should be noted, however, that the authors compare the effects of the inhibitor under different conditions, because on the one hand they use kidney slices, and on the other a partially purified preparation of brain hexokinase.

Ciccarone and Milani (1964) show that cystamine affects the anaerobic glycolysis of the ascite tumor cells (hepatoma Yoshida AH130). In the early stages, with cystamine present, a transitory increase in the production of lactic acid is noticed, followed by a period of decrease (Fig. 7). The authors consider that the formation of mixed disulfides between cystamine and the —SH groups present in the cell produces a certain amount of free MEA, which would be responsible for the increased production of lactic acid. A similar observation has already been made by McIlwain (1959), which shows that the presence of thiols increases the rate of aerobic glycolysis in slices of rat brain. This is also shown by Lelièvre

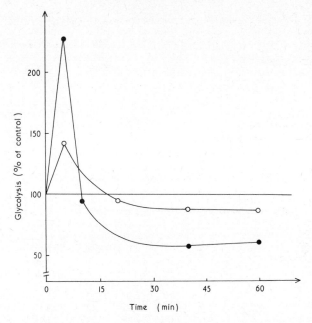

FIG. 7. Effect of cystamine on the glycolysis of Yoshida hepatoma ascites cells. o, 5 mM cystamine; ●, 30 mM cystamine. (Modified from Ciccarone and Milani, 1964.)

and Betz (1960), who observe slight activation of kidney and liver hexokinase in the presence of MEA. Ciccarone and Milani (1964) observe the early increase in production of lactic acid in anaerobiosis without increased consumption of exogenous glucose, and point to the endogenous origin of this lactic acid. This implies that the addition of cystamine creates MEA and also stimulates the activity of several enzyme systems of the glycolytic chain.

The inhibiting effect of cystamine on the hexokinase present in the slices or homogenates of the tissues is confirmed by experiments on purified hexokinase (Lelièvre, 1959). Yeast hexokinase, however, seems to be relatively more resistant to the effect of cystamine than is animal hexokinase. Quite high concentrations of cystamine are required to obtain strong inhibition. This is completely reversed by addition of thiols (Table 10).

6.4.1.2.2. Phosphofructokinase

The systematic study of the different metabolic stages of degradation of glycogen to fructose 1,6-bisphosphate has helped to show that

TABLE 10. INHIBITION OF YEAST HEXOKINASE (From Lelièvre, 1961a)

First addition	Inhibition (%) after second addition of		
	None	0.88 M cysteine	0.88 M MEA
None	100	101	101
0.22 M Cystamine	48	99	99
0.27 M Monoiodoacetate	61	61	—
1 mM *para*-Chloromercuribenzoate	0	75	—

TABLE 11. INHIBITION OF THE PHOSPHOFRUCTOKINASE ACTIVITY OF VARIOUS RAT ORGANS
(From Lelièvre, 1961a)
Triose phosphate formation was measured as the result of the combined action of phosphofructokinase, aldolase, and triosephosphate isomerase

Additions	Phosphofructokinase activity (μmol/mg protein nitrogen per 30 min) in					
	Liver	Kidney	Brain	Spleen	Testes	Thymus
None	4.59	6.03	7.47	1.93	0.91	1.44
9 mM Cysteine	4.68	5.85	7.29	1.82	0.90	1.47
9 mM MEA	4.69	5.94	7.47	1.87	0.92	1.43
15 mM Cystamine	3.15	4.05	5.67	1.53	0.72	1.12
1 mM Monoiodoacetate	3.42	4.59	6.30	1.62	0.72	1.22

cystamine also inhibits phosphofructokinase. In contrast, MEA and cysteine are inactive. Inhibition of phosphofructokinase by cystamine is less intense than that of hexokinase. This is why, for example, cystamine (3 mM) reduces the hexokinase activity of a kidney homogenate of a rat to less than 50% of its normal value; in contrast, a 15 mM concentration of cystamine causes only about 30% inhibition of phosphofructokinase (Lelièvre, 1961a) (Table 11). This effect of cystamine on phosphofructokinase has been confirmed by Froede *et al.* (1968), who observe inhibition of cardiac muscle phosphofructokinase in sheep in the presence of certain disulfides, particularly cystamine, GSSG and hydroxyethyldisulfide.

6.4.1.2.3. Glyceraldehyde-phosphate dehydrogenase

Inhibition of hexokinase and, to a lesser degree, of phosphofructokinase is not the only mechanism by which cystamine causes the slowing down of anaerobic glycolysis. In fact, cystamine added to the incubation medium containing fructose 1,6-bisphosphate as substrate slows down the production of lactic acid by homogenates prepared from the liver and brain of the rat. This slowing down of the anaerobic metabolism under such conditions is due to partial inhibition of phospho-glyceraldehyde dehydrogenase in the presence of cystamine (Lelièvre, 1961a). Cysteamine is inactive under the same conditions. Purified yeast phosphoglyceraldehyde dehydrogenase is inhibited by cystamine: in contrast, MEA or cysteine slightly activates the reaction. This is a reversible inhibition and the addition of thiols such as MEA or cysteine regenerates the initial activity after treatment by cystamine or by certain specific inhibitors of the —SH such as *para*-chloromercuribenzoate. Other specific inhibitors of the thiol functions, such as mono-iodoacetic acid or N-ethylmaleimide, also clearly inhibit phosphoglyceraldehyde dehydrogenase of purified yeast, but this inhibition is irreversible. The slight enzyme activity which reappears after treatment by the thiols of enzyme solutions treated with mono-iodoacetic acid or N-ethylmaleimide should be attributed to the fraction of the enzyme in the form of disulfide which could not react with the inhibitors, but which is released in —SH form by the reactivators.

Cystamine, added to phosphoglyceraldehyde dehydrogenase of yeast in solution, protects against the effects of X-rays (Lelièvre, 1961b).

The work of Pihl and Lange (1962) and Lange and Pihl (1961) partly confirms these results. These authors also observe the protective effect of cystamine on purified phosphoglyceraldehyde dehydrogenase of rabbit's muscle, irradiated in pure solution. The radioprotective effect is shared by other sulfur-containing compounds such as MEA, cysteine, or cystine. However, they did not observe an inhibitory effect by cystamine on the purified phosphoglyceraldehyde dehydrogenase of the rabbit's muscle *in vitro*. They attribute the action of the GSSG, which inhibits the activity of phosphoglyceraldehyde dehydrogenase *in vitro* (Labeyrie, 1949; Velick, 1955) to contamination by hydrogen peroxide. They did not observe any formation of mixed disulfide between cystamine and the phosphoglyceraldehyde dehydrogenase of the muscle rabbit. Other substances tested, particularly tetrathionate and cystamine sulfoxide, inhibit the activity of the phosphoglyceraldehyde dehydrogenase *in vitro*, and become fixed on the —SH groups, giving in the former case a sulfenyl-thiosulfate derivative, and in the latter case a mixed disulfide. These two substances, tetrathionate and cystamine sulfoxide, are not radioprotective agents (Langendorff and Koch, 1954). It seems difficult to reconcile these observations with the hypothesis of mixed disulfides proposed by Eldjarn and Pihl (1957, 1958), although it is possible *in vitro* to obtain mixed disulfides between cysteine and certain thiols such as thioglycolic acid, which is not a protective agent *in vivo*.

6.4.2. EFFECTS OF AET

In normal rats AET produces a considerable hepatic glycogenolysis, a hypoglycemia produced by stimulation of the secretion of insulin, and a significant increase in the level of lactic acid in the blood. These effects seem to depend on hormonal factors, because in rats rendered diabetic with alloxan, AET rapidly causes hyperglycemia, which is reduced by previous administration of ergotamine, or suppressed by adrenalectomy. Thus, it seems that, not only insulin, but also adrenergic factors or adrenal-cortical hormones, are implicated in such mechanisms. Zins *et al.* (1958a, 1959) attribute the increased blood lactate to inhibition of the aerobic metabolism stimulating the anaerobic glycolysis.

In vitro, slices of rat liver incubated in the presence of MEG produce more lactic acid than do the controls (Zins *et al.,* 1959). However, if the incubation is prolonged *in vitro*, aerobic glycolysis, after a brief stimulation, increases more slowly than it does in the controls. The authors draw the conclusion that inhibition is due not to MEG, but to an oxidation product. It is in fact known that this is guanidine-ethyl disulfide, and that this is the real inhibitor of glycolysis. In this respect, guanidine-ethyl disulfide behaves, in relation to MEG, in a manner very similar to that of cystamine with relation to MEA.

Although parenteral administration of radioprotective doses of MEG causes increased lactacidemia in rats, tissues taken from an animal so treated, and incubated *in vitro,* have normal glycolytic activity. This is particularly the case with homogenates prepared from the rat's brain taken 30 min after injection with the radioprotective agent. This is rather remarkable, because the particular symptoms of intoxication observed after heavy doses of MEG would seem to indicate an important effect at the level of the central nervous system (DuBois *et al.,* 1958a).

6.4.3. EFFECTS OF DIETHYLDITHIOCARBAMATE

6.4.3.1. *Hexokinase*

Strömme (1963a) shows that *N*-diethyldithiocarbamate, an excellent radioprotective agent (see Bacq, 1965), in high concentrations causes slight inhibition of the purified yeast hexokinase. This inhibition is greatly increased by adding oxidized cytochrome *c* to the incubation medium. Strömme shows that oxidized cytochrome *c* transforms the thiol compound diethyldithiocarbamate into its disulfide, disulfiram, which is, in fact, the inhibitor of yeast hexokinase (Fig. 8).

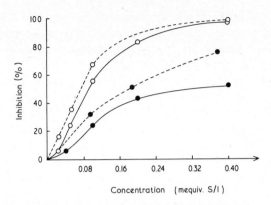

FIG. 8. Inhibition of yeast and brain hexokinases by disulfiram (———) and diethyldithiocarbamate (----), the latter in the presence of cytochrome *c*. ●, yeast hexokinase;
o, brain hexokinase. (Strömme, 1963a.)

Animal hexokinase, extracted from a calf's brain and partially purified, is much more sensitive than yeast hexokinase to the inhibitory effect of DEDTC. The addition of oxidized cytochrome *c* also increases the inhibition (Fig. 8).

This inhibition is prevented by the addition of GSH to the incubation medium. The inhibition caused by DEDTC in the presence of oxidized cytochrome *c* is reversible, and after addition of GSH a reactivation of the hexokinase is observed. Disulfiram blocks the sulfhydryl groups of hexokinase by a mechanism similar to that of cystamine with the formation of an inactive mixed disulfide.

Diethyldithiocarbamate, in spite of its inhibitory effect on hexokinase and other —SH-containing enzymes (Keilin and Hartree, 1940; Richert *et al.*, 1950; Nygaard and Sumner, 1952), may be administered with impunity during long periods as, for example, in the case of alcoholic detoxication cures, without producing any grave metabolic disorders. Strömme (1963a) suggests that the ingested disulfiram is reduced in the organism, and maintained in this non-toxic form. Ingestion of ethanol would cause reoxidation of the DEDTC in disulfiram. The intensity of this reoxidation would exceed the capacity of the organism to reduce the disulfide, and would lead to generalized metabolic poisoning.

Intact human erythrocytes incubated in the presence of glucose and DEDTC (below 10 mM) consume more glucose than do controls; this reaction remains linear longer than in the absence of DEDTC (Strömme, 1963b). This increased utilization of glucose is probably due to stimulation of the pentose phosphate shunt. In support of this hypothesis, it is known that other activating agents of the pentose phosphate shunt, such as methylene blue, also cause increased glucose utilization by the erythrocytes.

If the DEDTC content is increased (10 mM) proportional inhibition of the utilization of glucose is observed (Strömme, 1963b). Addition of DEDTC to the incubation medium is also observed to cause a drop in the GSH content of the erythrocytes, and the concentration of DEDTC necessary to bring about the total disappearance of GSH in the erythrocytes is also that which causes complete inhibition of glucose consumption. Weak concentrations of DEDTC which do not inhibit glucose utilization cause only a slight drop in GSH, rapidly followed by a return to normal values.

Erythrocytes treated with amyl nitrite and having an abnormally high proportion of methemoglobin behave like normal erythrocytes in the presence of DEDTC, but the concentrations of this thiol necessary

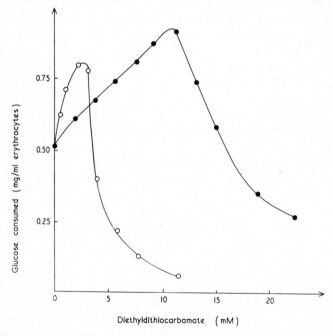

FIG. 9. Effect of diethyldithiocarbamate on glucose consumed by erythrocytes. ●, normal erythrocytes; o, erythrocytes pretreated with amyl nitrite. (Strömme, 1963b.)

to obtain the same effects are clearly less than those that must be used with normal red corpuscles (Strömme, 1963b). This observation indicates the active role played by methemoglobin in the mechanism of the transformation of DEDTC into disulfiram (Fig. 9).

It should be noted that, in the presence of DEDTC, normal red corpuscles always contain a certain amount of methemoglobin derived from auto-oxidation of hemoglobin catalyzed by the thiol (Strömme, 1963c).

The role of methemoglobin can be demonstrated by anaerobic incubation of the erythrocytes. Under such conditions, no methemoglobin is formed, and no variation may be observed either in glucose utilization, or in the GSH content in the presence of DEDTC. Against this, erythrocytes incubated anaerobically in the presence of preformed methemoglobin and DEDTC behave in the same way as red corpuscles incubated in the presence of O_2 and DEDTC. The methemoglobin enables the DEDTC to be converted to disulfiram, which is, in fact, the inhibitor of glucose consumption, and thus plays a role similar to that of oxidized cytochrome c (Strömme, 1963b). This role, is not, however, identical, because cytochrome c directly transforms DEDTC into disulfiram by transforming itself into reduced cytochrome c, whereas methemoglobin acts as a catalyst between the DEDTC and the O_2.

Here glutathione reductase also constitutes a protective mechanism against poisoning by disulfiram. The latter reacts spontaneously with

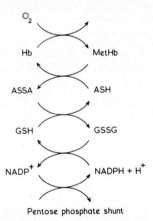

Fig. 10. Sequence of reactions explaining protection against disulfiram poisoning in erythrocytes. Hb, hemoglobin; MetHb, methemoglobin; ASH, diethyldithiocarbamate; ASSA, disulfiram. (Strömme, 1963b.)

GSH *in vitro*; the rapid disappearance of this thiol inside the erythrocytes in the presence of disulfiram shows that this reaction also occurs intracellularly. The GSSG is reduced by the glutathione reductase system (see graph on Fig. 10), resulting in accumulation of oxidized disulfiram, and therefore inhibition only from the moment the GSH is oxidized and cannot be further reduced.

The reducing capacity of the glutathione reductase system is extremely high: Strömme (1963b), allowing for the fact that the release of a CO_2 molecule accompanies the formation of two molecules of NAD(P)H, which are capable of reducing two molecules of disulfiram by the glutathione reductase system, calculated that the erythrocytes of an adult man can reduce about 50 g of disulfiram per day.

Strömme (1963b) also showed that disulfiram inhibits not only hexokinase but also other enzymatic systems of anaerobic glycolysis. He showed that, if the erythrocytes are first incubated with DEDTC in concentrations higher than 2.5 mM, without substrate and under conditions such that the protective effect of the glutathione reductase system is abolished, the addition of inosine, which prevents the participation of hexokinase, no longer re-establishes the production of lactic acid at a normal level. This indicates that DEDTC can cause inhibition of glycolysis beyond the hexokinase-catalyzed reaction.

The metabolic reduction of methemoglobin, which, in the presence of DEDTC, is mainly associated with the pentose phosphate shunt, is more affected by disulfiram than the production of lactate, which indicates that this shunt may be inhibited by concentrations of disulfiram slightly smaller than those necessary to inhibit the last stages of glycolysis (Strömme, 1963b). Concerning the activity of glucose-6-phosphate dehydrogenase, it should be mentioned that Chefurka (1957) showed that, in purified form, this enzyme is strongly inhibited by DEDTC at concentrations below 10 mM. Nevertheless, according to the experiments of Strömme (1963b), DEDTC, which might be expected to behave in a similar way to dimethyldithiocarbamate with regard to the same enzyme, does not appear to influence glucose-6-phosphate dehydrogenase of intact erythrocytes. Other radioprotective agents, such as AET, activate glucose-6-phosphate dehydrogenase in rat liver during the period of radioprotection (Sonka *et al.*, 1968). In contrast, GSH, GSSG, cysteine, MEA, and AET, incubated *in vitro* with human red corpuscles, only very slightly modify the activity of glucose-6-phosphate dehydrogenase. These results are in complete agreement with Strömme (1963b) concerning DEDTC.

6.4.3.2. *Glyceraldehyde-phosphate Dehydrogenase*

Nygaard and Sumner (1952), comparing 3-phosphoglyceraldehyde dehydrogenase of muscle and the aldehyde dehydrogenase of the liver, showed that disulfiram very strongly inhibits phosphoglyceraldehyde dehydrogenase, whether in pure solution or in a crude preparation. They noted that cysteine, added halfway through incubation, increased the activity of the phosphoglyceraldehyde dehydrogenase, and prevented its inhibition by disulfiram. An analogous observation is made by Graham (1951), concerning liver aldehyde dehydrogenase, its activity being inhibited by the GSSG. This inhibition is reversible, and the reduced reductase re-establishes the enzymatic activity. Such an observation obviously supports direct reaction of disulfiram with the essential thiol groups of the enzyme that are transformed into inactive disulfides. This hypothesis is taken up again by Johnston (1953), who concludes, at the end of his experiments, that disulfiram (tetraethylthiuram disulfide) and tetramethylthiuram disulfide probably cause oxidation of the —SH groups of phosphoglyceraldehyde dehydrogenase to disulfide. This mechanism seems more likely to be responsible for the inhibition observed, rather than competition between the disulfiram and the substrate for the enzyme, a mechanism suggested by Nygaard and Sumner (1952).

6.5. CELLULAR RESPIRATION AND OXIDATIVE PHOSPHORYLATION

Owing to their considerable reactivity with thiol or disulfide-containing enzymes, sulfur-containing radioprotective agents, as was to be expected, interfere with some of the essential enzymatic reactions of energy-producing oxidative metabolism.

6.5.1. EFFECTS OF MEA AND CYSTAMINE

6.5.1.1. In vitro *Addition*

Cystamine, added to the homogenates of organs of rats which have been incubated in the presence of pyruvate and fumarate, inhibits O_2 consumption (Lelièvre and Betz, 1960). The intensity of the inhibition varies according to the organ tested, and the cystamine content of the incubation medium. With equal concentrations of cystamine, the liver and thymus seem scarcely sensitive to this substance; on the other hand, homogenates of the kidney, spleen, and especially of the brain show

TABLE 12. OXYGEN CONSUMPTION AND OXIDATIVE PHOSPHORYLATION BY
MITOCHONDRIA FROM RAT ORGANS[a] (Modified from Lelièvre and Betz, 1963)

Organ	Cystamine concentration (mequiv. S/l)	Oxygen consumed (μatom/mg protein nitrogen per 30 min)	Phosphorus esterified (μatom/mg protein nitrogen per 30 min)	P/O ratio
Liver	0	4.6	12.1	2.5
	0.88	4.9	11.9	2.4
	4.44	4.4	9.2	2.1
	17.8	3.7	5.7	1.6
	71	0.8	0	0
Kidney	0	13.3	32.8	2.5
	0.88	15.9	33.2	2.1
	4.44	12.3	22.3	1.9
	17.8	5.8	8.6	1.5
	71	0.9	0	0
Brain	0	9.4	26.2	2.8
	0.88	8.4	20.4	2.4
	4.44	5.2	10.2	2.0
	17.8	4.5	7.4	1.7
	71	0.8	0.5	0.7

[a] Substrates: 5 mM pyruvate + 5 mM fumarate.

a considerable drop in O_2 consumption. Similar results are obtained by incubating with cystamine suspensions of mitochondria (Table 12) rather than homogenates prepared from liver, brain, or kidney of rat, in the presence of pyruvate and fumarate (Lelièvre and Betz, 1963: Lelièvre, 1965a).

A low concentration of cystamine, 0.88 m-equiv of sulfur per ml, causes a slight increase in O_2 consumption by liver mitochondria incubated in the presence of pyruvate and fumarate. In higher concentrations cystamine inhibits the O_2 consumption. Cysteamine is inactive under similar conditions.

The disappearance of pyruvate from the incubation medium parallels the O_2 consumption. In low concentrations, cystamine slightly increases pyruvate utilization by the mitochondria, whereas in higher concentrations the opposite effect is observed (Fig. 11).

The slight increase in O_2 consumption observed when incubating liver homogenates or suspensions of mitochondria in the presence of low cystamine concentrations is not due to the oxidation of the cystamine.

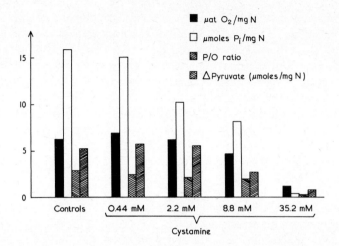

FIG. 11. Effect of cystamine on pyruvate metabolism in isolated rat liver mitochondria. Pyruvate and fumarate, 5 mM; 30 min incubation at 30°C. (Corrected from Lelièvre, 1965b.)

Specific determinations of disulfides show that cystamine is relatively stable in these experimental conditions, and that its oxidation is too small to explain the increase in O_2 consumption.

Cavallini *et al.* (1956a, b, 1957) point out that certain tissues, particularly rat liver, can metabolize cystamine to the same extent as other diamines, such as cadaverine or putrescine, by oxidative deamination with absorption of a certain amount of O_2.

The variations in O_2 consumption observed by Lelièvre (1965a), when incubating homogenates or mitochondria of rat liver in the presence of cystamine, could be the result of two distinct metabolic activities: on the one hand, a slowing down of cellular respiration; and on the other, a consumption of O_2 due to oxidative deamination. The results of Lelièvre (1965a) argue strongly against the participation of diamine oxidases in the observed changes. In fact, the O_2 consumption due to the activity of diamine oxidase in liver homogenates is very low, compared with the O_2 consumption of mitochondrial respiration. At the same time, the addition of specific inhibitors of diamine oxidases scarcely affects the variations in O_2 consumption of the homogenates or suspensions of mitochondria incubated in the presence of pyruvate, fumarate, and cystamine (Lelièvre, 1965b).

The increased O_2 consumption in the presence of low cystamine concentrations may be due to the ability of liver mitochondria to reduce certain disulfide compounds to sulfhydryl compounds in the presence of intermediates of the Krebs cycle, as shown by Eldjarn and Bremer (1963).

Bicheikina and Romantsev (1966b) showed that administration of radioprotective doses of mercaptopropylamine (MPA) does not alter the O_2 consumption of mitochondria prepared from the brain or liver of animals. *In vitro,* MPA (23 mM) stimulates the O_2 consumption of mitochondria from rabbit brain and liver; at higher concentrations (110 mM), it inhibits mitochondrial respiration.

Ciccarone and Milani (1964) observed that cystamine lowers the O_2 consumption of the ascite tumor cells (hepatoma Yoshida AH 130) incubated *in vitro* in the absence of added substrates. This inhibition of O_2 consumption in the presence of cystamine does not seem to be affected by the addition of intermediates of the tricarboxylic acid cycle, such as citric acid or succinic acid, to the incubation medium. The authors conclude that the drop in O_2 consumption is not due to the blocking of a stage of the aerobic oxidizing metabolism. Pre-incubation of the ascite tumor cells with glucose reduces the O_2 consumption (Crabtree effect), which then becomes insensitive to the action of cystamine, and remains unchanged in the presence of this substance. On the other hand, the addition of glucose to an incubation medium containing ascite tumor cells and cystamine causes inhibition of the consumption of O_2. From this, the authors conclude that the inhibition is caused by disulfide poisoning. The addition of glucose enables the cell thus poisoned to reduce and detoxicate the disulfides to some extent, by means of the system proposed by Nesbakken and Eldjarn (1963). The effect of glucose is to enable the cell to produce, by the pentose monophosphate shunt, the necessary NADPH for such a reduction.

6.5.1.2.   In vivo *Administration*

Ciccarone (1965) states that liver homogenates taken from mice that have received an i.v. dose of 170 mg/kg *in vitro,* in the presence of pyruvate, consume less O_2 than do the controls. The utilization of the pyruvate present in the incubation medium is also considerably slowed down. The maximum inhibition of O_2 consumption and of pyruvate utilization *in vitro* is observed in liver homogenates taken about 20 min after the administration of the radioprotective agent. At the moment, an accumulation of pyruvic acid and 2-oxoglutaric acid is seen in the liver taken from mice.

The addition of a thiol compound, such as 2-mercaptoethanol or reduced coenzyme A, partly removes the inhibition of O_2 consumption caused by the injection of cystamine. However, O_2 consumption in the presence of 2-mercaptoethanol or reduced coenzyme A remains lower than that of homogenates taken from uninjected animals treated and supplemented with the *in vitro* addition of the same thiol compounds.

Ciccarone and Bacq (1966) have shown that the O_2 consumption of liver homogenates is unaffected by the pre-injection (20 min) of doses of 2-mercaptoethanol equal in sulfur content to radioprotective doses of cystamine. The lowering of the O_2 consumption of the liver homogenates, taken from mice previously treated with cystamine and incubated in the presence of pyruvate, is not due to a specific property of the sulfur-containing radioprotective agents because 5-HT under the same conditions has a similar effect to cystamine. Ciccarone and Bacq (1966) observed, in fact, that homogenates of livers taken from rats which 20 min earlier had received an injection of 5-HT (80 mg/kg) consume less O_2 than do the controls.

However, it has not been possible to confirm these results in rats. Romantsev and Savitch (1958) measured the O_2 consumption of liver slices taken from rats having been pre-injected with 200 mg/kg MEA. These slices are taken from the animals at varying intervals after administration of the radioprotective agent. Some animals are given an injection of cysteine (in equimolecular dose) instead of MEA.

These authors observed an increase in O_2 consumption of liver slices incubated *in vitro* after the administration of MEA. The maximum activation of O_2 consumption is observed in slices of liver removed about 30 min after injection with the radioprotective agent. Cysteine in equimolecular dose is not very effective, causing only a slight increase in O_2 consumption 5 min after the injection. This increase is transitional, and disappears 25 min after the administration of cysteine.

Salerno and Friedell (1954) observed an analogous qualitative effect due to cysteine. Slices of liver, spleen, heart, and kidney, taken from rats that had previously been injected with a radioprotective dose of cysteine (1 g/kg), consumed more O_2 than did control slices incubated under the same conditions. As the dose of cysteine injected was greater than that used by Romantsev and Savitch, the effect was more quantitatively noticeable. The increase in O_2 consumption by the slices of liver, spleen, heart, and kidney was respectively 42, 45, 39 and 23% of the normal respiration.

Betz and Lelièvre (1969) obtained analogous results, after i.p. injection of cystamine (100 mg of the dihydrochloride/kg), measuring the O_2

consumption of liver homogenates taken from the animal at varying times after injection of the radioprotective compound. It was noted that 2 min after injection of cystamine, the O_2 consumption increased, and in the liver slices reached a maximum, 30–45 min after injection, and then decreased. Homogenates prepared from livers taken 90 min after administration of the protective agent still showed a clearly higher O_2 consumption than normal. The uptake of inorganic phosphate was also increased during the period in which the increase in O_2 consumption was observed. But this increase was proportionately less than that of the O_2 consumption, indicating a partial uncoupling of oxidative phosphorylation.

Benabid and Rinaldi (1966) also showed that MEA in a dose of 150 mg (base)/kg cause increased O_2 consumption in slices of liver, spleen, and brain taken from mice 15 min after injection with the radioprotective agent. On the other hand, slices of kidney or muscle isolated under the same conditions consume less O_2 than do controls not treated with a

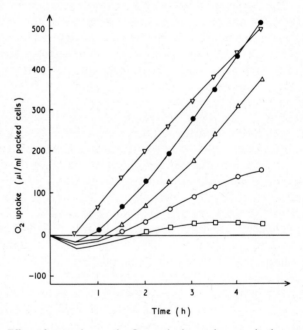

FIG. 12. Effect of cystamine on the O_2 uptake by erythrocytes in the presence of methylene blue. Glucose, 11 mM. Cystamine: ▽, none; ●, 1.5 mM; △, 3 mM; o, 6 mM; □, 10 mM. (Eldjarn and Bremer, 1962.)

radioprotective agent. Cysteine in 150 mg (base)/kg was less active than MEA, and causes a drop in O_2 consumption only in the spleen. Cysteamine or cystamine considerably reduces the O_2 consumption of pigeon and dog erythrocytes *in vitro* (Kuznetsov and Tank, 1964). The 5-mercapto-pentylamine, a non-radioprotective compound, in equimolecular concentrations, decreases the O_2 consumption of pigeon and dog erythrocytes.

Eldjarn and Bremer (1962) note a similar effect of cystamine incubated *in vitro* with human red corpuscles in the presence of glucose and methylene blue. Inhibition of O_2 consumption is proportional to the concentration of cystamine in the incubation medium, and is attributed by the authors to blocking the action of hexokinase by disulfide poisoning (Fig. 12).

In weak doses cystamine is reduced in erythrocytes by spontaneous exchange with GSH, which is then converted to GSSG. This is then reduced by glutathione reductase to GSH. However, in stronger concentrations, cystamine inhibits its own reduction (Eldjarn and Bremer, 1962), and the toxic effect of disulfide poisoning may be seen. Under similar conditions, MEA is inactive, and does not alter the O_2 consumption of human erythrocytes incubated *in vitro* in the presence of glucose and methylene blue.

If the glucose in the incubation medium is replaced by inosine, the inhibitory effect of cystamine on O_2 consumption disappears. Further-more, the addition of inosine in the presence of methylene blue to the incubation medium of erythrocytes previously poisoned by the cystamine and subsequently washed restores the O_2 consumption. The subsequent addition of glucose then re-establishes O_2 consumption comparable with that of the controls. Similarly, an —SH donor can reactivate the O_2 consumption of human erythrocytes previously blocked by cystamine. It seems that the effect of inosine is at the level of the pentose phosphate shunt: the metabolism of the pentoses produced from the inosine provides NADPH, which enables the glutathione reductase to reduce the cystamine and restore the O_2 consumption.

6.5.1.3. *Effects on Mitochondrial Enzymes*

In vitro cystamine strongly inhibits the acetylation of sulfanilamide by a bicarbonate extract of acetone powder of pigeon liver (Lelièvre, 1960). Other sulfur-containing radioprotective agents, such as MEA or cysteine, exercise *in vitro* the opposite effect, activating the acetylation.

Vandeberg (1961) observed that the administration of cystamine

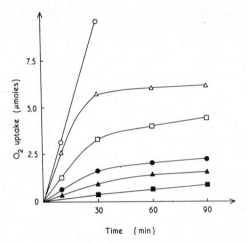

Fig. 13. Inhibition of citrate oxidation after pre-incubation with cystamine. Pre-incubation for 5 min with cystamine (o, none; △, 0.1 mM; □, 0.5 mM; ●, 1 mM; ▲, 2.5 mM; ■, 5 mM); citrate (6.7 mM) added immediately afterwards. (Skrede *et al.*, 1965.)

or MEA in radioprotective doses slows down the accumulation of fluoro-citrate in rat kidney and liver poisoned by fluoroacetate. Since it is known that the condensing enzyme is insensitive to the effect of these radio-protective agents (Betz and Lelièvre, 1969), one may logically suppose that, in the presence of MEA or cystamine, fluoroacetylation of coenzyme A is slowed down, thus causing a drop in accumulation of fluorocitrate.

Skrede *et al.* (1965) showed that cystamine and tetraethylcystamine cause marked inhibition of citrate oxidation in rat liver mitochondria (Fig. 13). Cysteamine, under the same conditions, is inactive, or causes a slight stimulation of O_2 consumption. Other sulfur-containing sub-stances, such as GSSG or oxidized mercaptoethanol, are inactive. This inactivity is attributed by the author to the fact that these substances penetrate the biological membranes very slowly.

The results obtained after pre-incubation of rat liver mitochondria with varying quantities of cystamine indicate that respiration continues normally, as long as the capacity to reduce cystamine is greater than the rate of diffusion of cystamine across the mitochondrial membrane. As soon as the reducing capacity of the mitochondria is exceeded, rapid disulfide poisoning occurs, and O_2 consumption drops rapidly.

On the other hand, cystamine strongly inhibits pyridine-dependent oxidations in mitochondria. In fact, Skrede *et al.* (1965) showed that

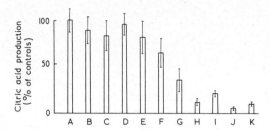

FIG. 14. Citrate production from pyruvate and oxaloacetate in rat liver mitochondria in the presence of various additions (4.4 mequiv. S/l except for EDTA, 4.4 mM). A, cysteine; B, MEA; C, MEG; D, GSH; E, 2-mercaptoethanol; F, EDTA; G, thiourea; H, cystamine; I, GSSG; J, GED; K, diethyldithiocarbamate. (Betz and Lelièvre, unpublished graph; cf. Betz and Lelièvre, 1969.)

rat liver mitochondria incubated in the presence of cystamine and various intermediates of the tricarboxylic acid cycle, oxidation of which is NAD-dependent, consume less O_2 than do the controls. Betz and Lelièvre (1969) have confirmed this in studying the conversion of pyruvate to citrate (Fig. 14); sulfur-containing radioprotective agents, such as MEA and MEG, have no effect.

Cystamine does not inhibit the oxidation of succinate or NADH itself, which indicates that disulfides do not interfere with the electron transport chain. Inhibition by cystamine of oxidation linked to pyridine nucleotides would be caused by preventing the flow of electrons before formation of NADH (Skrede *et al.*, 1965).

Mitochondria from rat liver pre-incubated in the presence of cystamine appear incapable of utilizing intermediates of the tricarboxylic acid cycle, the oxidation of which is linked with pyridine nucleotides. The addition of NAD^+ alone cannot remove this inhibition caused by cystamine. However, the addition of NAD^+, MEA, and thiolated Sephadex, which counteracts the auto-oxidation of the thiols, partially or totally restores the initial metabolic activity (Table 13). These results suggest that cystamine, in addition to swelling of the mitochondria (which facilitates the loss of oxidized NAD^+ (see below)), interferes with the association of the pyridine nucleotides with the mitochondria, probably at the level of the —SH groups essential to this association, and releases a certain amount of reduced pyridine nucleotides. The requirement of a thiol (MEA) in addition to NAD^+ to reactivate the oxidation of the 2-oxoglutarate after treatment with cystamine indicates inhibition of the 2-oxoglutarate dehydrogenase complex by the disulfides, in addition to the loss of pyridine nucleotides.

TABLE 13. REACTIVATION OF NAD⁺-DEPENDENT MITOCHONDRIAL OXIDATIONS AFTER INHIBITION BY CYSTAMINE (Modified from Skrede *et al.*, 1965)

Mitochondria were pre-incubated with 2 mM cystamine for 7 min at 30°C. Substrates and re-activators added after pre-incubation at the following concentrations: substrates (6.7 mM, except for DL-3-hydroxybutyrate, 13.3 mM); MEA (5 mM), NAD⁺ (2 mM); thiolated Sephadex (40 mg/3 ml)

Substrate added	Uninhibited control	Reactivators added to inhibited mitochondria (μmol O_2 taken up 120 min after addition of substrate)				
		None	NAD⁺	MEA +thiolated Sephadex	MEA +NAD⁺	MEA +NAD⁺ +thiolated Sephadex
—	5.8	0	0.6	0.9	0.6	1.6
2-Oxoglutarate	23.7	1	2.6	3.1	4.7	24.8
Pyruvate	23.2	1	2.6	1.8	5.0	9.9
3-Hydroxybutyrate	19.0	1.4	7.9	3.0	10.5	10.5

In this enzymatic complex, a certain number of substances are found such as lipoic acid, lipoyl dehydrogenase, and coenzyme A, which are indispensable for enzymatic activity and, since they contain the essential —SH groups, are very reactive with regard to the disulfides and especially to cystamine. This is especially the case with coenzyme A, which easily forms mixed disulfides in the presence of cystamine (Jaenicke and Lynen, 1960), with a more or less pronounced inactivation of the acetylation (Norum, 1965; Lelièvre, 1960).

Lipoyl dehydrogenase possesses a disulfide/dithiol group essential for the exchange of electrons between the flavoproteins and the pyridine nucleotides. After reducing the disulfide group with NADH, the enzyme becomes sensitive to arsenite; the inhibition can be lifted by 2,3-dimercaptopropanol. Cystamine can also, at this stage, inactivate lipoyl dehydrogenase. Finally, lipoic acid easily forms mixed disulfides with cystamine and MEA (Reed *et al.,* 1953).

For this reason it may be considered that inhibition of the 2-oxoglutarate dehydrogenase complex by cystamine is caused not only by the loss of NADH, but also by the formation of mixed disulfides between cystamine on the one hand and lipoic acid, lipoyl dehydrogenase, and coenzyme A on the other.

Inhibition of pyruvate oxidation by cystamine is probably due to a mechanism similar to that which inhibits the oxidation of the 2-oxoglutarate, because of the strong analogy that exists between these two dehydrogenases.

6.5.1.4. *Oxidative Phosphorylation*

Park *et al.* (1956) showed that certain sulfur-containing compounds, particularly MEA and cystamine, incubated *in vitro* with hamster liver mitochondria uncouple the oxidative phosphorylation in the presence of the 3-hydroxybutyrate. Park also states that the uncoupling activity of these two compounds is very different: cystamine is much more efficient than MEA. The uncoupling activity of the latter is attributed by Park and his coworkers to auto-oxidation during incubation, leading to the formation of cystamine, which is the true uncoupling agent. This suggestion had already been made by Lardy and Maley (1954), who, observing a slight uncoupling of oxidative phosphorylation in the presence of cysteine, attributed this action to cystine.

Lelièvre and Betz (1963) measured simultaneously the consumption of oxygen and the coupled oxidative phosphorylation by the mitochondria of rat liver in the presence of pyruvate plus fumarate and observed that these two metabolic activities are inhibited by cystamine. In the presence of low cystamine content, consumption of oxygen remains unchanged or increases slightly. If the concentration of cystamine is increased, the O_2 consumption is inhibited. The oxidative phosphorylation is inhibited whatever the content of cystamine. In all cases, at equal disulfide concentration, esterification of the inorganic phosphate is proportionally slower than the consumption of O_2, so that the ratio esterified phosphate/oxygen consumed (P/O ratio) varies inversely with the concentration of cystamine in the incubation medium (Fig. 11). Cysteamine is inactive under similar conditions.

Similar results were obtained by Skrede (1966), incubating rat liver mitochondria in the presence of succinate, with either MEA or cystamine. Uncoupling of the oxidative phosphorylation was not observed under the influence of MEA and thiolated Sephadex (which prevents oxidation of the —SH compound into disulfide).

It is known that, in the presence of intermediates of the tricarboxylic acid cycle, rat liver mitochondria can reduce certain disulfides of low molecular weight, particularly cystamine. Skrede *et al.* (1965), pre-incubating the mitochondria with cystamine, blocked the reducing capacity of rat liver mitochondria with respect to disulfides. Mitochondria treated in this way cannot reduce cystamine, when it is added to the incubation medium containing succinate. In the absence of —SH groups, a much more pronounced uncoupling is observed than that obtained by adding cystamine to the mitochondrial suspension containing succinate; in this case the cystamine is likely to be partially reduced to MEA which is

TABLE 14. EFFECT OF CYSTAMINE ON OXIDATIVE PHOSPHORYLATION
(Modified from Skrede *et al.*, 1965)

Experimental conditions	Cystamine (mM)	Oxygen uptake (μatom per 10 min)	Phosphate esterified (μmol per 10 min)	P/O ratio
Cystamine added with succinate	—	9.7	18.1	1.9
	0.5	9.6	17.0	1.8
	1.0	10.0	14.0	1.4
	2.5	9.0	16.7	1.8
	5.0	10.3	16.5	1.6
Cystamine added 7 min before succinate	—	10.3	21.7	2.1
	0.5	9.9	18.0	1.8
	1.0	7.6	12.4	1.6
	2.5	7.7	2.7	0.3
	5.0	7.4	0	0

inactive as an uncoupling agent (Table 14).

Oxygen consumption under these conditions is slightly lowered. It is possible that cystamine, like dinitrophenol, because of its uncoupling activity, causes an accumulation of oxaloacetate (Slater and Hulsmann, 1961), a powerful inhibitor of succinate oxidation.

Skrede (1966) also showed that cystamine unmasks the activity of the adenosine triphosphatase in freshly prepared mitochondria, releases intramitochondrial magnesium, and slows down the phosphate exchange reaction between adenosine triphosphate (ATP) and inorganic phosphate.

Certain observations suggest that the mechanisms by which cystamine and dinitrophenol uncouple oxidative phosphorylation are different. Whereas dinitrophenol uncouples by reacting with certain energy-rich intermediates (Hemker, 1964), it seems that the uncoupling action of cystamine may be due to alteration of the permeability of the mitochondrial membrane.

The effect of cystamine on the mitochondrial permeability cannot be directly associated with its swelling effect, because MEA from this point of view is almost as active as cystamine (Neubert and Lehninger, 1962), without, however, producing the effects of the latter in regard to adenosine triphosphatase and coupled oxidative phosphorylation.

Skrede (1966) showed that the association of cystamine with mitochondrial proteins varies according to the metabolic state of the mitochondria. Subsequently, Skrede (1968) showed that the mitochondrial membrane is impermeable to cystamine in the metabolic states 1 and 4 as defined by Chance and Williams (1956). This permeability barrier seems to reflect a state of high energy in the membrane. The energy required to maintain this barrier could be provided either by the respiratory chain or by the exogenous ATP. This permeability barrier can be abolished by uncoupling agents, by inhibitors of the respiratory chain, by anaerobiosis, or by phosphate. It is probably located at the internal membrane of the mitochondria, because the external membrane appears easily permeable to various substances of low molecular weight (Klingenberg and Pfaff, 1966). Some —SH groups capable of reacting with cystamine are apparently located on the outside of this permeability barrier. When —SH groups in the saccharose space combine with cystamine to form disulfides after state 1 incubation of the mitochondria, no lowering of oxidative phosphorylation is observed.

When cystamine can easily penetrate the mitochondria, for example in state 2, the disulfides easily react with the thiol groups of the membrane, and the permeability of the membrane to endogenous nucleotides, and to ions such as magnesium, is greatly increased (Skrede *et al.,* 1965; Skrede, 1966). The uncoupling effect of cystamine which follows may be explained either by a change in the structure of the membrane, or by a blockage of a specific protein support taking part in the formation of an energy-rich intermediate.

It seems that inorganic phosphate facilitates the passage of cystamine into the interior of the mitochondria by causing the latter to swell. However, it should be noted that although ATP and succinate increase the swelling effect of inorganic phosphate, these two substances prevent the passage of cystamine into the mitochondria. Certain uncoupling agents such as antimycin A lift the mitochondrial permeability barrier to cystamine without inducing swelling, which indicates that swelling is not the general mechanism that assists penetration of the disulfide into the intramitochondrial space (Skrede, 1966). Cystamine causes uncoupling of oxidative phosphorylation in mitochondria at metabolic states 2 and 5, but is inactive at states 1, 3, and 4. The uncoupling effect depends strongly on the state of phosphorylation: ATP counteracts uncoupling, unlike adenosine diphosphate (ADP). The experiments of Skrede (1968) seem to suggest that the permeability barrier with regard to cystamine in the internal membrane of mitochondria in metabolic states 1 and 4 is a barrier of electric charge, exercising its effect on the positively charged disulfides. It is true that, in metabolic states 1 and 4,

TABLE 15. DISAPPEARANCE OF THIOL GROUPS IN MATRIX PROTEINS AS AN INDEX OF THE PENETRATION OF $NNN'N'$-TETRAMETHYLCYSTAMINE AND CYSTAMINE[a] (Modified from Skrede, 1968)

Addition of	SH in matrix proteins (nmol/mg of protein) of mitochondria incubated with		
	—	Antimycin A	Dinitrophenol
—	74	71	74
Me$_4$-Cystamine	73	48	53
Cystamine	71	46	54

[a] Thiol groups determined by silver titration.

TABLE 16. PENETRATION OF DIACETYLCYSTAMINE AND CYSTAMINE INTO RAT LIVER MITOCHONDRIA (Modified from Skrede, 1968)

Additions	Disulfide sulfur bound (natom/mg of protein)
NN'-Diacetyl [^{35}S] cystamine	4.0
NN'-Diacetyl [^{35}S] cystamine + 2,4-DNP[a]	4.4
[^{35}S] Cystamine	13.6
[^{35}S] Cystamine + 2,4-DNP[a]	43.4

[a] DNP = dinitrophenol.

the mitochondrial membrane opposes the passage of cystamine and of $NNN'N'$-tetramethylcystamine, whereas the neutral derivate, NN'-diacetylcystamine, has free access to the intramitochondrial space (Tables 15 and 16).

As it is set out, the hypothesis of a charge barrier advanced by Skrede (1968) is not easily reconcilable with the chemi-osmotic theory of oxidative phosphorylation proposed by Mitchell (1961, 1966a, b), according to which the permeable cations are accumulated in the mitochondria by an exchange process with hydrogen ions during electron transfer. Such a mechanism would imply that the cystamine would have to be accumulated during states 1 and 4 and not repelled by a charge barrier. If such a charge barrier is a transmembrane potential, the direction is opposite to that proposed by Mitchell. The results of Skrede (1968) give no conclusive indication of the creation of such a transmembrane potential, which would interfere with the passage of the positively charged disulfides. The lowered permeability of these cations in a high energy state might also depend on fixed charges in the membrane without relation to the state of equilibrium on both sides of the mitochondrial membrane.

6.5.2. EFFECTS OF AET

Zins *et al.* (1958b) determined the effect of AET on the metabolism of substrates of the tricarboxylic acid cycle. In their experiments, they estimated the activity of AET by directly measuring the utilization of substrates by homogenates of rat organs rather than by the consumption of O_2, the exact measurement of which presents certain difficulties in the presence of easily oxidizable sulfur-containing radioprotective agents.

TABLE 17. EFFECT OF ADDED RADIOPROTECTIVE AGENTS ON THE UTILIZATION OF PYRUVATE BY HOMOGENATES OF RAT LIVER AND KIDNEY
(Modified from Zins *et al.*, 1958a)

Addition (1 mм)	Pyruvate utilization (%) by homogenates of	
	Liver	Kidney
None	100	100
MEA	90	69
2-Mercaptoethanol	100	100
AET	55	45
GED	55	27
3-Aminopropylisothiourea	31	31
4-Aminobutylisothiourea	89	100
DEDTC	19	2
para-Aminopropiophenone	84	88

TABLE 18. EFFECT OF INJECTED RADIOPROTECTIVE AGENTS ON THE UTILIZATION OF PYRUVATE BY HOMOGENATES OF RAT LIVER AND KIDNEY[a]
(Modified from Zins *et al.*, 1958a, b)

Compound injected	Dose injected (mg/kg)	Pyruvate utilization (%) by homogenates of	
		Liver	Kidney
None	—	100	100
MEA	77	87	75
2-Mercaptoethanol	78	100	92
AET	190	49	42
GED	118	81	80
3-Aminopropylisothiourea	206	58	37
4-Aminobutylisothiourea	309	100	100
DEDTC (sodium salt)	225	47	86
para-Aminopropiophenone	30	100	93
NaAsO$_2$	5	52	0

[a] The compounds tested are injected 30 min before sacrifice. The dose is 1 mequiv. S/kg for the first seven compounds; it is lower for the last two which are too toxic.

The addition of 225 mg/l AET to the incubation medium significantly reduces pyruvate utilization by rat liver or kidney homogenates. This inhibition is observed *in vitro* in the presence of MEG, and also guanidine ethyldisulfide (Table 17). Another *S*-alkylated derivative, β-aminopropyl-isothiourea, also inhibits the utilization of pyruvate under the same conditions. However, 4-aminobutylisothiourea, a non-radioprotective compound, causes a slight inhibition in the liver homogenates, but is inactive in homogenates of the kidney.

Intraperitoneal administration of AET 30 min before removal of the organs used for preparation of the homogenates also inhibits the activity of the latter with regard to pyruvate utilization (Table 18). In this case also, the non-protective 4-aminobutylisothiourea is inactive. It is also seen that MEA in radioprotective doses exerts a less marked inhibitory effect than AET, in relation to the same enzymatic systems. The authors noted a certain correlation between the development of radio-protective action after injection with AET and the development of inhibition of certain metabolic processes in the living animal (observed by measuring the metabolic activity of the homogenates of organs removed at varying times after the administration of the radioprotective agent). There is also a correlation between the extent of the inhibition and the intensity of the symptoms of intoxication that follow injections with AET.

In higher concentrations, MEG and guanidine ethyldisulfide (GED) inhibit *in vitro* other enzymes that participate in the functioning of the tricarboxylic acid cycle, especially succinate dehydrogenase (Fig. 15), malate dehydrogenase and cytochrome oxidase (Fig. 16); MEG has a

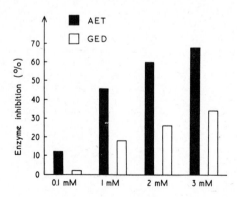

FIG. 15. Inhibition of succinate dehydrogenase *in vitro* by AET and GED. (Zins *et al.*, 1958b.)

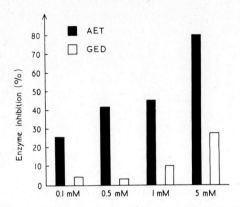

FIG. 16. Inhibition of cytochrome oxidase *in vitro* by AET and GED. (Zins *et al.*, 1958b.)

more significant effect than GED (Zins *et al.*, 1958a).

Scaife (1965) confirmed the results of Zins *et al.* (1958a), and observed intense inhibition of oxidation of 2-oxoglutarate by an homogenate of rat liver in the presence of 2 mM MEG. Scaife determined the metabolic activity by measuring the consumption of oxygen, and also observed that an appreciable quantity of MEG is oxidized during incubation, in the absence or in the presence of 2-oxoglutarate. The degree of inhibition by AET is increased if, before adding the substrate, the homogenate is incubated with the radioprotective agent. The inhibition increases in intensity in an oxygen-rich atmosphere. This observation suggests, as does the development of the inhibition curve obtained by incubating liver homogenates in the presence of 2-oxoglutarate and MEG, that an oxidizing mechanism is implicated in the inhibition of O_2 consumption. In other words, the disulfides exercise a more marked inhibitory effect than the corresponding thiols. Scaife showed that the extent of inhibition produced by different disulfides is significantly greater than that corresponding to the thiol in the same intervals of time.

Aminoethylisothiourea, in the form of MEG, does not seem to uncouple the oxidative phosphorylation in the presence of 2-oxoglutarate *in vitro*. It also causes inhibition of O_2 consumption of homogenates of rat liver incubated in the presence of other intermediates of the tricarboxylic acid cycle, especially pyruvate, malate, fumarate, 3-hydroxybutyrate, and glutamate. However, inhibition observed with these substrates is less than that obtained in the presence of equimolecular quantities of

2-oxoglutarate. Scaife (1965) showed that there is no correlation between the radioprotective effect of a thiol or disulfide and its ability to reduce cytochrome *c,* and from this concluded that inhibition of the oxidation of the 2-oxoglutarate *in vitro* is probably not due to interference of the electron transport chain by the inhibitor.

At the same time, there is a good correlation between the radioprotective effects of certain sulfur-containing compounds in the disulfide form and their inhibiting activities with regard to the oxidation of 2-oxoglutarate by rat liver homogenate.

DuBois *et al.* (1958b) observed a certain cumulative effect of AET from the point of view of enzymatic inhibition. Rats were given a daily dose of 100, 200, or 300 mg/kg of AET. This treatment was continued for several days and, 24 hr after the last dose, the animal was sacrificed, and the oxidation capacity of their liver or kidney homogenates measured in the presence of pyruvate. No inhibiting effect was observed on the oxidation of pyruvate in the liver or kidney of animals having received a daily dose of 100 mg/kg AET. On the other hand, higher doses of the order of 300 mg/kg daily caused significant inhibition of the pyruvate oxidation in homogenates of the kidney.

6.5.3. EFFECTS OF DIETHYLDITHIOCARBAMATE (DEDTC)

Diethyldithiocarbamate (112 mg/l) added to a homogenate of rat liver or kidney causes significant inhibition of the pyruvate utilization. This inhibition is of the order of 81 % for liver, and 98 % for kidney (Table 17) (Zins *et al.,* 1958b). These authors observed the same effect when the homogenate was prepared from organs taken from animals who, 30 min previously, had received an i.p. radioprotective dose of 225 mg/kg DEDTC. It is seen that DEDTC (in the form of the diethylamine salt) causes 53 % inhibition of the pyruvate utilization in liver preparations and 14 % inhibition in kidney preparations (Table 18).

Liver and kidney seem to behave in a slightly different way *in vivo,* with regard to dimethyldithiocarbamate (DuBois *et al.,* 1961). These authors administered different i.p. doses of dimethyldithiocarbamate to groups of rats during several successive days. The daily doses were of the order of 200, 300, and 400 mg/kg. Twenty-four hours after the last dose, the animals were killed, and the utilization of pyruvate by the homogenates prepared from liver and kidney was measured. There did not appear to be any cumulative effect on pyruvate utilization by the kidney preparation. At the same time, repeated doses of dimethyldithiocarbamate progressively increased the inhibitory effect on the utilization of pyruvate by the liver homogenates. When animals had been pretreated for several days with 200, 300, or 400 mg/kg of dimethyldithiocarbamate administered by i.p. injection, and the sharp activity immediately produced by a 100-mg dose of dimethyldithiocarbamate was measured, it was observed that the liver had become much more sensitive. This single dose of 100 mg of dimethyldithiocarbamate (which in a whole animal produced just a moderate inhibition of pyruvate oxidation *in vitro*) caused, in an animal which had received several days' prior treatment, very serious inhibition of pyruvate utilization. Under the same conditions kidney does not show this hypersensitivity phenomenon.

DuBois *et al.* (1961) showed that dimethyldithiocarbamate and DEDTC (in the form of diethylamine salts), sodium diethyldithiocarbamate and dimethyldithiocarbamate disulfide caused *in vitro* a significant inhibition of O_2 consumption, pyruvate utilization, and citrate synthesis in liver and kidney homogenates of rats, mice, or guinea-pigs.

Thiols exercise a different effect from that of the sulfide derivatives if administered *in vivo* in massive tolerated doses (500 mg/kg for dimethyl-dithiocarbamate of diethylamine; 150 mg/kg for the corresponding disulfide). Pretreatment of animals with dimethyldithiocarbamate results in *in vitro* inhibition of pyruvate utilization by liver or kidney homogenates taken from the treated animals. At the same time, the corresponding disulfide injected in the animal in no way altered the oxidative metabolic capacity of homogenates of these same organs incubated *in vitro*. The same observations have been made by these authors concerning the activity of other dehydrogenases, particularly 2-oxoglutaric dehydro-genase and succinic dehydrogenase. The thiol derivative, dimethyl-dithiocarbamate, reduces *in vitro* and *in vivo* the capacity of the homogenates to utilize 2-oxoglutarate and succinate. The corresponding disulfide exerts an inhibitory effect *in vitro*, but is inefficient *in vivo* (DuBois *et al.*, 1961).

Mercaptoethyldithiocarbamate (DuBois *et al.*, 1961) inhibits 2-oxoglutaric and succinic dehydrogenases *in vitro*. However, a strong dose (400 mg/kg) injected into the animal scarcely affects the metabolic activity of the tissues, measured *in vitro*, and affects neither glycolysis nor the respiration of brain homogenates.

DuBois *et al.* (1961) described a cumulative effect, from the enzymatic point of view, of dimethyldithiocarbamate and AET. They showed that AET and dimethyldithiocarbamate administered separately at 100 mg/kg for several days do not alter the capacity of liver homogenates, prepared

from these animals, to utilize pyruvate. At the same time, daily administration of 100 mg of AET and 100 mg of dimethyldithiocarbamate after
6-day treatment results in inhibition of the activity of the pyruvic dehydrogenase of between 13 and 35 % on the basis of decrease in O_2 consumption,
and between 20 and 35 % on the basis of inhibition of pyruvate utilization.
This inhibition subsequently reaches a maximum which does not increase
further during the following 20 days. Kidney homogenates prepared
from animals so treated (receiving 100 mg/kg per day AET or dimethyldithiocarbamate, for several days) showed no effect on pyruvic dehydrogenase activity. At the same time, simultaneous administration of these
two substances in the same animal and at the same dose causes, after
6-day treatment, a decrease of metabolic activity with regard to pyruvate.
Kidney homogenates from these animals show inhibition of the pyruvic
dehydrogenase of between 7 and 16 % on the basis of oxygen consumption,
and of 10–30 % on the basis of pyruvate utilization. After 20-day treatment
inhibition of renal tissue activity reaches 37% on the basis of oxygen
consumption and 45 % on the basis of pyruvate.

Daily doses of 200 mg/kg of AET and dimethyldithiocarbamate,
to the same animal, cause significant and extremely rapid inhibition of
enzyme activity in the liver and kidney. From the second day, inhibition
of pyruvate utilization of the order of 44% in the liver homogenates
and 49% in kidney preparations may be seen. Prolonging such treatment
soon causes a very high mortality, whereas the daily injection of 400 mg
of dimethyldithiocarbamate for several weeks has no effect on the survival
of the animals (DuBois and Raymund, 1958).

Disulfiram in a concentration of 0.14 mM totally inhibits the O_2
consumption of a suspension of rat liver mitochondria incubated in
the presence of 3-hydroxybutyrate (Hassinen, 1966). In the presence of
pyruvate or malate, the inhibition caused by disulfiram (0.27 mM) is
only 26%. Finally, the activity of the succinic dehydrogenase is not
affected by the presence of disulfiram in the incubation medium.

Oxidation of NADH in the submitochondrial sonicated particles is
seriously inhibited by disulfiram. Dimethyldithiocarbamate on the contrary, in the same conditions, is inactive, and does not affect O_2 consumption of the mitochondria in the presence of different substrates.
The inhibitory effect of disulfiram may be prevented by the addition, to
the incubation medium containing the mitochondria, of an —SH donor
such as 2-mercaptoethanol before the addition of disulfiram.

The disulfiram seems to become strongly fixed, and profoundly affects
the respiratory system associated with the oxidation of pyruvate and

3-hydroxybutyrate. Intensive washing of mitochondria pre-incubated with disulfiram cannot restore enzymatic activity. Similarly, treatment of the mitochondria blocked in this way by the use of an —SH donor such as 2-mercaptoethanol cannot remove the inhibition produced by disulfiram, even if the quantities of 2-mercaptoethanol used are four times greater than that sufficient to prevent inhibition, which would be caused by the subsequent addition of disulfiram (Hassinen, 1966).

Following treatment with dinitrophenol and uncoupling of oxidative phosphorylation, the mitochondria are less sensitive to the effect of the disulfiram, and about double concentrations are necessary to obtain an inhibitory effect corresponding to that obtained with intact mitochondria (Hassinen, 1966). Inhibition of activated adenosine triphosphatase in the presence of dinitrophenol is also observed whereas the adenosine triphosphatase activated in the presence of magnesium is only slightly inhibited. Disulfiram in a concentration of 0.1 mM caused about 50 % inhibition of the exchange reaction between ATP and inorganic phosphate.

The author suggests that the inhibitory effect of disulfiram may be due to interaction of this compound with adjacent thiol groups on the enzyme. This hypothesis is supported by certain observations, particularly the similarity between the inhibition of 3-hydroxybutyrate oxidation caused by disulfiram and that induced by bivalent cadmium and arsenite in the presence of 2,3-dimercaptopropanol (Hassinen, 1966); such inhibition is considered as indicating the presence of adjacent thiol groups on the enzyme (Lehninger *et al.*, 1960; Sekuzu *et al.*, 1963). Subsequently, Hassinen and Hallmann (1967) have shown that disulfiram inhibits the action of NADH oxidase, without affecting the dehydrogenase activity. Disulfiram also inhibits reduction of cytochrome *b* by NADH, without affecting reduction by succinate. These authors have shown that the site of action of disulfiram, as well as that of arsenite, in the presence of dimercaptopropanol is located at the level of the ubiquinone fraction of the system ubiquinone–NADH reductase. This site could be made up of dithiol groups present on the "ubiquinone factor", as suggested by analogy of the behavior of disulfiram and arsenite in the presence of dimercaptopropanol, considered as a specific reagent of the dithiols (Stocken and Thompson, 1946).

6.6. PERMEABILITY CHANGES AND LIPID PEROXIDATION

6.6.1. SWELLING OF MITOCHONDRIA

6.6.1.1. *Introduction*

As is shown in Chapter 4 of this volume, administration of sulfur-containing radioprotective agents in animals entails changes of the structure of mitochondria *in vivo,* which can be seen with the aid of the electron microscope. According to Bacq *et al.* (1965b), it may be suggested that the radioprotective agents react with the proteins of the mitochondrial membranes, modify their permeability, and, in this way distort their normal functioning. The non-radioprotective thiols do not visibly alter the structure of the mitochondria.

Frederic (1958) showed with the help of chicken fibroblast cultures that mitochondria of living cells can undergo changes of size and structure in the presence of pharmacological agents (such as inhibitors of respiration). Mitochondria in such cells treated with MEA seem to be thicker and shorter than usual, and also less mobile (Chèvremont-Comhaire and Chèvremont, 1953).

Changes in volume of isolated mitochondria have already been studied (see particularly Raaflaub, 1953a, b) by measuring the variations of the light scattering by their suspensions at a neutral wavelength that is isosbestic for oxidized and reduced forms of the respiratory catalysts. It has been observed that the change of volume could be passive, caused by a change in the osmotic pressure of the medium, or active, because of changed respiratory activity, in the presence of high-energy compounds or compounds affecting the metabolism, such as dinitrophenol or thyroxine (for reviews, see Lehninger, 1962, 1964). Only mitochondria respiring in the presence of oxidizable substrates and oxygen, but with limiting amounts of ADP or ATP (state 4 of Chance and Williams, 1956), swell.

6.6.1.2. *Effects of Thiols*

Glutathione, in concentrations similar to those found in the tissues, produces swelling of the mitochondria (Lehninger and Schneider, 1959), but this is different from the kinetic point of view from that produced by thyroxine (Fig. 17). It is produced after a longer lag phase, is not prevented by dinitrophenol, nor by amytal or antimycin A; however, it is counteracted by ATP, EDTA, or Mn^{2+} (not Mg^{2+}).

Figure 17 and Table 19 show that these effects can be produced by

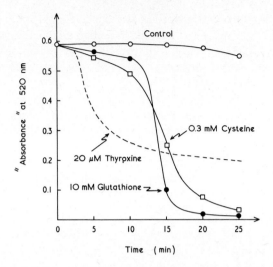

FIG. 17. Swelling of rat liver mitochondria in the presence of GSH or cysteine. Swelling is registered as a decrease in "absorbance" at 520 nm. (Modified from Lehninger and Schneider, 1959.)

TABLE 19. SWELLING OF MITOCHONDRIA IN THE PRESENCE OF THIOLS AND DISULFIDES (Modified from Neubert and Lehninger, 1962)

Addition (1 mM)	Change in absorbance $(10^3 \times \Delta A_{520}/50 \text{ min})$
L-Cysteine	− 60
D-Cysteine	− 15
L-Cysteine methyl ester	− 50
L-Cysteinylglycine	− 50
GSH	− 10
Thioglycolate	− 10
MEA	−135
2-Mercaptoethanol	−115
Dithiocarbamate	− 30
GSSG	− 20
Dithiodiglycolate	−150
Cystamine	−190
2-Hydroxyethyl disulfide	−160
Disulfiram[a]	−160
Oxidized thioctic acid	− 35

[a] Disulfiram at 0.1 mM only.

cysteine and some of its derivatives whose efficiency is greater than that of GSH. They are even more marked (Neubert and Lehninger, 1962) in the presence of MEA and of 2-mercaptoethanol (the latter, a non-radio-protective compound, does not alter the appearance of mitochondria if injected into the animal).

It is not certain that GSH, cysteine, and MEA act by the same mechanism. In fact, mitochondria that have swelled in the presence of cysteine or MEA can contract again under the influence of ATP, whereas those that swelled under the effect of GSH have lost a factor (Factor C) that enables them to contract again under the influence of ATP. This factor contains catalase and glutathione peroxidase (Neubert and Lehninger, 1962).

6.6.1.3. *Effect of Disulfides*

Disulfides, GSSH, 2-hydroxyethyl disulfide, and above all disulfiram, are more efficient than the corresponding thiols (Table 19) and the combinations of GSH and disulfides are even more efficient (Table 20).

It may be observed that disulfide-containing hormones (oxytocin, vasopressin, and insulin) are, mole for mole, 50–100 times more efficient than GSSG. Their potency is further increased about 10-fold by the addition of very low concentrations of GSH insufficient by themselves (Lehninger and Neubert, 1961).

A mechanism for the interpretation of the interaction of a disulfide with a protein structure carrying —SH groups has been suggested by

TABLE 20. MITOCHONDRIAL SWELLING BY DISULFIDES. POTENTIATION BY GSH
(Modified from Lehninger and Neubert, 1961 and Neubert and Lehninger, 1962)

Disulfide	Concentration (mM)	Change in absorbance ($10^3 \times \Delta A_{520}$/hr) in the presence of GSH at the following concentrations (μM)				
		0	2–3	20	300–500	1000
GSSG	1	0				− 70
Dithiodiglycolate	1	− 50				−150
Cystine	0.3	− 90			−280	
2-Hydroxyethyl disulfide	1	−250				−110
Oxytocin	0.016	− 10			−115	
Oxytocin	0.05	− 50	−160			
Vasopressin	0.024	− 10	−120	− 80		
Insulin	0.01	0				−130
Insulin	0.03	−140				−220

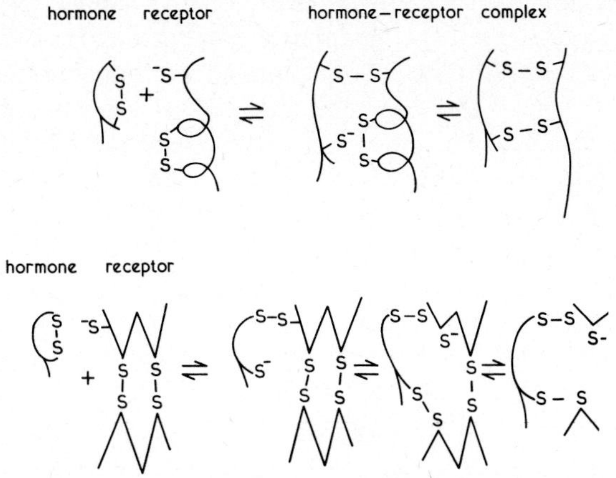

FIG. 18. Hypothetical mechanism for the combination of vasopressin with a receptor. This may bring about conformational changes (upper part) or linear propagation of a series of thiol-disulfide interchanges producing a separation of fibrillar elements in a protein diffusion barrier. (Schwartz *et al.*, 1960.) Although this mechanism may well apply to many biological actions and to the action of some hormones, it has been found not to be obligatory for the action of vasopressin. (Schwartz *et al.*, 1964.)

Schwartz *et al.* (1960) to explain the action of the vasopressin. It is illustrated in Fig. 18.

Apparently there are two categories of —SH groups in the mitochondrial membrane; one is very sensitive to Ag^+, and the titration of these —SH groups causes immediate swelling. These —SH groups are no longer titratable by the Ag^+ if the mitochondria have been previously incubated in the presence of GSSG (Riley and Lehninger, 1964), which demonstrates that a thiol–disulfide interaction between the GSSG and the mitochondrial membrane has occurred.

The swelling observed *in vitro,* in the presence of the mixture GSSG + GSH, leads to the complete disintegration of the mitochondria (Gebicki and Hunter, 1964).

6.6.1.4. *Discussion*

It is not possible to extrapolate the observations made *in vitro* to those made *in vivo,* following administration of radioprotectors (see Chapter 4). The number of factors likely to affect these phenomena, in one direction or another, and even in a different direction according to the experimental conditions, is unfortunately considerable (for a discussion of this, refer to the reviews of Lehninger, 1962, 1964).

It has already been mentioned that mercaptoethanol causes swelling *in vitro,* and not *in vivo.* The observations on swelling *in vitro* were mostly carried out on very dilute suspensions. Under the conditions used for measuring the respiratory activity in the Warburg apparatus, it seems difficult to correlate the inhibition of respiration of the mitochondria and the changes in the light scattering of their suspensions associated with swelling. This is particularly evident in the publications of Bicheikina and Romantsev (1966a, b) concerning brain and liver mitochondria following the addition or injection of MPA or MEA.

Other changes in the permeability of membranes by thiols and disulfides have been described, for example: release of enzymes and formation of protoplasts under the influence of mercaptoethanol in *Saccharomyces fragilis* (Davies and Elvin, 1964), or the increased concentration of certain intercellular enzymes in the blood of rats following injection of MEA (Plomteux *et al.,* 1966, 1967).

6.6.2. LIPID PEROXIDATION AND GLUTATHIONE PEROXIDASE

6.6.2.1. *Swelling and Peroxidation of Lipids*

The swelling of mitochondria observed in the presence of a mixture of GSSG + GSH is accompanied by the formation of lipid peroxides, measured by the thiobarbituric acid test. The accelerators and inhibitors of GSH-induced swelling affect the formation of peroxides in a similar

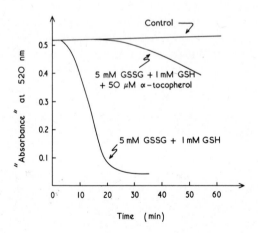

FIG. 19. Inhibition of the (GSSG + GSH)-induced swelling by α-tocopherol. (Hunter *et al.,* 1964.)

manner (Hunter *et al.,* 1964). It is in this way that the antioxidants such as α-tocopherol inhibit the two phenomena (Fig. 19).

It is observed, moreover, that a suspension of pure methyl arachidonate, without mitochondria, produces lipid peroxides in the presence of GSH and GSSG, in the concentrations used in the experiments on isolated mitochondria (Fig. 20); GSH or GSSG added alone has hardly any effect at all.

Cystamine, in moderate concentrations (maximum effect at 0.5 mM),

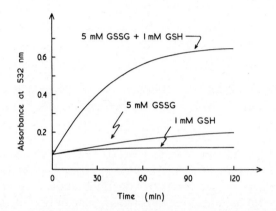

FIG. 20. Formation of lipid peroxides from methyl arachidonate in the presence of (GSSG + GSH). The malonylaldehyde formed during peroxidation is estimated by the thiobarbituric-acid method. (Hunder *et al.,* 1964.)

TABLE 21. FORMATION OF LIPID PEROXIDES IN RAT LIVER MITOCHONDRIA
(From Skrede and Christophersen, 1966)

Addition	Malonylaldehyde formed (nmol/hr per 10 mg protein)
None	1.9
10 mM Cystamine	9.2
5 mM MEA	39.1
5 mM MEA + 40 mg thiolated Sephadex[a]	4.3
5 mM MEA + 10 mM Cystamine	17.8
10 mM GSSG	10.5
5 mM GSH	6.0
5 mM GSH + 40 mg thiolated Sephadex[a]	3.1
5 mM GSH + 10 mM GSSG	80.8
10 mM Cystamine + 5 mM EDTA	0

[a] To counteract auto-oxidation.

also stimulates peroxidation of lipids in the mitochondria (Table 21). Cysteamine and GSH do so only if their auto-oxidation is not prevented (Skrede and Christophersen, 1966). Simultaneous release of mitochondrial proteins in the medium is observed.

6.6.2.2.   *Role of Thiols in Lipid Peroxidation*

The formation of lipid peroxides is not a phenomenon exclusively linked with the oxidation of the thiols in mitochondria. It is also observed when isolated subcellular fractions are aerobically incubated in the presence of cysteine (Meyerhof, 1923; Christophersen, 1968a, b), of heme derivatives (Tappel and Zalkin, 1960), or of ascorbate (Ottolenghi, 1959; Thiele and Huff, 1960). The oxidizable metallic cations, the Fe^{2+} in particular, catalyze the formation of lipid peroxides *in vitro* (Ottolenghi, 1959).

The formation of lipid peroxides is also observed during E-avitaminosis (Tappel and Zalkin, 1959; Bieri and Anderson, 1960; Corwin, 1962), because of the antioxidizing character of α-tocopherol, but this is contested by El-Khatib *et al.* (1964).

Ultraviolet irradiation (Wilbur *et al.*, 1949) or X-ray irradiation (Horgan and Philpot, 1954, 1962, 1964) is another source of lipid peroxides, as shown by the reaction with thiobarbituric acid. Wills and Wilkinson (1966) observed that direct irradiation of lysosomes by X-rays caused the formation of lipid peroxides and the release of enzymes; they think that the two phenomena are linked (Skrede and Christophersen, 1966: see Table 21). Direct injection of lipid peroxides is itself very toxic (Horgan *et al.*, 1957). Administration of sulfur-containing radioprotective agents reduces the peroxide content in the tissues of irradiated animals (Romantsev and Zhulanova, 1961).

Thiol oxidation with lipid peroxides is much more rapid with hydrogen peroxide (Little and O'Brien, 1968a). Enzymes may be inactivated in this way (Little and O'Brien, 1966), and the glycolytic activity of extracts of guinea-pig cortex is 50% inhibited by as little as 27 mmol/mg linoleic acid hydroperoxide (Little and O'Brien, 1967).

NADPH-induced peroxidation of lipids catalyzed by ADP has also been described in rat liver microsomes (Hochstein and Ernster, 1963); this system is involved in the so-called drug metabolism of liver cells (see Fig. 22). Its K_m for oxygen was found by Lumper *et al.* (1968) to be $30 \mu M$ (corresponding to a partial O_2 pressure of about 15 mmHg), i.e. 15–20 times higher than the K_m of cytochrome oxidase for O_2. This source of lipid peroxides therefore mainly depends on the partial O_2

pressure in the tissues, so perhaps it is not surprising that hypoxia reduces lipid peroxide formation in irradiated animals (Romantsev and Zhulanova, 1961).

Liver homogenates produce lipid peroxides from the moment they no longer contain any GSH and this production can be stopped by further addition of GSH (Christophersen, 1966). Lipid peroxides are transformed by GSH into non-toxic hydroxylated fatty acids (Christophersen, 1968a), in agreement with the following equation:

$$ROOH + 2GSH \longrightarrow ROH + GSSG + H_2O$$

This reaction, similar to that catalyzed by glutathione peroxidase, is no doubt enzymatic, because GSH ceases to inhibit the ascorbate-induced production of lipid peroxides in microsomal and mitochondrial preparations if these have been heat-denatured (Table 22). Cysteamine (see also Bernheim, 1964) remains inhibitory in the presence of heat-denatured suspensions, no doubt because of its high affinity for the metallic cations (in this case Fe^{2+}). Thioglycollate and mercaptoethanol have no effect, whereas cysteine and homocysteine stimulate production of lipid peroxides, even in the absence of ascorbate.

Thiols, it would seem, then, can act in different ways at this level: (a) their auto-oxidation (cysteine and homocysteine) produces lipid peroxides, which GSH can enzymatically detoxicate, and (b) MEA and DEDTC reduce the formation of peroxides by complexing Fe^{2+}.

TABLE 22. EFFECT OF THIOLS ON THE ASCORBATE-INDUCED PEROXIDATION OF FRESH AND BOILED MICROSOMAL FRACTIONS[a] (From Christophersen, 1968b)

Addition (1 mM)	Microsomal fraction (nmol/hr per 8 mg protein)	
	Fresh	Boiled
None	30	58
GSH	4	51
MEA	10	2
DEDTC	0	8
Thioglycolate	36	63
Mercaptoethanol	33	57
L-Cysteine	32	55
	16[a]	26[a]
DL-Homocysteine	38	57
	43[a]	78[a]

[a] In the absence of ascorbate (otherwise 0.2 mM).

6.6.2.3. *Enzymes Acting on GSH/GSSG*

Aebi *et al.* (1964) showed that the destruction of small amounts of hydrogen peroxide in the red cells is an effect of the glutathione peroxidase: catalase only participates in the presence of higher concentrations of hydrogen peroxide.

Glutathione peroxidase allows the red cells to maintain the iron of their hemoglobin in the reduced state (Mills, 1957: Mills and Randall, 1958). This enzyme has been purified (Mills, 1959), and its properties have been analyzed (Schneider and Flohé, 1967). It is present in a large number of tissues (Mills, 1960; Pirie, 1965).

In fact, this enzyme is more active in the presence of linoleic acid hydroperoxide than in the presence of hydrogen peroxide (O'Brien and Little, 1967). It is found in the mitochondrial fraction, and in the supernatant fraction after centrifugation of the microsomes (Little and O'Brien, 1968b). Cysteamine and cysteine can be substituted for GSH but the velocity of the reaction is reduced to about 40 and 20% of that in the presence of GSH.

The reduction of GSSH into GSH is effected by NAD(P)H in the presence of glutathione reductase (Meldrum and Tarr, 1935; Francoeur and Denstedt, 1954; Scott *et al.*, 1963). This enzyme thus catalyzes the reduction of GSSG, at the expense of electrons provided by the NAD(P)-linked dehydrogenases, such as glucose-6-phosphate dehydrogenase (Fig. 21).

That this is an important mechanism maintaining GSH in the reduced state is shown by the rapid disappearance of GSH in erythrocytes of individuals with glucose-6-phosphate dehydrogenase deficiency (Cohen and Hochstein, 1961).

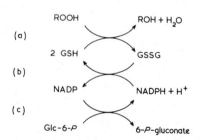

Fig. 21. Detoxication of lipid peroxides in animal cells. Enzymes involved are: (a) glutathione peroxidase, (b) glutathione reductase, (c) glucose-6-phosphate dehydrogenase (or other NAD P-linked dehydrogenase). ROOH, lipid peroxide; Glc-6-P, glucose-6-phosphate.

Other enzymes catalyze the oxidation of GSH *in vitro*: glutathione-homocystine transhydrogenase (Racker, 1954, 1955), nitroglycerol reductase (Heppel and Hilmoe, 1950), cytochrome *c*–cytochrome oxidase (Stotz *et al.*, 1937–8; Keilin and Hartree, 1938), and catalase (Boeri and Bonnichsen, 1952; see, however, Keilin and Nicholls, 1958). It is not known whether these enzymes oxidize GSH *in vivo*.

Glutathione can also reduce the disulfide bridges of several proteins, insulin in particular. This reaction is observed in the absence of enzyme but GSH-insulin-transhydrogenase accelerates the reaction (Katzen *et al.*, 1963). Several other thiols, such as cysteine, MEA, thioglycollate, and mercaptoethanol, can replace GSH (Schneider *et al.*, 1967).

Glutathione can also be coupled with epoxides in the presence of an *S*-epoxide transferase (Boyland and Williams, 1965):

$$GSH + R -CH-CH-R'' \longrightarrow GS-CHR'-CHR''OH$$
$$O$$

In this reaction, cysteine cannot replace GSH.

Finally GSH reacts with compounds containing active double bonds (Boyland and Chasseaud, 1966), under the effect of an enzyme different from *S*-aryltransferase (Booth *et al.*, 1960, 1961; Grover and Sims, 1964).

6.6.3. DRUG METABOLISM

Administration of MEA prolongs the duration of anesthesia produced by barbiturates (Della Bella and Bacq, 1953; Varagić *et al.*, 1962). This fact is no doubt related to the inhibition of barbiturate metabolism in the liver. This organ contains an enzymatic system capable of detoxicating a number of drugs (for a review, see Brodie *et al.*, 1958). This system is localized in the microsomes, and requires the presence of O_2 and NADPH.

Hydroxylation of drugs and peroxidation of lipids by the hepatic microsomes are linked phenomena. The oxidative demethylation (of the compound RCH_3 in Fig. 22) inhibits the peroxidation of lipids, by competing for the flow of electrons (Orrenius *et al.*, 1964a). Carbon monoxide, on the other hand, combines with cytochrome *P*-450, inhibiting NADPH oxidase, and drug metabolism, without affecting the formation of lipid peroxides (Estabrook *et al.*, 1963; Orrenius, 1965). Liébecq *et al.* (1964) have shown that oxidation of hexobarbital by a rat-liver homogenate free of nuclei and mitochondria is about 50% inhibited by 1.5 mM cystamine; it has also been observed that oxidation of NADPH is

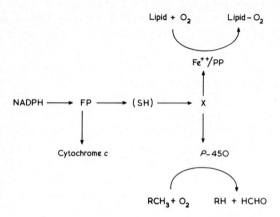

FIG. 22. Lipid peroxidation and drug metabolism in rat-liver microsomes. FP, flavoprotein; PP, pyrophosphate; P-450, a CO-binding cytochrome. (Modified from Slater, 1968.)

inhibited by the same concentration of cystamine. Cysteamine is about 5 times less efficient on the metabolism of hexobarbital, and only inhibits NADPH oxidase after a lag period of about 15 min, during which time it is probably oxidized into cystamine.

Cystamine presumably inhibits the transfer of electrons between the flavoprotein FP (of Fig. 22) and the cytochrome P-450 where the presence of a thiol group reacting with *para*-chloromercuribenzoate has been shown by Orrenius *et al.* (1964b).

Similar observations have been reported by Mizrahi and Emmelot (1963), concerning demethylation of dimethylnitrosamine, and by Liébecq (1966), concerning the hydroxylation of antipyrine.

REFERENCES

AEBI, H., HEINIGER, J. P. and LAUBER, E. (1964) Methämoglobinbildung in Erythrocyten durch Peroxideinwirkung. Versuche zur Beurteilung der Schutzfunktion von Katalase und Glutathionperoxydase. *Helv. chim. Acta* **47**: 1428–40.

BACQ, Z. M. (1965) *Chemical Protection against Ionizing Radiation,* C. C. Thomas Publ., Springfield, Ill., U.S.A.

BACQ, Z. M. (1966) La protection chimique contre les radiations ionisantes chez les Mammifères. *Bull. Acad. r. Méd. Belg.* (7e série) **6**: 115–41.

BACQ, Z. M. and ALEXANDER, P. (1955) *Principes de radiobiologie.* Masson et Cie, Paris.

BACQ, Z. M. and ALEXANDER, P. (1961) *Fundamentals of Radiobiology.* 2nd ed., Pergamon Press, Oxford.

BACQ, Z. M. and FISCHER, P. (1953) The action of cysteamine on liver glycogen. *Arch. int. Physiol.* **61**: 417–18.

BACQ, Z. M., CUYPERS, Y., EVRARD, E. and SOETENS, R. (1955) Action de la cystamine sur la résistance du rat à la dépression barométrique. *C.r. Séanc. Soc. Biol.* **149**: 2014–17.

BACQ, Z. M., LIÉBECQ-HUTTER, S. and LIÉBECQ, C. (1960) Protection against irradiation afforded by sodium fluoroacetate. *Radiat. Res.* **13**: 286–97.

BACQ, Z. M., BEAUMARIAGE, M. L. and LIÉBECQ-HUTTER, S. (1965a) Relation entre la radio-protection et l'hypothermie induite par certaines substances chimiques. *Int. J. Radiat. Biol.* **9**: 175–8.

BACQ, Z. M., BEAUMARIAGE, M. L., VAN CANEGHEM, P. and CICCARONE, P. (1965b) Impor-tance for radioprotective effect in mammals of pharmacological and biochemical actions of cysteamine and related substances. *Ann. Ist. super. Sanità* **1**: 639–45.

BEKKUM, D. W. VAN and ZAALBERG, O. B. (1960) Mechanisms of chemical protection against ionizing radiation in living organisms. *Int. J. Radiat. Biol. Suppl.* **1**: 155–61.

BELOKONSKII, I. S. (1959) Oxygen consumption by rats with changed radioresistance during their irradiation with X-rays. *Med. Radiol.* **4**: 27–31 (in Russian).

BENABID, Y. and RINALDI, R. (1966) Influence de certains composés hétérocycliques radio-protecteurs ou non sur la consommation d'oxygène dans différents tissus. *C.r. hebd. Séanc. Acad. Sci., Paris* **263**: 683–6.

BERNHEIM, F. (1964) Effect of 2-mercaptoethylamine on the peroxidation in microsomes of unsaturated lipids catalysed by cysteine or thiolactic acid and ultraviolet light. *Radiat. Res.* **23**: 454–60.

BETZ, E. H. and LELIÈVRE, P. (1969) Metabolic effect of sulfur containing radioprotecting drugs. In: *Book of Abstracts. Second International Symposium on Radiosensitizing and Radioprotective Drugs, Rome, 6–8 May*, p. 22.

BETZ, E. H., LELIÈVRE, P. and SMOLIAR, V. (1967) Protective effectiveness of some sulfur-containing substances and oxygen uptake in the rat. *Int. J. Radiat. Biol.* **12**: 163–8.

BETZ, E. H., MEWISSEN, D. J. and LELIÈVRE, P. (1962) Protective effectiveness of cystamine *versus* delay of exposure, body temperature and protein linkage. *Int. J. Radiat. Biol.* **4**: 231–7.

BICHEIKINA, N. I. and ROMANTSEV, E. F. (1966a) Influence of some radioprotectors on respiration of mitochondria of healthy and irradiated tissues. *Radiobiologiya* **6**: 598–600 (in Russian).

BICHEIKINA, N. I. and ROMANTSEV, E. F. (1966b) Effect of radioprotective agents on res-piration of rabbit liver and brain mitochondria. *Radiobiologiya* **6**: 880–2 (in Russian).

BIERI, J. G. and ANDERSON, A. A. (1960) Peroxidation of lipids in tissue homogenates as related to vitamin E. *Arch. Biochem. Biophys.* **90**: 105–10.

BOERI, E. and BONNICHSEN, R. K. (1952) Oxidation of thiol groups by catalase. *Acta chem. scand.* **6**: 968–70.

BOOTH, J., BOYLAND, E. and SIMS, P. (1960) Metabolism of polycyclic compounds, 15. The conversion of naphthalene into a derivative of glutathione by rat-liver slices. *Bio-chem. J.* **74**: 117–22.

BOOTH, J., BOYLAND, E. and SIMS, P. (1961) An enzyme from rat liver catalyzing conjuga-tions with glutathione. *Biochem. J.* **79**: 516–24.

BOYLAND, E. and CHASSEAUD, L. F. (1966) An enzyme catalysing the reaction of glutathione with unsaturated compounds. *Biochem. J.* **99**: 13–14P.

BOYLAND, E. and WILLIAMS, K. (1965) An enzyme catalyzing the conjugation of epoxides with glutathione. *Biochem. J.* **94**: 190–7.

BRODIE, B. B., GILLETTE, J. R. and LA DU, B. N. (1958) Enzymatic metabolism of drugs and other foreign compounds. *Ann. Rev. Biochem.* **27**: 427–54.

BÜCHER, T. and KLINGENBERG, M. (1958) Wege des Wasserstoffs in der lebendigen Organi-sation. *Angew. Chem.* **70**: 552–70.

CATER, D. B. (1960) Oxygen tension and oxido-reduction potentials in living tissues. *Prog. Biophys.* **10:** 153–60.

CAVALLINI, D., DE MARCO, C. and MONDOVI, B. (1956a) The oxidation of cystamine and other sulfur diamines by diamine-oxidase preparations. *Experientia* **12:** 377–84.

CAVALLINI, D., DE MARCO, C. and MONDOVI, B. (1956b) Alcune aspetti del metabolismo della cistamina *in vitro*. *Boll. Soc. ital. Biol. sper.* **32:** 1145–7.

CAVALLINI, D., DE MARCO, C. and MONDOVI, B. (1957) Cystaldimine: the product of oxidation of cystamine by diaminooxidases. *Biochim. biophys. Acta* **24:** 353–8.

CHANCE, B. (1957) Cellular oxygen requirements. *Fedn Proc. Fedn Am. Socs exp. Biol.* **16:** 671–80.

CHANCE, B. and WILLIAMS, G. R. (1956) The respiratory chain and oxidative phosphorylation. *Adv. Enzymol.* **17:** 65–134.

CHANCE, B., COHEN, P., JOBSIS, F. and SCHOENER, B. (1962a) Intracellular oxidation–reduction states *in vivo*. *Science* **137:** 499–508.

CHANCE, B., LEGALLAIS, V. and SCHOENER, B. (1962b) Metabolically linked changes in fluorescence, emission spectra of cortex of rat brain, kidney, and adrenal gland. *Nature (Lond.)* **195:** 1073–5.

CHANCE, B., SCHOENER, B. and SCHINDLER, F. (1964) The intracellular oxidation–reduction state. In: *Oxygen in the Animal Organism*. DICKENS, F. and NEIL, E. (eds.). Pergamon Press, Oxford, pp. 367–92.

CHANCE, B., WILLIAMSON, J. R., JAMIESON, D. and SCHOENER, B. (1965) Properties and kinetics of reduced pyridine nucleotide fluorescence of the isolated and *in vivo* rat heart. *Biochem. Z.* **341:** 357–77.

CHARLIER, R. (1954) Effects of cysteamine and cysteine on cardiac output and oxygen content of venous blood. *Proc. Soc. exp. Biol. Med.* **86:** 290–3.

CHEFURKA, W. (1957) Oxidative metabolism of carbohydrates in insects. II. Glucose-6-phosphate dehydrogenase and 6-phosphogluconate dehydrogenase in the housefly. *Enzymologia* **18:** 209–27.

CHÈVREMONT-COMHAIRE, S. and CHÈVREMONT, M. (1953) Action de la β-mercaptoéthylamine sur la croissance et la mitose dans des cultures de fibroblastes et myoblastes. *C.R. Assoc. Anat.* (40e réunion): 127–31.

CHRISTOPHERSEN, B. O. (1966) Oxidation of reduced glutathione by subcellular fractions of rat liver. *Biochem. J.* **100:** 95–101.

CHRISTOPHERSEN, B. O. (1968a) Formation of monohydroxy-polyenic fatty acids from lipid peroxides by a glutathione peroxidase. *Biochim. biophys. Acta* **164:** 35–46.

CHRISTOPHERSEN, B. O. (1968b) The inhibitory effect of reduced glutathione on the lipid peroxidation of the microsomal fraction and mitochondria. *Biochem. J.* **106:** 515–22.

CICCARONE, P. (1965) Some metabolic aspects of cystamine treated mice. *Prog. Biochem. Pharmacol.* **1:** 522–7.

CICCARONE, P. and BACQ, Z. M. (1966) Inhibition of oxygen consumption in liver homogenates from mice injected with radioprotectors in the presence of pyruvate. *Nature (Lond.)* **210:** 648–9.

CICCARONE, P. and MILANI, R. (1964) Effects of cystamine on the metabolism of Yoshida hepatoma ascites cells *in vitro*. *Biochem. Pharmacol.* **13:** 183–91.

COHEN, G. and HOCHSTEIN, P. (1961) Glucose-6-phosphate dehydrogenase and detoxification of hydrogen peroxide in human erythrocytes. *Science* **134:** 1756–7.

COOPERSTEIN, S. J. (1963a) The effect of disulfide bond reagents on cytochrome oxidase. *Biochim. biophys. Acta* **73:** 343–6.

COOPERSTEIN, S. J. (1963b) Reversible inactivation of cytochrome oxidase by disulfide bond reagents. *J. biol. Chem.* **238:** 3606–10.

CORWIN, L. M. (1962) Studies on peroxidation in vitamin-E deficient rat liver homogenates. *Arch. Biochem. Biophys.* **97:** 51–8.

DAVIES, R. and ELVIN, P. A. (1964) The effect of β-mercaptoethanol on release of invertase and formation of protoplasts of *Saccharomyces fragilis*. *Biochem. J.* **93**: 8–9P.

DELLA BELLA, D. and BACQ, Z. M. (1953) Unpublished observations, quoted in LIÉBECQ *et al.* (1964).

DIEMER, K. (1963) Eine verbesserte Modellvorstellung zur Sauerstoffversorgung des Gehirns. *Naturwissenschaften* **50**: 617–18.

DIEMER, K. (1965a) Ueber die Sauerstoffdiffusion im Gehirn. I. Räumliche Vorstellung und Berechnung der Sauerstoffdiffusion. *Pflüger's Arch. ges. Physiol.* **285**: 99–108.

DIEMER, K. (1965b) Ueber die Sauerstoffdiffusion im Gehirn. II. Die Sauerstoffdiffusion bei O_2-Mangelzuständen. *Pflüger's Arch. ges. Physiol.* **285**: 109–18.

DOBROVOLSKII, N. M. (1967) Change of oxygen tension and redox potential in various mouse organs by the action of radioprotectors. *Radiobiologiya* **7**: 240–2 (in Russian).

DUBOIS, K. P. and RAYMUND, A. B. (1958a and b) Effect of ionizing radiation on the biochemistry of mammalian tissues. I. Effect of single and repeated doses of sulfur containing radioprotective agents on intermediary carbohydrate metabolism. *Univ. Chicago U.S.A.F. Radiation Lab. Quart. Progr. Rep.* **27**: 1–14 and **28**: 1–15.

DUBOIS, K. P., RAYMUND, A. B. and HIETBRINK, B. E. (1961) Inhibitory action of *N*-diethyldithiocarbamate on enzymes of animal tissues. *Toxicol. appl. Pharmacol.* **3**: 236–55.

DUYCKAERTS, C. and LIÉBECQ, C. (1970) Blood redox potentials of rats and mice injected with cystamine. In: *Radiation Protection and Sensitization*, MOROSON, H. L. and QUINTILIANI, M. (eds.). Taylor & Francis Ltd., London, pp. 429–32.

DUYCKAERTS, C., BLEIMAN, C., WINAND-DEVIGNE, J. and LIÉBECQ, C. (1969) Potentiel d'oxydo-réduction du sang du rat et de la souris. *Archs int. Physiol. Biochim.* **77**: 374–6.

DUYCKAERTS, C., GILLES, R. and LIÉBECQ, C. (1971) Activation de la glycogénolyse par la cystamine. *J. Physiol. Paris* **63**: 207A.

ELDJARN, L. and BREMER, J. (1962) The inhibitory effect at the hexokinase level of disulfides on glucose metabolism in human erythrocytes. *Biochem. J.* **84**: 286–91.

ELDJARN, L. and BREMER, J. (1963) The disulfide reducing capacity of liver mitochondria. *Acta chem. scand.* **17**: 59–66.

ELDJARN, L. and PIHL, A. (1957) On the mode of action of X-rays protective agents. Interaction between biologically important thiols and disulfides. *J. biol. Chem.* **225**: 499–507.

ELDJARN, L. and PIHL, A. (1958) Mechanisms of protective and sensitizing action. In: *25th Anniversary Publication from the Norwegian Radium Hospital*. Avhandlinger Utgitt Norske Videnskaps Akademi, Oslo, pp. 253–88.

EL-KHATIB, S., CHENAU, U. A., CARPENTIER, M. P., TRUCCO, R. E. and CAPUTTO, R. (1964) Possible presence of lipid peroxides in tissues of tocopherol-deficient animals. *Nature (Lond.)* **201**: 188–9.

EMMELOT, P., MIZRAHI, I. J., NACCARATO, R. and BENEDETTI, L. (1962) Changes in function and structure of the endoplasmic reticulum of rat liver cells after administration of cysteine. *J. Cell Biol.* **12**: 177–84.

ESTABROOK, R. W., COOPER, D. Y. and ROSENTHAL, O. (1963) The light reversible carbon monoxide inhibition of the steroid C21-hydroxylase system of the adrenal cortex. *Biochem. Z.* **338**: 741–55.

FIRKET, H. and LELIÈVRE, P. (1966) Effet de la cystamine sur la respiration, la phosphorylation oxydative et l'ultrastructure des mitochondries de rat. *Int. J. Radiat. Biol.* **10**: 403–15.

FISCHER, P. (1954) Glycogène hépatique, rayons X et cystéamine. *Archs int. Physiol.* **62**: 134–6.

FISCHER, P. (1956) Elimination urinaire d'acides organiques après administration de cystéamine, cystamine et cyanure. *Archs int. Physiol.* **64**: 130–2.

FRANCOEUR, M. and DENSTEDT, O. F. (1954) Metabolism of mammalian erythrocytes. VII. The glutathione reductase of the mammalian erythrocyte. *Can. J. Biochem. Physiol.* **32:** 663–9.

FREDERIC, J. (1958) *Recherches cytologiques sur le chondriome normal ou soumis à l'expérimentation dans des cellules vivantes cultivées* in vitro. Thèse d'agrégation de l'enseignement supérieur, Université de Liège.

FROEDE, H. C., GERASI, G. and MANSOUR, T. E. (1968) Studies on heart phosphofructokinase. *J. biol. Chem.* **243:** 6021–9.

FUMIGALLI, P. and MALASPINA, A. (1958) The effect of cysteamine, a radioprotector, on the hepatic glycogen of the rat after whole body irradiation with mortal dose. *Radiobiol. latina* **1:** 28–39.

GALEOTTI, T., MAYER, D. and VAN ROSSUM, G. (1969) Spectrofluorimetric detection of free and bound forms of NAD(P)H in intact cells. *Abstracts 6th FEBS Meeting, Madrid,* p. 763.

GEBICKI, J. M. and HUNTER, F. E. JR. (1964) Determination of swelling and disintegration of mitochondria with an electronic particle counter. *J. biol. Chem.* **239:** 631–9.

GRAHAM, W. D. (1951) *In vitro* inhibition of liver aldehyde dehydrogenase by tetraethylthiuram disulfide. *J. Pharm. Pharmacol.* **3:** 160–8.

GRAY, L. H. (1956) A method for oxygen assay applied to a study of the removal of dissolved oxygen by cysteine and cysteamine. In: *Progress in Radiobiology.* MITCHELL, J. S., HOLMES, B. E. and SMITH, C. L. (eds.). Oliver & Boyd, Edinburgh, pp. 267–78.

GRAY, L. H. and SCOTT, C. A. (1964) Oxygen tension and radiosensitivity of tumours. In: *Oxygen in the Animal Organism.* DICKENS, F. and NEIL, E. (eds.), Pergamon Press, Oxford, pp. 537–53.

GRAYEVSKY, E. Y., SHAPIRO, I. M., KONSTANTINOVA, M. M. and BARAKINA, N. F. (1961) The role of cellular damage in the mammalian radiation syndrome. In: *The Initial Effects of Ionizing Radiations on Cells.* HARRIS, R. J. C. (ed.). Academic Press, New York, pp. 237–55.

GRAYEVSKY, E. Y., BARAKINA, N. F., KONSTANTINOVA, M. M. and SMIRNOVA, I. B. (1962) Investigations on radioprotection in mammals. In: *Radiation Effects in Physics, Chemistry and Biology.* Proc. 2nd Int. Congr. Radiation Res., Harrogate 1962. EBERT, M. and HOWARD, A. (eds.). North–Holland Publ. Co., Amsterdam, pp. 294–304.

GROVER, P. L. and SIMS, P. (1964) Conjugations with glutathione: Distribution of glutathione S-aryltransferase in vertebrate species. *Biochem. J.* **90:** 603–6.

GUDBJARNASON, S. and BING, R. J. (1962) The redox-pontential of the lactate–pyruvate system in blood as an indicator of the functional state of cellular oxidation. *Biochim. biophys. Acta* **60:** 158–62.

HASSINEN, I. (1966) Effect of disulfiram (tetraethylthiuram disulfide) on mitochondrial oxidation. *Biochem. Pharmacol.* **15:** 1147–53.

HASSINEN, I. and HALLMANN, M. (1967) Comparison of the effects of disulfiram and dimercaptopropanol arsenite on mitochondrial structure and function. *Biochem. Pharmacol.* **16:** 2155–66.

HEIFFER, M. H., MUNDY, R. L. and MEHLMAN, B. (1961) Plasma catecholamine levels and adrenal ascorbic acid content following β-mercaptoethylamine administration. *Endocrinology* **69:** 746–52.

HEIFFER, M. H., MUNDY, R. L., and MEHLMAN, B. (1962) The pharmacology of radioprotective chemicals. On some of the effects of cysteamine and cystamine in the rat. *Radiat. Res.* **16:** 165–74.

HEMKER, H. C. (1964) Inhibition of adenosine triphosphatase and respiration of rat liver mitochondria by dinitrophenols. *Biochim. biophys. Acta* **81:** 1–9.

HEPPEL, L. A. and HILMOE, R. J. (1950) Metabolism of inorganic nitrite and nitrate esters. II. The enzymatic reduction of nitroglycerine and erythritol tetranitrate by glutathione. *J. biol. Chem.* **183:** 129–38.

HIETBRINK, B. E., RAYMUND, A. B. and RYAN, B. A. (1959) The effect of ionizing radiations on the biochemistry of mammalian tissues. III. The influence of various chemical compounds on radiation induced changes in enzyme activities in certain rat tissues. *Univ. Chicago U.S.A.F. Radiation Lab. Quart. Progr. Rep.* **22**: 1–14.

HOCHSTEIN, P. and ERNSTER, L. (1963) ADP-activated lipid peroxidation coupled to the TPNH oxidase system of microsomes. *Biochem. biophys. Res. Commun.* **12**: 388–94.

HOHORST, H. J., KREUTZ, F. H. and BÜCHER, T. (1959) Ueber Metabolitgehalte und Metabolit-Konzentration in der Leber der Ratte. *Biochem. Z.* **332**: 18–46.

HOHORST, H. J., KREUTZ, F. H., REIM, H. and HÜBENER, H. J. (1961) The oxidation/reduction state of the extramitochondrial DPN$^+$/DPNH system in rat liver and the hormonal control of substrate levels *in vivo*. *Biochem. biophys. Res. Commun.* **4**: 163–8.

HOLLAENDER, A. and STAPLETON, G. E. (1953) Fundamental aspect of radiation protection from a microbiological point of view. *Physiol. Rev.* **33**: 77–80.

HORGAN, V. J. and PHILPOT, J. ST. L. (1954) The chemistry of biological after-effects of ultraviolet and ionizing radiations. VII. Attempted estimation of organic peroxides in X-irradiated mice. *Br. J. Radiol.* **27**: 63–72.

HORGAN, V. L. and PHILPOT, J. ST. L. (1962) The apparent peroxide content of irradiated and alarmed mice. *Int. J. Radiat. Biol.* **5**: 167–81.

HORGAN, V. J. and PHILPOT, J. ST. L. (1964) Apparent peroxide ("problue") in organs of irradiated and alarmed mice. *Int. J. Radiat. Biol.* **8**: 165–76.

HORGAN, V. J., PHILPOT, J. ST. L., PORTER, B. W. and ROODYN, D. B. (1957) Toxicity of autoxidized squalene and linoleic acid, and of simpler peroxides, in relation to toxicity of radiation. *Biochem. J.* **67**: 551–8.

HUGON, J., MAISIN, J. R. and BORGERS, M. (1964) Effets de l'AET sur les ultrastructures des cryptes duodénales de la souris. *C.r. Séanc. Soc. Biol.* **158**: 201–5.

HUNTER, F. E. JR., SCOTT, A., HOFFSTEN, P. E., GEBICKI, J. M., WEINSTEIN, J. and SCHNEIDER, A. (1964) Studies on the mechanism of swelling, lysis and disintegration of isolated liver mitochondria exposed to mixtures of oxidized and reduced glutathione. *J. biol. Chem.* **239**: 614–21.

JAENICKE, L. and LYNEN, F. (1960) Coenzyme A. In: *The Enzymes.* 2nd ed. BOYER, P. D., LARDY, H. and MYRBÄCK, K. (eds.). Academic Press, New York, pp. 3–103.

JAMIESON, D. and VAN DEN BRENK, H. A. S. (1966) Studies of mechanisms of chemical radiation protection *in vivo*. III. Changes in fluorescence of intracellular pyridine nucleotides and modification by excellular hypoxia. *Int. J. Radiat. Biol.* **10**: 223–41.

JOHNSTON, C. D. (1953) The *in vitro* reaction between tetraethylthiuramdisulfide (antabuse) and glutathione. *Arch. Biochem. Biophys.* **44**: 249–59.

KATZEN, H. M., TIETZE, F. and STETTEN, D., JR. (1963) Further studies on the properties of hepatic glutathione-insulin transhydrogenase. *J. biol. Chem.* **238**: 1006–11.

KEILIN, D. and HARTREE, E. F. (1938) Cytochrome oxidase. *Proc. R. Soc. B.* **125**: 171–86.

KEILIN, D. and HARTREE, E. F. (1940) Succinic dehydrogenase—cytochrome system of cells. Intracellular respiratory system catalysing aerobic oxidation of succinic acid. *Proc. R. Soc. B.* **129**: 277–306.

KEILIN, D. and NICHOLLS, P. (1958) On the supposed catalytic oxidation of thiol groups by catalase. *Biochim. biophys. Acta* **28**: 225.

KESSLER, M. (1968) Unpublished observations quoted in LÜBBERS (1968).

KESSLER, M. and LÜBBERS, D. W. (1964) Bestimmung des kritischen Sauerstoffdruckes an isolierten Lebermitochondrien. *Pflüger's Arch. ges. Physiol.* **281**: 50.

KLINGENBERG, M. and BÜCHER, T. (1960) Biological oxidations. *Ann. Rev. Biochem.* **29**: 669–708.

KLINGENBERG, M. and LIÉBECQ, C. (1963) Unpublished observations quoted in LIÉBECQ (1964).

KLINGENBERG, M. and PFAFF, E. (1966) Structural and functional compartmentation in mitochondria. In: *Regulation of Metabolic Processes in Mitochondria.* TAGER, J. M.,

PAPA, S., QUAGLIARIELLO, E. and SLATER, E. C. (eds.), Elsevier Publ. Co., Amsterdam, pp. 180–201.

KOHN, H. T. and GUNTER, S. E. (1959) Factors influencing the radioprotective activity of cysteine. Effects in *Escherichia coli* due to drug concentration, temperature, time, and pH. *Radiat. Res.* **11:** 732–7.

KOHN, H. T. and GUNTER, S. E. (1960) Cysteine protection against X-rays and the factor of oxygen tension. *Radiat. Res.* **13:** 250–8.

KONOPOLYANIKOV, A. G., KUDRYASHOV, Y. B. and MEKHTIEVA, S. M. (1966) Use of redox potential measurements in animal tissues during selection of effective radioprotectors for mice irradiated by high-energy protons (660 MeV). In: *Zashchita i Vosstanovlenie pri Luchvykh Povrezhdeniyakh.* GRAEVSKI, E. Y., IVANOV, V. I. and KOROGODIN, V. I. (eds.), Izdatel'stvo Nauka, Moscow, pp. 177–182 (in Russian). In: *Chem. Abstr.* (1967), 626s.

KUZNETSOV, V. I. and KUSHAKOVSKII, M. S. (1963) The mechanism of action of anti-irradiation agents. *Med. Radiol.* **6:** 27–32 (in Russian).

KUZNETSOV, V. I. and TANK, L. I. (1964) Changes in the oxygen consumption of the erythrocytes due to the action of cysteamine. *Radiobiologiya* **4:** 284–8 (in Russian).

LABEYRIE, F. (1949) Rôle du coenzyme dans les réactions d'oxydation et de réduction des groupes sulfhydryles des triosephosphate déshydrogénases. *Bull. Soc. Chim. biol.* **31:** 1624–34.

LANGE, R. and PIHL, A. (1961) The radiosensitizing effect of thioglycolic acid, dithioglycolic acid and homocysteine on muscle glyceraldehyde-3-phosphate dehydrogenase. *Int. J. Radiat. Biol.* **3:** 249–57.

LANGENDORFF, H. and KOCH, R. (1954) Untersuchungen über einen biologischen Strahlenschutz. IX. Zur Wirkung von SH Blockern auf die Strahlenempfindlichkeit. *Strahlentherapie* **95:** 542–5.

LARDY, H. A. and MALEY, G. F. (1954) Metabolic effect of thyroid hormone *in vitro*. *Recent Prog. Horm. Res.* **10:** 129–55.

LECOMTE, J. (1952) Propriétés pharmacodynamiques de la cystinamine. *Archs int. Physiol.* **60:** 179–85.

LEHNINGER, A. L. (1962) Water uptake and extrusion by mitochondria in relation to oxidative phosphorylation. *Physiol. Rev.* **42:** 467–517.

LEHNINGER, A. L. (1964) *The Mitochondrion. Molecular Basis of Structure and Function.* W. A. Benjamin, Inc., New York, pp. 180–204.

LEHNINGER, A. L. and NEUBERT, D. (1961) Effect of oxytocin, vasopressin, and other disulfide hormones on uptake and extrusion of water by mitochondria. *Proc. natn. Acad. Sci., U.S.A.* **47:** 1929–36.

LEHNINGER, A. L. and SCHNEIDER, M. (1959) Mitochondrial swelling induced by glutathione. *J. biophys. biochem. Cytol.* **5:** 109–16.

LEHNINGER, A. L., SUDDUTH, H. C. and WIESE, J. B. (1960) D-β-Hydroxybutyric dehydrogenase of mitochondria. *J. biol. Chem.* **235:** 2450–5.

LELIÈVRE, P. (1959) Action de la cystamine sur l'hexokinase et la phosphoglycéraldéhyde déshydrogénase. *C.r. Séanc. Soc. Biol.* **153:** 1879–83.

LELIÈVRE, P. (1960) Action de la cystéamine et de la cystamine sur l'acétylation de la sulfanilamide *in vitro*. *C.r. Séanc. Soc. Biol.* **154:** 1890–3.

LELIÈVRE, P. (1961a) *Contribution à l'étude de l'interaction cystamine protéines sulfhydrylées. Quelques conséquences sur le plan biologique.* Thèse de doctorat, Université de Liège.

LELIÈVRE, P. (1961b) Unpublished observations.

LELIÈVRE, P. (1965a) Action de la cystamine et de la cystéamine sur la consommation d'oxygène et la phosphorylation oxydative couplée de mitochondries de foie de rat. *Int. J. Radiat. Biol.* **9:** 107–13.

LELIÈVRE, P. (1965b) Consommation d'oxygène par le foie de rat en présence de cystamine. Rôle des diamino-oxydases. *Int. J. Radiat. Biol.* **9:** 261–7.

LELIÈVRE, P. (1965c) Oxygen consumption after administration of various radioprotective substances in the rat. *Int. J. Radiat. Biol.,* **10**: 296–7.

LELIÈVRE, P. and BETZ, E. H. (1959) Variations de la teneur des tissus en cystamine libre et fixée après injection de cette substance. *C.r. Séanc. Biol.* **153**: 181–5.

LELIÈVRE, P. and BETZ, E. H. (1960) Action de la cystamine et de la cystéamine sur la glycolyse anaérobie et la consommation d'oxygène tissulaire d'organes de rat. *C.r. Séanc. Soc. Biol.* **154**: 466–8.

LELIÈVRE, P. and BETZ, E. H. (1963) Action de la cystamine sur la consommation d'oxygène et la phosphorylation couplée des mitochondries d'organes de rat. *C.r. Séanc. Soc. Biol.* **157**: 693–6.

LELIÈVRE, P., FIRKET, H. and SMOLIAR, V. (1963) Distribution précoce de la radioactivité dans les organes du rat après injection de cystamine ^{35}S et de cystéamine ^{35}S. II. Dosage de la radioactivité et conclusions. *C.r. Séanc. Soc. Biol.* **157**: 690–3.

LELIÈVRE, P., SMOLIAR, V. and BETZ, E. H. (1969) Influence de certains radioprotecteurs soufrés sur la tension d'oxygène dans la rate du rat. *Atomkernenergie* **14**: 445–7.

LIÉBECQ, C. (1964) Discussion on radiosensitivity and cellular redox potential. In: *Oxygen in the Animal Organism.* DICKENS, F. and NEIL, E. (eds.), Pergamon Press, Oxford, pp. 535–6.

LIÉBECQ, C. (1966) Influence des thiols et disulfures sur l'hydroxylation de l'antipyrine par les microsomes hépatiques. *Int. J. Radiat. Biol.* **10**: 297.

LIÉBECQ, C., BACQ, Z. M. and THOMOU, A. (1964) Effet de quelques radioprotecteurs sur le système enzymatique des microsomes hépatiques dégradant l'hexobarbital. *Biochem. Pharmacol.* **13**: 51–8.

LITTLE, C. and O'BRIEN, P. J. (1966) Inactivation of glyceraldehyde 3-phosphate dehydrogenase by linoleic acid hydroperoxide. *Biochem. J.* **101**: 13P.

LITTLE, C. and O'BRIEN, P. J. (1967) Thiol oxidation in subcellular fractions and inhibition of glycolysis by a lipid peroxide. *Biochem. J.* **102**: 29–30P.

LITTLE, C. and O'BRIEN, P. J. (1968a) The effectiveness of a lipid peroxide in oxidizing protein and non-protein thiols. *Biochem. J.* **106**: 419–23.

LITTLE, C. and O'BRIEN, P. J. (1968b) An intracellular GSH-peroxidase with a lipid peroxide substrate. *Biochem. biophys. Res. Commun.* **31**: 145–50.

LOCKER, A. and PANY, J. E. (1964) Die Wirkung von Cysteamin und AET auf den Sauerstoffverbrauch und die Körpertemperatur der Maus. *Z. ges. exp. Med.* **138**: 331–7.

LÜBBERS, D. W. (1968) Intercapillärer O_2-Transport und intracelluläre Sauerstoffkonzentration. In: *Biochemie des Sauerstoffes.* HESS, B. and STAUDINGER, H. (eds.). Springer Verlag, Berlin, pp. 67–92.

LUMPER, L., PLOCK, H. J. and STAUDINGER, H. (1968) Untersuchungen zur Abhängigkeit der Lipidperoxydation in Rattenlebermikrosomen vom Sauerstoffpartialdruck. *Hoppe-Seyler's Z. physiol. Chem.* **349**: 1185–90.

MAISIN, J. R., HUGON, J. and LÉONARD, A. (1964) Radiation protectors and cancers. In: *Panel on the Molecular Basis of Radiosensitivity.* International Atomic Energy Agency, Vienna, PL 11574.

MCILWAIN, H. (1959) Thiols and the control of carbohydrate metabolism in cerebral tissue. *Biochem. J.* **71**: 281–5.

MCKEE, R. W. (1952) Effects of X-irradiation on liver glycogen and blood sugar. *Fedn Proc. Fedn. Socs exp. Biol.* **11**: 256–61.

MELDRUM, N. U. and TARR, H. L. A. (1935) The reduction of glutathione by the Warburg–Christian system. *Biochem. J.* **29**: 108–15.

MEYERHOF, O. (1923) Ueber Blausäure Hemmung in autoxydablen Sulphhydrilsystemen. *Pflüger's Arch. ges. Physiol.* **200**: 1–10.

MILLS, G. C. (1957) Hemoglobin catabolism. I. Glutathione peroxydase, an erythrocyte enzyme which protects hemoglobin from oxidative breakdown. *J. biol. Chem.* **229**: 189–97.

MILLS, G. C. (1959) The purification and properties of glutathione peroxidase of erythrocytes. *J. biol. Chem.* **234**: 502–6.

MILLS, G. C. (1960) Glutathione peroxidase and the destruction of hydrogen peroxide in animal tissues. *Arch. Biochem. Biophys* **86**: 1–5.

MILLS, G. C. and RANDALL, H. P. (1958) Hemoglobin catabolism. II. The protection of hemoglobin from oxidative breakdown in the intact erythrocyte. *J. biol. Chem.* **232**: 589–98.

MITCHELL, P. (1961) Coupling of phosphorylation to electron and hydrogen transfer by a chemiosmotic type of mechanism. *Nature (Lond.)* **191**: 144–8.

MITCHELL, P. (1966a) Metabolic flow in the mitochondrial multiphase system: an appraisal of the chemi-osmotic theory of oxidative phosphorylation. In: *Regulation of Metabolic Processes in Mitochondria.* TAGER, J. M., PAPA, S., QUAGLIARIELLO, E. and SLATER, E. C. (eds.), Elsevier Publ. Co., Amsterdam, pp. 65–85.

MITCHELL, P. (1966b) Chemiosmotic coupling in oxidative and photosynthetic phosphorylation. *Biol. Rev.* **41**: 445–502.

MIZRAHI, I. J. and EMMELOT, P. (1963) Counteraction by sulphydril compounds of the enzymic conversion of and the metabolic lesions produced by two carcinogenic N-nitrosodialkylamines in rat liver. *Biochem. Pharmacol* **12**: 55–63.

NESBAKKEN, R. and ELDJARN, L. (1963) The inhibition of hexokinase by disulfide. *Biochem. J.* **87**: 526–32.

NEUBERT, D. and LEHNINGER, A. L. (1962) The effect of thiols and disulfides on water uptake and extrusion by rat liver mitochondria. *J. biol. Chem.* **237**: 952–8.

NORUM, K. (1965) Palmityl coenzyme A: carnitine palmityl transferase. Demonstration of essential sulfhydryl group on the enzyme. *Biochim. biophys. Acta* **105**: 505–6.

NOVAK, L. (1958) Adaptation metabolism as an indication of the degree of radiation injury to the organism. *Physiol. bohemsl.* **7**: 150–8.

NOVAK, L. (1966) The effect of radioprotectors on the course of some metabolic processes in whole mammals. *Bull. Acad. r. Belg. Cl. Sci.* **52**: 633–50.

NOVAK, L. and VACEK, A. (1959) Changes in adaptive oxygen consumption in mice subjected to the action of cysteine and irradiation. *Folia biol., Praha* **5**: 134–44.

NOVAK, L., ROTKOVSKA, D., HOSEK, B. and MISUSKOVA, J. (1967) A contribution to the radioprotective effect of cysteine, cystamine and fluoroacetate. *Studia biophys., Berlin* **6**: 1–9.

NYGAARD, A. P. and SUMNER, J. B. (1952) D-Glyceraldehyde-3-phosphate dehydrogenase. A comparison with liver aldehyde dehydrogenase. *Arch. Biochem. Biophys.* **39**: 119–27.

O'BRIEN, P. J. and LITTLE, C. (1967) An intracellular glutathione peroxidase with a lipid peroxide as substrate. *Biochem. J,* **103**: 31P.

OPITZ, E. and SCHNEIDER, M. (1950) Über die Sauerstoffversorgung des Gehirns und den Mechanismus von Mangelwirkungen. *Ergebn. Physiol.* **46**: 126–260.

ORRENIUS, S. (1965) On the mechanism of drug hydroxylation in rat liver microsomes. *J. Cell Biol.* **26**: 713–23.

ORRENIUS, S., DALLNER, G. and ERNSTER, L. (1964a) Inhibition of the TPNH-linked lipid peroxidation of liver microsomes by drugs undergoing oxidative demethylation. *Biochem. biophys. Res. Commun.* **14**: 329–34.

ORRENIUS, S., DALLNER, G. and ERNSTER, L. (1964b) Microsomal NADPH oxidase: catalytic components and functional aspects. In: *Abstr. 1st FEBS Meeting (London)*, pp. 13–14.

OTTOLENGHI, A. (1959) Interaction of ascorbic acid and mitochondrial lipids. *Arch. Biochem. Biophys.* **79**: 355–63.

PARK, J. H., MERIWETHER, B. P., PARK, C. R., MUDD, S. H. and LIPMAN, F. (1956) Glutathione and EDTA antagonism of uncoupling of oxidative phosphorylation. *Biochim. biophys. Acta* **22**: 403–4.

PATT, H. M., STRAUBE, R. L., BLACKFORD, M. E. and SMITH, D. E. (1950) Nature of cysteine induced radioresistance, sulfhydryl levels and distribution of cysteine sulfur. *Am. J. Physiol.* **163**: 740–52.

PETERS, R. A. (1952) Lethal synthesis. *Proc. R. Soc. B.* **139**: 143–70.

PIHL, A. and LANGE, R. (1962) The interaction of oxidized glutathione, cystamine monosulfoxide and tetrathionate with the SH group of rabbit muscle D-glyceraldehyde-3-phosphate dehydrogenase. *J. biol. Chem.* **237**: 1356–62.

PIRIE, A. (1965) Glutathione peroxidase in lens and a source of hydrogen peroxide in aqueous humour. *Biochem. J.* **96**: 244–53.

PLOMTEUX, G., BEAUMARIAGE, M. L., HEUSGHEM, C. and BACQ, Z. M. (1966) Augmentation de certains enzymes dans le plasma du rat après injection d'une dose radioprotectrice de cystéamine. *Archs int. Pharmacodyn. Thérap.* **163**: 230–1.

PLOMTEUX, G., BEAUMARIAGE, M. L., BACQ, Z. M. and HEUSGHEM, C. (1967) Variations enzymatiques dans le plasma du rat après injection d'une dose radioprotectrice de cystéamine. *Biochem. Pharmacol.* **16**: 1601–7.

POSPÍŠIL, M. and NOVAK, L. (1957) Der Verlauf der Adaptation auf unspezifische Reizung bei kleinen Laboratoriumstieren. *Z. ges. exp. Med.* **129**: 385–91.

RAAFLAUB, J. (1953a) Die Schwellung isolierter Leberzellmitochondrien und ihre physikalisch-chemische Beeinflussbarkeit. *Helv. physiol. pharmacol. Acta* **11**: 142–56.

RAAFLAUB, J. (1953b) Ueber den Wirkungsmechanismus von Adenosintriphosphat (ATP) als Cofaktor isolierter Mitochondrien. *Helv. physiol. pharmacol. Acta* **11**: 157–65.

RACKER, E. (1954) Glutathione as a coenzyme in intermediary metabolism. In: *Glutathione*. COLOWICK, S. P., LAZAROW, A., RACKER, E., SCHWARZ, D. R., STADTMAN, E. and WAELSCH, H. (eds.), Academic Press, New York, pp. 165–83.

RACKER, E. (1955) Glutathione-homocystine transhydrogenase. *J. biol. Chem.* **217**: 867–74.

RALL, T. W. and LEHNINGER, A. L. (1952) Glutathione reductase of animal tissues. *J. biol. Chem.* **194**: 119–31.

REED, L. J., DE BUSK, B. G., HORNBERGER, C. S. JR. and GUNSALUS, I. C. (1953) Interrelationships of lipoïc acids. *J. Am. chem. Soc.* **75**: 1271–3.

RICHERT, D. A., VANDERLINDE, R. and WESTERFELD, W. W. (1950) The composition of rat liver xanthine oxidase and its inhibition by antabuse. *J. biol. Chem.* **186**: 261–74.

RILEY, M. V. and LEHNINGER, A. L. (1964) Changes in sulfhydryl groups of rat liver mitochondria during swelling and contraction. *J. biol. Chem.* **239**: 2083–9.

ROMANTSEV, E. F. and SAVITCH, A. V. (1958) *Chemical Protection from Ionizing Radiation.* Medgiz, Moscow, pp. 71–92 (in Russian).

ROMANTSEV, E. F. and ZHULANOVA, Z. I. (1961) Effect of protective substances upon the formation of organic peroxides. *Radiobiologiya* **1**: 73–7 (in Russian).

ROSS, M. H. and ELY, J. O. (1951) Radiation effects on liver glycogen in the rat. *J. cell. compar. Physiol.* **37**: 163–71.

SALERNO, P. R. and FRIEDELL, H. L. (1954) Further studies on the relationship between oxygen tension and the protective action of cysteine, mercaptoethylamine, and *para*-aminopropiophenone. *Radiat. Res.* **1**: 559.

SALERNO, P. R., UYEKI, E. and FRIEDELL, H. L. (1955) On the mechanism of the protective action of cysteine and pitressine against X-irradiation injury in mice and rats. *Radiat. Res.* **3**: 344–50.

SCAIFE, J. F. (1965) An enzymatic evaluation of thiol radioprotectors. *Can. J. Biochem.* **44**: 319–30.

SCHNEIDER, F. and FLOHÉ, L. (1967) Untersuchungen über die Glutathion: H_2O_2-Oxydoreductase (Glutathion-Peroxydase). *Hoppe-Seyler's Z. physiol. Chem.* **348**: 540–52.

SCHNEIDER, F., SCHAUER, R., MARTINI, O. and HAHN, J. (1967) Reversibilität der Glutathion-Insulin-Transhydrogenierung (Proteindisulfid-Reduktase-Reaktion). *Hoppe-Seyler's Z. physiol. Chem.* **348**: 391–400.

SCHWARTZ, I. L., RASMUSSEN, H., SCHOESSLER, M. A., SILVER, L. and FONG, C. T. O. (1960) Relation of chemical attachment to physiological action of vasopressin. *Proc. natn Acad. Sci. U.S.A.* **46**: 1288–98.

SCHWARTZ, I. L., RASMUSSEN, H. and RUDINGER, J. (1964) Activity of neurohypophysial hormone analogues lacking a disulfide bridge. *Proc. natn. Acad. Sci. U.S.A.* **52**: 1044–5.

SCOTT, E. M., DUNCAN, I. W. and EKSTRAND, V. (1963) Purification and properties of glutathione reductase of human erythrocytes. *J. biol. Chem.* **238**: 3928–33.

SEKUZU, I., JURTSHUK, P. and GREEN, D. E. (1963) Studies on the electron transfer system. II. Isolation and characterization of the D-β-hydroxybutyric apodehydrogenase from beef and heart mitochondria. *J. biol. Chem.* **238**: 975–82.

SKREDE, S. (1966) Effects of cystamine and cysteamine on the adenosinetriphosphatase activity and oxidative phosphorylation of rat liver mitochondria. *Biochem. J.* **98**: 702–10.

SKREDE, S. (1968) A permeability barrier in mitochondria in "high energy state" against positively charged disulphides. *Biochem. J.* **107**: 645–53.

SKREDE, S. and CHRISTOPHERSEN, B. O. (1966) Effects of cystamine and cysteamine on the peroxidation of lipids and the release of proteins from mitochondria. *Biochem. J.* **101**: 37–41.

SKREDE, S., BREMER, J. and ELDJARN, L. (1965) The effects of disulphides on mitochondrial oxidations. *Biochem. J.* **95**: 838–46.

SLATER, E. C. and HULSMANN, W. C. (1961) The requirement of energy for respiration in mitochondria. *Proc. natn Acad. Sci. U.S.A.* **47**: 1109–12.

SLATER, T. F. (1968) Aspects of cellular injury and recovery. In: *The Biological Basis of Medicine*. BITTAR, E. E. and BITTAR, N. (eds.), Academic Press, London and New York, Vol. 1, pp. 369–414.

SMOLIAR, V. and BETZ, E. H. (1962) Survie des rats irradiés à des délais variables après injection de cystéamine. *C.r. Séanc. Soc. Biol.* **156**: 1202–8.

SOKAL, J. E., SARCIONE, E. J. and GERSZI, K. E. (1959) Glycogenolytic action of mercapto-ethylamine. *Am. J. Physiol.* **196**: 261–4.

SONKA, J., SOCHOROVA, M. and HILGERTOVA, J. (1968) Effets des substances radioprotectrices sur la glucose-6-phosphate déshydrogénase. *Agressologie* **4**: 513–18.

STARLINGER, H. and LÜBBERS, D. W. (1973) Polarographic measurements of the oxygen pressure performed simultaneously with optical measurements of the redox state of the respiratory chain in suspensions of mitochondria under steady-state conditions at low oxygen tensions. *Pflügers Arch.* **341**: 15–22.

STOCKEN, L. A. and THOMPSON, R. H. S. (1946) British anti-Lewisite. Arsenic derivatives of thiol proteins. *Biochem. J.* **40**: 529–35.

STOTZ, E., HARRER, C. J., SCHULTZE, M. O. and KING, C. G. (1937–8) The oxidation of ascorbic acid in the presence of guinea-pig liver. *J. biol. Chem.* **122**: 407–18.

STRÖMME, J. H. (1963a) Inhibition of hexokinase by disulfiram and diethyldithiocarbamate. *Biochem. Pharmacol.* **12**: 157–66.

STRÖMME, J. H. (1963b) Effects of diethyldithiocarbamate and disulfiram on glucose metabolism and glutathione content of human erythrocytes. *Biochem. Pharmacol.* **12**: 705–15.

STRÖMME, J. H. (1963c) Methaemoglobin formation induced by thiols. *Biochem. Pharmacol.* **12**: 937–48.

SUMARUKOV, G. V. and KUDRYASHOV, Y. B. (1963) Potentiometric determination of the efficacy of the protective action of cysteamine in mice. *Med. Radiol.* **8**: 42–4 (in Russian).

TAPPEL, A. L. and ZALKIN, H. (1959) Inhibition of lipid peroxidation in mitochondria by vitamin E. *Arch. Biochem. Biophys.* **80**: 333–6.

TAPPEL, A. L. and ZALKIN, H. (1960) Inhibition of lipid peroxidation in microsomes by vitamin E. *Nature (Lond.)* **185**: 35.

THIELE, E. H. and HUFF, J. W. (1960) Quantitative measurements of lipid peroxide formation by normal liver mitochondria under various conditions. *Arch. Biochem. Biophys.* **88**: 203–7.

THORS, M. B. and JACKSON, F. L. (1959) Interaction of non-specific reducing and oxidizing agents with the cytochrome system in heart muscle preparations. *Biochim. biophys. Acta* **35**: 65–76.

VANDEBERG, A. (1961) Action of cysteamine and cystamine on metabolism in the liver and kidney of male rat poisoned with sodium fluoroacetate. *Archs. int. Physiol. Biochim.* **69**: 235–50.

VAN DER MEER, C. and VAN BEKKUM, D. W. (1959) The mechanism of radiation protection by histamine and other biological amines. *Int. J. Radiat. Biol.* **1**: 5–23.

VAN DER MEER, C. and VAN BEKKUM, D. W. (1961) A study on the mechanism of radiation protection by 5-hydroxytryptamine and tryptamine. *Int. J. Radiat. Biol.* **4**: 105–12.

VAN DER MEER, C., VALKENBURG, P. W. and REMMELTS, M. (1961) Effects of radioprotective sulfhydryl compounds on the oxygen tension in the spleen of mice. *Nature* (*Lond.*) **189**: 588–9.

VAN DER MEER, C., BROCADES-ZAALBERG, O., VOS, O., VERGROESEN, A. J. and VAN BEKKUM, D. W. (1962) On the mechanism of the radioprotective action of cyanide. *Int. J. Radiat. Biol.* **4**: 311–19.

VARAGIĆ, V., STEPANOVIĆ, S. and HAJDUKOVIĆ, S. (1962) The effect of X-irradiation and cysteamine on the barbiturate sleeping time in rats. *Archs int. Pharmacodyn. Therap.* **138**: 113–19.

VELICK, S. F. (1955) Glyceraldehyde 3-phosphate dehydrogenase from muscle. In: *Methods in Enzymology.* COLOWICK, S. P. and KAPLAN, N. O. (eds.), Academic Press, New York, Vol. I, pp. 401–6.

VERLY, W. G. (1955) Le métabolisme de la cystéamine. *Bull. Acad. r. Méd. Belg.* (6e série) **10**: 447–64.

WILBUR, K. M., BERNHEIM, F. and SHAPIRO, O. W. (1949) The thiobarbituric acid reagent as a test for the oxidation of unsaturated fatty acids by various agents. *Arch. Biochem.* **24**: 305–13.

WILLIAMSON, D. H., LUND, P. and KREBS, H. A. (1967) The redox state of free nicotinamide-adenine dinucleotide in the cytoplasm and mitochondria of rat liver. *Biochem. J.* **103**: 514–27.

WILLS, E. D. and WILKINSON, A. E. (1966) Release of enzymes from lysosomes by irradiation and the relation of lipid peroxide formation to enzyme release. *Biochem. J.* **99**: 657–66.

ZEITOUNIAN, K. A., KONSTANTINOVA, M. H. and SEMENOV, L. F. (1962) Effects of certain chemical protectors on the oxygen tension in the tissues in relation with their influence on the radiosensitivity of animals. *Radiobiologiya* **2**: 616–24 (in Russian).

ZINS, G. R., RAYMUND, A. B. and DuBOIS, K. P. (1958a) The inhibitory action of some radioprotective compounds on oxidative reactions in rat tissues. *Univ. Chicago U.S.A.F. Radiation Lab. Quart. Progr. Rep.* **28**: 129–40.

ZINS, G. R., RAYMUND, A. B. and DuBOIS, K. P. (1958b) The effects of some radioprotective agents and X-irradiation on certain enzymes in animal tissues. *Univ. Chicago U.S.A.F. Radiation Lab. Quart. Progr. Rep.* **29**: 1–14.

ZINS, G. R., RAYMUND, A. B. and DuBOIS, K. P. (1959) Effect of aminoethylisothiourea (AET) on enzymes in animal tissues. *Toxicol. appl. Pharmacol.* **1**: 8–27.

CHAPTER 7

EFFECTS ON CELL GROWTH PROCESSES (MITOSIS, SYNTHESIS OF NUCLEIC ACIDS AND OF PROTEINS)

R. Goutier

Liège, Belgium

THE depressive effects of SH-containing chemical radioprotective agents on many metabolic reactions (see previous chapters) have also been observed in the processes of nucleic acid synthesis leading to cell division. This chapter is devoted to the interference of —SH protective agents with cell division and with the processes of nucleic acid and protein synthesis which are a prerequisite for mitosis. Much of the work discussed below has been included in several recent reviews mainly concerned with its importance in the phenomenon of radioprotective action (see Bacq, 1965; Bacq and Liébecq, 1965; Bacq and Goutier, 1967).

7.1. MITOTIC INHIBITION

Inhibition of cell division has been described in animal and plant cells and in bacteria.

7.1.1. ANIMAL CELLS

7.1.1.1. *Cells in Culture*

The action of —SH protective agents on cells in culture depends on the concentration of the substance and on the time of incubation.

Concentration factor

When survival curves are determined for increasing concentrations of various thiol protective agents, it is surprising to observe that

283

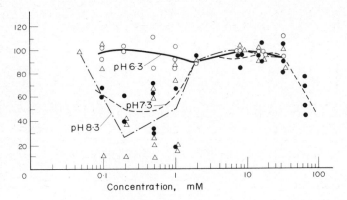

FIG. 1. Survival of human kidney cells after incubation for 20 min with different concentrations of MEA at pH 6.3 (o), 7.3 (•), and 8.3 (△). The lines are drawn through the means of different estimations at one concentration and pH. (From Vergroesen *et al.*, 1967.) Ordinates = % survival.

intermediate concentrations exert a maximal toxic effect. Using human kidney cells, Vergroesen *et al.* (1967) found not only that the toxicity of several thiol protective agents was highest for intermediate concentrations and decreased at greater concentrations, but also that it depended on the pH of the incubation mixture, the toxicity being greater at higher pH

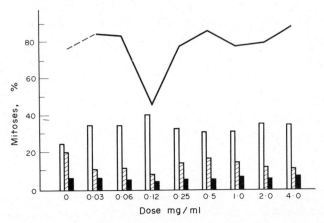

FIG. 2. Mitotic index and proportion of the various mitotic phases in Chinese hamster fibroblasts as a function of MEA concentration. White bars: prophases; hatched bars: metaphases; black bars: terminal phases. (From Delrez and Firket, 1968.)

values (8.3 > 7.3 > 6.3); all these observations were made after incubation for 20 min [Fig. 1 for cysteamine (MEA)].

At higher pH values, enhanced oxidation of thiols is thought to be responsible for increased toxicity, because the survival rate goes back to an almost normal level after the addition of KCN, 1 mM.

A similar relationship is obtained when the mitotic index is measured. On Chinese hamster fibroblasts, MEA produced a drop in the mitotic index, after incubation for 1 hr, with concentrations ranging from 0.5 to 2 mM; the index was almost unchanged for lower and higher concentrations (Delrez and Firket, 1968). Careful examination of the mitotic figures, however, revealed that the mitoses were abnormal in the higher concentration range, although the number of mitotic figures was not necessarily decreased; the proportion of prophases was always higher in the MEA treated cells, as shown in Fig. 2 (Delrez and Firket, 1968).

A comparison of the toxicities of MEA, cysteine, and aminoethylisothiourea (AET) after incubation periods of 10–30 min is given in Table 1 for human kidney cells (Vos *et al.*, 1962); AET appeared to be less toxic than the other compounds.

TABLE 1. TOXICITY OF MEA, CYSTEINE, AND AET ON HUMAN KIDNEY CELLS IN CULTURES[a]
(Vos *et al.*, 1962)

Concentration (mM)	MEA	Cysteine	AET
1/16	66	—	—
1/8	41	74	96
1/4	15	39	83
1/2	18	22	54
1	18	52	48
2	62	42	72
4	84	88	97
8	97	99	103
64	59	81	47

[a] Survival in percent of controls. Incubation time 10–30 min.

Time factor

Thiols are unstable in solution and are oxidized rapidly. In fact, a 20 min incubation of T-cells in a 25 min old solution of MEA at pH 8.3 gave a much lower survival rate than incubation in a freshly prepared solution. This is shown in Table 2 (from Vergroesen *et al.*, 1967) for two different concentrations of MEA, the higher concentration being less toxic. This factor should be taken into account but its incidence is hard to evaluate

TABLE 2. TOXICITY OF AGED (25 MIN) AND FRESH SOLUTIONS OF MEA ON HUMAN KIDNEY CELLS (Vergroesen *et al.*, 1967)

Concentration (mM)	Type of solution	Survival percent
0.5	Fresh	59.7
0.5	Aged	28.5
1.0	Fresh	73.2
1.0	Aged	62.7

^a Incubation: pH 8.3, 20 min. Survival in percent of control values.

quantitatively in the many experiments in which the thiol protective agent is incubated for hours in the presence of cells, which, moreover, do not metabolize the compound. Prolonged incubation may result in recovery after a transient inhibition of mitotic activity. After 30 hr incubation with 0.3 mM MEA the mitotic index of chicken fibroblasts in culture dropped from 16 (controls) to 5 % (treated cells); after 48 hr, however, it came back to an almost normal level (Chèvremont and Chèvremont, 1953; Bassleer and Chèvremont-Comhaire, 1960; Chèvremont, 1961). By counting cells in L-cell cultures incubated with MEA or cystamine for 1 to several days, Therkelsen (1961) observed that the increase in cell counts was only 53 % of the control value after 3 days in cystamine (0.125 mM), but reached 84% of the control value on the fifth day. From these cell count data, it appears that cystamine is about four times more toxic than MEA, in conditions of prolonged incubation.

The growth of Chang cells (human hepatic cells) and of L-cells was inhibited by incubation in cystamine (0.25 to 1 mM) for 24–48 hr (Eker *et al.*, 1964).

7.1.1.2. *Mammalian Tissues*

Mitotic inhibition in various mammalian tissues has also been reported following injection of thiol radioprotective agents. Intravenous injection of cysteine (less than 1 g/kg) in rabbits resulted in complete arrest of mitotic activity in the lens epithelium from 24 hr to 4 days after injection (Pirie and Lajtha, 1959). The first synchronous wave of mitoses, which is normally observed in regenerating rat liver 27 hr after partial hepatectomy, was delayed for 24 hr when AET (150 mg/kg) was injected intraperitoneally (i.p.) 1 hr before partial hepatectomy as shown in Fig. 3 (Goutier *et al.*, 1966). An increase in the proportion of prophases in mouse intestinal mucosa has been observed by Maisin (1968) after injection of AET (8 mg/mouse); the total number of mitotic figures, however, remained unchanged.

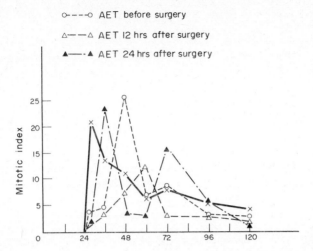

o— — —o AET before surgery

△— —△ AET 12 hrs after surgery

▲——·▲ AET 24 hrs after surgery

FIG. 3. Mitotic indexes in rat regenerating liver when a single dose of AET (Br, HBr) (150 mg/kg) is injected 1 hr before partial hepatectomy, 12 hr after surgery, or 24 hr after surgery. Full line=controls, Abscissae: time in hours after partial hepatectomy. (From Goutier *et al.*, 1966.)

Similarly in the thymus cells of mice, injection of MEA produced an increase in the proportion of prophases within 1 hr and, within 6 hr, an increase in the proportion of metaphases (Kobayashi *et al.*, 1965b). It is conceivable that the accumulation of mitotic figures (which could be linked to a slowing down of the mitotic cycle) may give the impression of increased mitotic activity; this was observed by Kobayashi *et al.* (1965a) in bone-marrow and thymus cells of mice injected with AET (20–40 mg/100 g body-weight) or MEA (20 mg/100 g body-weight), and in ascites tumor cells of rats and mice after MEA injections (12–20 mg/100 g body-weight). The rate of the mitotic cycle was evaluated by Maisin (1968) in mouse intestinal crypt cells, by counting the labeled mitoses at various times following injection of labeled thymidine. It is clear from his results that after injection of AET (8 mg/mouse) the first mitotic cycle lasts longer, due mainly to the increased duration of the S and G2 phases; the second cycle on the contrary seemed to have a shortened G1 period, so that the delay observed during the first cycle had completely disappeared when the third cycle began.

Similarly, Irwin (1964) observed that 10 min after i.p. injection of 10 mmol/kg cysteine in mice and guinea-pigs, metaphase figures accumulated in the ileum during the first 20 min, then rapidly decreased.

7.1.2. PLANT CELLS

When roots of *Allium cepa* were dipped into a 0.5% solution of cyste-amine, the cells rapidly died; mitotic activity stopped within 24 hr in 0.1% MEA; a progressive decrease in mitotic activity was seen after the third day in 0.05% MEA. On the same material, cystamine was found to be less toxic than MEA, the mitotic index being almost normal for concentrations of 0.05 and 1% (Deysson and Truhaut, 1953).

Mitotic anomalies with decreased mitotic activities have been reported in roots of *Oriza sativa* and *Pisum sativum* treated with MEA 0.01% (1.3 mM) and 0.05% (6.5 mM); a concentration of 0.001% (0.13 mM) MEA did not affect the mitoses (Horvath and Gilles, 1962).

7.1.3. BACTERIA

Cysteamine at a concentration of 44 mM forced a logarithmic culture of *E. coli* (strain 15 TAU-bar) into the stationary phase; a normal growth rate was resumed after removal of MEA (Fig. 4; Ginsberg, 1966). The

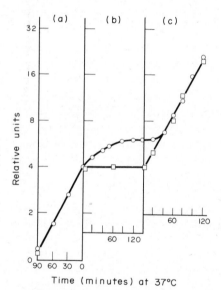

FIG. 4. Growth of a logarithmic-phase culture of *E. coli* in: (a) supplemented minimal medium; (b) supplemented minimal medium with 0.044 M MEA; (c) supplemented minimal medium after removal of MEA; $\circ$ = radioactivity incorporated in DNA (1 unit = 160 ^{14}C counts/min/ml of culture); $\square$ = washed dry mass (1 unit = 0.025 mg/ml of culture). (From Ginsberg, 1966.)

growth of *E. coli* B was similarly inhibited by 0.2 mM cysteine; this effect was quite specific for cysteine and could not be reproduced by any other amino acid even at concentrations of 10 mM (Kovács *et al.*, 1968).

7.2. NUCLEIC ACIDS

7.2.1. EFFECTS ON THE SYNTHESIS

Inhibition of the synthesis of nucleic acids by —SH radioprotective substances has been observed with many different materials.

7.2.1.1. *Cultures of Cells and Bacteria*

In lymphatic cells *in vitro,* the uptake of ^{32}P into DNA and RNA was inhibited by 50% after the addition of AET 0.2 mg/ml (0.7 mM); MEA at a concentration of 0.2 mg/ml (1.7 mM) did not inhibit but at 2 mg/ml (17 mM) concentration decreased ^{32}P uptake into DNA by 86% (Honjo *et al.*, 1963).

La Salle and Billen (1964) made a similar observation using murine bone-marrow cells treated with AET or MEA. When added to suspensions of cells *in vitro* the chemical protective compound resulted in a decrease in the labeling level of DNA in each labeled cell, whereas injection of the protective agent into the animal resulted in a decrease in the number of labeled cells; the inhibition was reversible in both cases.

On chicken embryo intestine *in vitro,* however, the addition of MEA at concentrations of 16 or 64 mM did not seem to affect the proportion of nuclei labeled with ^3H-thymidine (Kirrmann, 1967). It should be remembered, however, that such high doses of MEA have been observed to be less toxic in cell cultures than lower doses (see Chapter 7.1). In *E. coli* 15 T–, the synthesis of RNA was inhibited by cysteine (1 mM), although DNA synthesis in these conditions was relatively unaffected (Nagy *et al.,* 1968). In a medium supplemented with 44 mM MEA, however, the synthesis of DNA in *E. coli* 15 TAU-bar continued at a slower rate for about 90 min, whereas increase in dry mass was completely abolished (Fig. 4; Ginsberg, 1966). Unbalanced growth preceded the cessation of growth, as in the case of cysteine (Nagy *et al.,* 1968). Measurements of DNA content using cytophotometric techniques on embryonic fibroblasts indicated that after 30 hr, 0.3 mM MEA inhibited DNA synthesis, since the proportion of tetraploid nuclei was very much decreased (from 12 in the controls to 4 in the treated cultures), the values for diploid nuclei being unchanged. Later, however, DNA synthesis

TABLE 3. EFFECT OF CYSTAMINE ON THE CELLULAR CONTENT OF PROTEIN, DNA, AND RNA OF HUMAN LIVER CELLS (CHANG CELLS) AND MOUSE FIBROBLASTS (L-CELLS) IN CULTURES[a] (Eker *et al.*, 1964)

Strain	Cystamine concentration (mM)	Amount per cell in percent of untreated cells					
		Protein		DNA		RNA	
		24	48	24	48	24	48
Chang-cells	0.5	93	110	84	78	85	76
	1.0	100	95	87	24[b]	88	24
L-cells	0.25	92	111	95	110	95	96
	0.50	97	104	92	83	93	100

[a] Incubation time 24 or 48 hr.
[b] Cells showed pronounced morphological signs of degeneration.

seemed to be resumed, even in the presence of 0.3 mM MEA; the proportion of tetraploid nuclei after 48 hr reached 26 as against 10 for the controls (Bassleer and Chèvremont-Comhaire, 1960).

The amounts of RNA and protein per cell in Chang liver cells and in L-cells were slightly decreased by incubation with cystamine (0.5 mM or higher) as shown in Table 3 (Eker *et al.*, 1964); the drop in the amount of DNA in Chang cells is linked to pronounced morphological signs of degeneration.

In human leucocytes stimulated by phyto-hemagglutinin *in vitro*, however, 1 mM MEA produced polyploidy, an effect which is quite similar to that of X-ray irradiation (Jackson and Lindahl-Kiessling, 1964).

7.2.1.2. *Mammalian Tissues*

In the intestinal crypt cells of mice injected with 8 mg AET (Br, HBr) the number of grains per nucleus and, to a smaller extent, the percentage of labeled nuclei were decreased by about 10% within 1 hr (Maisin *et al.*, 1965); in these experiments, ^{3}H-thymidine was injected at times ranging from 0 min to 3 hr after administration of AET and the mice were killed 1 hr after thymidine injection. Table 4 shows results obtained by Maisin (1968) from nuclear labeling of intestinal crypt cells when glutathione or AET or a mixture of both was injected. Clearly, the number of grains per nucleus was decreased in all cases but the percentage of labeled nuclei was depressed only after injection of a mixture of GSH + AET. Simons and Davis (1966) observed a marked decrease of the proportion of labeled cells and of the grain counts per cell in the bone-marrow of mice 15 min after subcutaneous injection of AET (Br, HBr) (8 mg/mouse) or MEA

TABLE 4. PERCENT LABELED NUCLEI AND NUMBER OF GRAINS PER NUCLEUS IN INTESTINAL CRYPT CELLS IN MICE TREATED WITH GLUTATHIONE (16 mg/mouse, oral administration) OR AET (8 mg/mouse, i.p. injection) OR A MIXTURE OF BOTH[a] (Maisin, 1968)

	Percent labeled nuclei	Grains per nucleus
Controls	22.8	12.7
Glutathione	24.9	10.2[b]
AET	23	9.8[b]
Glutathione + AET	17.9	8.8[b]

[a] 3H-Thymidine is injected 30 min after the protector, and the animal sacrificed 1 hr later.
[b] $P < 0.001$ (treated animals compared with controls).

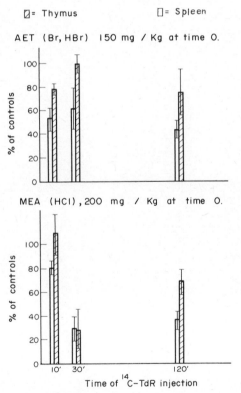

FIG. 5. Effect of i.p. injection of AET or MEA on 14C-thymidine uptake into rat spleen and thymus DNA. 14C-thymidine is i.v. injected 10, 30, or 120 min after the protector; the animals are killed 45 min after thymidine injection. Ordinates: specific radioactivity of DNA in the injected animals as percent of that of non-injected animals. (From Goutier and Baugnet-Mahieu, 1968.)

(4 mg/mouse); the grain counts were only 30% of the control value after AET and 44% of the control after MEA. When the specific radioactivity of DNA was measured, it could be shown (Fig. 5) that the incorporation of labeled thymidine into rat spleen and thymus DNA was decreased within 10 min after administration of the protective agent (Goutier *et al.*, 1967, 1968). A delay in the first wave of DNA synthesis has been observed in regenerating liver when AET was injected 1 hr before partial hepatectomy (Goutier *et al.*, 1966); this shift is due to a delay in the increased synthesis of nuclear RNA-polymerase (Vandergoten and Goutier, 1966) and the subsequent formation of the enzymes thymidine kinase and thymidylic kinase (Baugnet-Mahieu *et al.*, 1967) and probably DNA polymerase which allow DNA synthesis to proceed. Figure 6 shows the thymidine kinase activities measured at various times after partial hepatectomy in normal rats and in rats injected with AET (150 mg/kg) 1 hr before surgery; peak enzyme activity in the injected rats appeared after a 16 hr delay. The chemical protective agent acts on regenerating liver as if it prevented the genetic derepression phenomenon which is triggered by the partial hepatectomy. On this material, as with

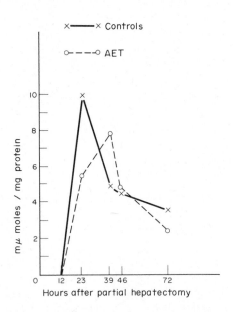

Fig. 6. Thymidine kinase activities measured at various times after partial hepatectomy in normal rats and in rats injected with AET (150 mg/kg) 1 hr before surgery. (From Baugnet-Mahieu *et al.*, 1967.)

all others discussed here, the radioprotective agent paradoxically exerts radiomimetic effects; the explanation of this apparent paradox is rather simple but does not concern us here (see Chapter 9).

Cysteamine injected into rats inhibited the activity of thymidine kinase in the thymus; when added to thymus homogenates *in vitro*, however, MEA failed to produce any inhibition of enzyme activity, a fact which strongly suggests that the inhibition observed *in vivo* results from interference with enzyme synthesis and not with the activity of preformed enzyme molecules (Romantsev *et al.*, 1968).

Synthesis of RNA (uptake of labeled uracil) was decreased in rat thymus within a few minutes after injection of MEA, AET, and cysteine (Romantsev *et al.*, 1968).

7.2.2. EFFECTS ON THE STRUCTURE OF DNA AND NUCLEOPROTEIN

Interactions between sulfhydryl radioprotective agents and free DNA or nucleoprotein *in vitro* have been studied by various authors. Two types of interaction may be considered:

1. Interaction with free DNA as well as the DNA moiety of nucleoprotein *in vitro*, shown only by the disulfide form of the protective agent which acts as a diamine, binding through its two terminal NH_3^+ groups to the negatively charged groups of DNA. This type of interaction is similar to that of cadaverine, or of the polyamines spermine or sperm-

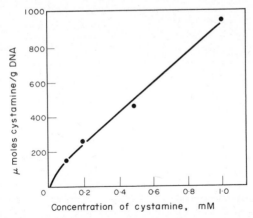

FIG. 7. Amounts of cystamine bound to calf thymus DNA with increasing concentrations of cystamine in the medium. (From Jellum, 1965.)

idine. Cystamine, bis(2-guanidoethyl) disulfide (GED), dimethylcystamine, tetramethylcystamine, tetraethylcystamine, cystine dimethylester and cystine diethylester all become reversibly bound to calf thymus DNA, *E. coli* RNA, and to calf-thymus and rat liver nucleoproteins (Jellum, 1965; Brown, 1968). Figure 7 shows the relatively high capacity of purified DNA to bind cystamine.

The molar ratios of bound agent to average nucleotides in the DNA were found to be 1/8 for GED, 1/22 for cystamine, and 1/16 for oxidized glutathione, all three agents being at the concentration of 1 mM (Kollmann *et al.*, 1967). The binding of the disulfide to DNA results in increased stability of the double helix; the melting temperature (temperature at which the two chains of the double helix separate) is increased to an extent which is proportional to the extent of binding (see Fig. 8). When a DNA–cystamine complex is filtered on a Sephadex gel it decomposes and the DNA eluted has recovered its normal melting temperature (Jellum, 1965); the binding of cystamine to DNA is therefore reversible. Nucleoproteins are precipitated by the disulfide form of the protective agents. Here again, the protective agent acts as a diamine (dication) and precipitation occurs from binding of the substance with the DNA moiety of the nucleohistone (Jellum, 1965); thiols are devoid of precipitating action.

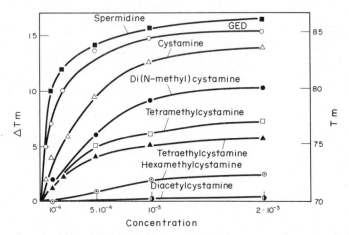

Fig. 8. Dependence of the melting temperatures (T_m, right ordinates) of calf thymus DNA on the concentration of various disulfides and spermidine in standard saline citrate. The increases in the melting temperatures (ΔT_m) are reported on the left ordinates. (From Jellum, 1965.)

Recently, however, electron spin resonance studies by Milvy and Pullman (1968) suggest that MEA (the thiol form) also binds to the phosphate group of the nucleotides of DNA through its amino group.

2. The presence of —SH groups on histone has been detected by Deakin *et al.* (1963). Jellum and Eldjarn (1965) observed that mixed disulfide formation may occur between cystamine or even MEA and isolated rat liver nucleoprotein. The arginine-rich (F 3) histones are rich in —SH groups and therefore particularly able to form mixed disulfides with S—S protective agents (Jellum, 1966).

It is not known to what extent such complexes between the protective agent and DNA or nucleoprotein also occur *in vivo*. Undoubtedly the protective agent becomes rapidly attached by covalent and non-covalent binding to almost all subcellular structures (see Chapter 5). Mixed disulfide formation is a well-documented type of covalent linkage to proteins (see Chapter 5) but the kind of binding with DNA and RNA *in vivo* is not identified although chemical fractionation of liver homogenates following injection of ^{35}S-mercaptoethylguanidine in rats reveals the presence of non-dialyzable label in the nucleic acid containing fractions (Bradford *et al.*, 1961). The difficulty of interpreting the results of such fractionation experiments has been stressed by Bacq (1965). The protective agent probably reaches the cell nucleus in the thiol form, and not as disulfide, since all cells contain a glutathione reductase as well as the mitochondrial reducing system, which would very efficiently reduce the disulfides (Eldjarn and Bremer, 1963). Indeed, after injection of MEA, cystamine, or cysteine into animals, increases in the level of non-protein bound —SH compounds have been observed (Sørbo, 1962); the cellular glutathione level increases by 20% after 10 min incubation of a suspension of ascites cells in an MEA or AET (6 mM) containing medium (Modig and Révész, 1967). However, an interaction of the thiol compound with DNA would be in agreement with the observation that the —SH protective agent maintains the DNA in a repressed state, i.e. temporarily prevents the transcription of messenger RNA and inhibits induced enzyme synthesis (Vandergoten and Goutier, 1966; Baugnet-Mahieu *et al.*, 1967). In order to try to reconcile both aspects of the problem, Brown (1967) postulated that the thiol protective agent may become bound to the DNA through its amino group and that this labile linkage would be stabilized by the formation of a mixed disulfide bond on the other end with a neighboring thiol group of the histone.

7.3. PROTEIN

Although less extensively studied than DNA synthesis inhibition, a depression of protein synthesis has been observed in several instances and participates in the more general inhibition of growth processes. In bacteria (*E. coli*), the increase in dry mass ceases immediately with the addition of MEA (44 mM) (Ginsberg, 1966) (Fig. 4). The growth-inhibiting action of cysteine at concentrations higher than 0.1 mM in *E. coli* is characterized, according to Kovács *et al.* (1968), by an immediate cessation of protein and RNA synthesis. In view of the fact that the growth-inhibiting action of cysteine is counteracted completely by addition of caseine hydrolysate, Kovács *et al.* (1968) postulate that cysteine might inhibit the synthesis of some amino acids, the shortage of which would cause inhibition of protein synthesis.

In regenerating rat liver, the increases in thymidine kinase (Fausto and Van Lancker, 1965) and RNA polymerase (Tsukada and Lieberman, 1965) activities induced by partial hepatectomy are due to a neosynthesis of enzyme molecules. The injection of AET (150 mg/kg) into rats 1 hr before surgery delays the induced synthesis of kinases (Fig. 6; Baugnet-Mahieu *et al.*, 1967) and of RNA polymerase (Vandergoten and Goutier, 1966). It is not known whether the —SH protective agent acts at a transcriptional or translational level. The wide reactivity of thiols would make it likely that both steps are affected. Indeed, on the one hand, inhibition of RNA synthesis has been observed (see above) and on the other, polysome preparations from liver of rats injected with AET (150 mg/kg) incorporate ^{14}C leucine less readily into acid-insoluble material *in vitro* than do control preparations (Baeyens and Goutier, unpublished experiments). In connection with these considerations, it must be remembered that in a study of the intracellular distribution of thiol radioprotective agents Bradford *et al.* (1961) put a special emphasis on the presence of rather tightly bound mercaptoalkylguanidine on the microsome fraction.

7.4. CONCLUSIONS AND SUMMARY

At radioprotective doses, the thiol radioprotective agents inhibit the mitotic activity equally as well in mammalian tissues as in cultured cells, plant cells, and bacteria. With cultured cells, the toxicity and the antimitotic activity are found to be at their highest level for intermediate concentrations of the compound and decrease for lower and higher concentrations.

Although the mechanism of this antimitotic action has not been systematically investigated, it is conceivable that the inhibition of mitotic activity originates from the decreased rate of DNA synthesis observed in many different cell types, and the inhibition of protein synthesis. In some cases, however (see Eker *et al.*, 1964), a marked inhibition of multiplication has been observed in cell cultures, the cells of which still retained a nearly normal amount of protein and a slightly decreased amount of DNA; although the fact that synthesis of new material is inhibited cannot be excluded in these experiments, it has been postulated that inhibition of mitosis might occur by mechanisms other than the inhibition of DNA and protein synthesis.

ADDENDUM

The following works were published after this article had been written. They provide more detailed information about the interaction between sulfhydryl protective substances and proteins and nucleic acids.

Sawada and Okada (1970) observed that incubation of mouse leukemic cells (strain L 5178 Y) for 30 min in the presence of MEA produced single-strand breaks in the DNA; the number of breaks was greater (5×10^3 breaks per cell) in the presence of 0.5 mM MEA than in the presence of 50 mM MEA. Therefore, the toxicity of MEA may be attributed, in part, to lesion of DNA molecules, since the lower concentration, more toxic than the higher with regard to killing effect, also produces more single-strand breaks in DNA.

Interference of MEA or cystamine by mixed disulfide formation with enzymes involved in nucleic acid synthesis has been observed *in vitro* and *in vivo*.

Addition of ^{35}S-cystamine to a purified preparation of RNA-polymerase from *E. coli* produced an inhibition of enzyme activity, in relation to the concentration of the drug and to the number of ^{35}S—R groups bound per enzyme molecule. Complete loss of enzyme activity occurred at a concentration of 10 mM cystamine, which blocked twelve —SH groups (Sümegi *et al.*, 1971).

Similarly, D-ribose-transferase (involved in deoxycytidine formation), partially purified from rat thymus, was inhibited by the addition of MEA or cystamine *in vitro*, with the formation of mixed disulfides. Fifteen minutes after intraperitoneal (i.p.) injection of ^{35}S-MEA to rats, labeled D-ribose-transferase could be purified from the thymus, the specific radioactivity increasing with increasing purity of the enzyme preparation; the enzyme activity, which was only 40% of the control preparation, could be partly restored by addition of dithiothreitol (Filippovitch *et al.*, 1971).

The same team (Filippovitch *et al.*, 1973) recently compared the effects of cysteine and of its isomer, isocysteine. When administered to mice in doses of 300, 600, or 1000 mg/kg 10–15 min before total body irradiation with 600 r γ rays, isocysteine was found to be devoid of protective action, whereas cysteine is a well-known radioprotector.

A dose of 1000 mg/kg cysteine given to rats markedly inhibited (50%) the thymidine kinase activity measured *in vitro* on extracts of spleen removed 15 min after injection. A similar test performed with the same dose (100 mg/kg) of isocysteine only produced a small inhibition of enzyme activity (15%). The observations that thymidine kinase activity in spleen or thymus extract and the activity of partially purified thymidine-cytosine deoxyribosyl transferase were more inhibited in the presence of cysteine than in the presence of equimolar amounts of isocysteine and that only the cysteine-inhibited enzymes would be partly reactivated by addition of dithiothreitol led the authors to conclude that only the protective substance—cysteine—can form mixed disulfides with enzymatic proteins and that the enzymatic inhibitions observed as well as the radioprotection afforded originate from the formation of the mixed disulfides.

The inhibition of nucleic acid synthesis exerted by MEA therefore seems to originate from direct inactivation of the enzymes involved and from single-strand breaks on the DNA molecule. Modig *et al.* (1972) observed that Ehrlich ascites-tumor cells incubated for 30 min in the presence of 10 mM ^{35}S-MEA bound about 12% of the radioactivity to their proteins in the form of mixed disulfides. When the proteins of the tumor cells were themselves pre-labeled with [35]S (by i.p. injecting 50 mcCi ^{35}S-cysteine into mice, 24 hr before harvesting the cells), the same authors could show that treatment of these labeled cells with MEA produced the release of labeled glutathione in proportion to the amount of MEA which became bound to the proteins. They concluded that protein-bound glutathione, which they consider as a possible reservoir of endogenous radioprotective substance, is released by MEA treatment in an exchange reaction.

In agreement with these observations, Graevsky *et al.* (1969) showed that non-protein-bound —SH was increased by 15.8% in the hemato-poietic tissues of mice injected with a protective dose of MEA 15 min before sacrifice.

The formation of mixed disulfides has also been shown to occur when proteins are treated *in vitro* with AET. Horvath *et al.* (1972) established a correlation between the amount of ^{14}C-AET bound *in vitro* to various molecules of enzymes (trypsin, ribonuclease), hormone (insulin), and oxygen carriers (hemoglobin) and the loss of biological activity incurred by these proteins.

REFERENCES

BACQ, Z. M. (1965) *Chemical Protection against Ionizing Radiations.* Ch. C. Thomas, Spring-field, Illinois, U.S.A.

BACQ, Z. M. and GOUTIER, R. (1967) Mechanism of action of sulfur-containing radio-protectors, pp. 241–60. In: *Recovery and Repair Mechanisms in Radiobiology.* Brook-haven Symposia in Biology, No. 20.

BACQ, Z. M. and LIÉBECQ, C. (1965) Effets métaboliques de quelques radioprotecteurs. pp. 11–142. In: *Drugs and Enzymes, Proc. 2nd Int. Pharmacol. Meeting,* Pergamon Press, London.

BASSLEER, R. and CHÈVREMONT-COMHAIRE, S. (1960) Etude cytophotométrique des ADN dans des cultures de fibroblastes traitées par la cystéamine. *Bull. Acad. Roy. Méd. Belg.* **25:** 709–33.

BAUGNET-MAHIEU, L., GOUTIER, R. and SEMAL, M. (1967) Effects of total-body X-irradiation and AET on the activity of thymidine-phosphorylating kinases during liver regeneration. *Radiation Res.* **31:** 808–25.

BRADFORD, R. H., SHAPIRA, R. and DOHERTY, D. G. (1961) The intracellular distribution and binding of radiation protective mercaptoalkylguanidine. *Int. J. Radiat. Biol.* **3:** 595–608.

BROWN, P. E. (1967) Mechanism of action of aminothiol radioprotectors. *Nature* **213:** 363–4.

BROWN, P. E. (1968) Some effects of binding agents on the X-irradiation of DNA. *Radiation Res.* **34:** 24–35.

CHÈVREMONT, M. (1961) Le mécanisme de l'action antimitotique. *Path. Biol.* **9:** 973–1004.

CHÈVREMONT, S. and CHÈVREMONT, M. (1953) Action de la β-mercaptoéthylamine sur la croissance et la mitose en culture de tissus. *C.R. Soc. Biol.* **147:** 164–6.

DEAKIN, G., ORD, M. G. and STOCKEN, L. A. (1963) Glucose-6-phosphate dehydrogenase activity and thiol content of thymus nuclei from control and X-irradiated rats. *Biochem. J.* **89:** 296–304.

DELREZ, M. and FIRKET, H. (1968) Action paradoxale d'un radioprotecteur sur la mitose et les chromosomes *in vitro. Biochem. Pharmacol.* **17:** 1893–9.

DEYSSON, G. and TRUHAUT, R. (1953) Recherches sur l'action cytotoxique des composés dits radiomimétiques. Protection exercée par la MEA vis-à-vis des effets toxiques de la trichloroéthylamine. *Bull. Soc. Chim. Biol.* **35:** 1019–26.

EKER, P., WAALER, P. E. and PIHL, A. (1964) Effect of cystamine on mammalian cells in culture. *Biochem. Pharmacol.* **13:** 1167–71.

ELDJARN, L. and BREMER, J. (1963) The disulphide reducing capacity of liver mitochondria. *Acta Chem. Scand.* suppl. 1, **17:** 59–66.

FAUSTO, N. and VAN LANCKER, J. L. (1965) Thymidylic kinase and DNA-polymerase activities in normal and regenerating liver. *J. Biol. Chem.* **240:** 1247–55.

FILIPPOVITCH, I. V., SHEREMETYENSKAYA, T. N. and ROMANTSEV, E. F. (1971) Mechanism of biochemical shock. II. Direct demonstration of mixed disulfide involvement in the inhibition of deoxycytidine formation in rat thymus *in vivo*. *Biochem. Pharmacol.* **20:** 135–9.

FILIPPOVITCH, I. V., KOLESNIKOV, E. E., SHEREMETYEVSKAYA, T. N., TARASENKO, A. T. and ROMANTSEV, E. F. (1973) Mechanisms of "Biochemical Shock". III. Comparative study of biochemical effects induced by a radioprotective and a non-radioprotective compound of isomer structure. *Biochem. Pharmacol.* **22:** 815–25.

GINSBERG, D. M. (1966) Effects of MEA on growth and radiation sensitivity of *E. coli* strain 15 TAU-bar. *Radiation Res.* **28:** 708–16.

GOUTIER, R. and BAUGNET-MAHIEU, L. (1968) Action of SH-containing radioprotectors on nucleic acid metabolism. In: *Radiation Damage and Sulphydryl Compounds.* International Atomic Energy Agency, Vienna, 1969, pp. 103–9.

GOUTIER, R., MAISIN, J. R., LÉONARD, A. and LAMBIET, M. (1966) Influence de l'AET sur l'activité mitotique et sur la synthèse du DNA dans le foie de rat en regénération irradié. *Rev. Fr. Et. Clin. Biol.* **11:** 1001–6.

GOUTIER, R., BAUGNET-MAHIEU, L. and BERG, T. L. (1967) Action des radiations ionisantes et des substances radioprotectrices sulphydrylées sur la synthèse des acides nucléiques. *Bull. Acad. Roy. Med. Belg.* **7:** 795–837.

GRAEVSKY, E. Y., KONSTANTINOVA, M. M. and TARASENKO, A. G. (1969) Sulfhydryl group and radiosensitivity. *Studia Biophysica, Berlin* **15/16:** 163–80.

HONJO, I., TCHOE, Y.-T., TAKAMORI, Y. and AKABOSHI, M. (1963) Chemical protection for the incorporation of ^{32}P into nucleic acids of lymphatic cells against γ-irradiation. *Nature* **197:** 914–15.

HORVATH, F. and GILLES, A. (1962) Radioprotection et altérations induites par la cysteamine. *Bull. Acad. Roy. Belg., Cl. Sc.* **48:** 1315–17.

HORVATH, M., FÖRIS, G., CSAGOLY, E., SZTANYIK, L. and DALOS, B. (1972) The binding of radioprotective AET to proteins. *Intern. J. Rad. Biol.* **21:** 263–78.

IRWIN, R. L. (1964) The effects of radioprotectants on mitotic kinetics. *Radiation Res.* **22:** 200.

JACKSON, J. F. and LINDAHL-KIESSLING, K. (1964) Action of SH compounds on human leukocyte mitosis *in vitro*. *Exptl. Cell. Res.* **34:** 515–24.

JELLUM, E. (1965) Interaction of cystamine and cystamine derivatives with nucleic acids and nucleoproteins. *Int. J. Rad. Biol.* **9:** 185–200.

JELLUM, E. (1966) Thiol content of calf thymus histone fractions. *Biochim. Biophys. Acta* **115:** 95–102.

JELLUM, E. and ELDJARN, L. (1965) Isolation of SH-containing DNA-nucleo-proteins by chromatography on organomercurial polysaccharide. *Biochim. Biophys. Acta* **100:** 144–53.

KIRRMANN, J. M. (1967) Protection chimique contre les effets précoces des rayons X sur l'incorporation de thymidine tritiée dans l'intestin embryonnaire de Poulet cultivé *in vitro*. *C.R. Acad. Sc. Paris* **265:** 1419–21.

KOBAYASHI, J., KATAYAMA, E., KITAJIMA, T. and KAWAMURA, F. (1965a) Cytological effects of AET on the tumor cells, bone-marrow and thymus cells. *Tokushima J. Exper. Med.* **12:** 40–4.

KOBAYASHI, J., KITAJIMA, T., KATAYAMA, E. and KAWAMURA, F. (1965b) Cytological effects of MEA on bone marrow and thymus cells. *Tokushima J. Exper. Med.* **12:** 35–9.

KOLLMANN, G., SHAPIRO, B. and MARTIN, D. (1967) Mechanism of the protective action of GED against radiation damage to DNA. *Radiation Res.* **31:** 721–31.

KOVÁCS, P., KARI, G., NAGY, ZS. and HERNÁDI, F. (1968) Possible explanation for the metabolic radioprotective effect of cysteine on *E. coli* B. *Radiation Res.* **36:** 217–24.

LA SALLE, M. and BILLEN, D. (1964) Inhibition of DNA synthesis in murine bone-marrow cells by AET and cysteamine. *Ann. N.Y. Acad. Sc.* **114:** 622–9.

MAISIN, J. R. (1968) Influence of radioprotectors on regeneration of the mucosa of the small intestine of the mouse after X-irradiation. In: *Effects of Radiation on Cellular Proliferation and Differentiation*. International Atomic Energy Agency, Vienna, pp. 541–56.

MAISIN, J. R., LÉONARD, A. and HUGON, J. (1965) Tissue and cellular distribution of tritium-labeled AET in mice. *J. Natl. Cancer Inst.* **35:** 103–12.

MILVY, P. and PULLMAN, I. (1968) ESR studies of spin transfer in irradiated nucleic acid-cysteamine systems. *Radiation Res.* **34:** 265–86.

MODIG, H. G. and RÉVÉSZ, L. (1967) Non-protein SH and glutathione content of Ehrlich ascites tumor cells after treatment with the radioprotectors AET, MEA and gluta-thione. *Int. J. Radiat. Biol.* **13:** 469–77.

MODIG, H. G., EDGREN, M. and RÉVÉSZ, L. (1972) Release of thiols from cellular mixed disulfides and its possible role in radiation protection. *Intern. J. Rad. Biol.* **22:** 257–68.

NAGY, ZS., HERNÁDI, F., KOVÁCS, P. and VÁLIY-NAGY, T. (1968) Radiosensitivity of *E. coli* 15 T and the metabolic effect of cysteine. *Radiation Res.* **35:** 652–60.

PIRIE, A. and LAJTHA, L. C. (1959) Possible mechanisms of cysteine protection against radiation cataract. *Nature* **184:** 1125–7.

ROMANTSEV, E. PH., PHILIPPOVITCH, I. V. and KOCHTCHEENKO, N. N. (1968) Protectors and change in the radiosensitive biochemical processes. In: *Radiation Damage and Sulphy-dryl Compounds*. International Atomic Agency, Vienna, 1969, pp. 169–75.

SAWADA, S. and OKADA, S. (1970) Cysteamine, cystamine, and single-strand breaks of DNA in cultured mammalian cells. *Radiation Res.* **44:** 116–32.

SIMONS, H. A. B. and DAVIS, E. M. (1966) The effect of radioprotective compounds on the incorporation of ^{3}H-thymidine into mammalian cells. *Int. J. Radiat. Biol.* **10:** 343–52.

SØRBO, B. (1962) The effect of radioprotective agents on tissue non protection SH and disulfide levels. *Arch. Biochem. Biophys.* **98:** 342–4.

SÜMEGI, J., SANNER, T. and PIHL, A. (1971) Involvement of highly reactive sulfhydryl groups in the action of RNA-polymerase from *E. coli. FEBS Letters* **16:** 125–7.

THERKELSEN, A. J. (1961) Protection of cells in tissue culture by means of cysteamine and cystamine against the action of nitrogen mustard and X-rays. *Biochem. Pharmacol.* **8:** 269–79.

TSUKADA, K. and LIEBERMAN, I. (1965) Liver nuclear RNA polymerase formed after partial hepatectomy. *J. Biol. Chem.* **240:** 1731–6.

VANDERGOTEN, R. and GOUTIER, R. (1966) Effects of total body X-irradiation and of chemical protector AET administration on the activity of nuclear RNA-polymerase in regene-rating rat liver. *Int. J. Rad. Biol.* **11:** 449–54.

VERGROESEN, A. J., BUDKE, M. and VOS, O. (1967) Protection against X-irradiation by SH-compounds. II. Studies on the relation between chemical structure and protective action for tissue culture cells. *Int. J. Rad. Biol.* **13:** 77–92.

VOS, O., BUDKE, L. and VERGROESEN, A. J. (1962) Protection of tissue-culture cells against ionizing radiation. I. The effects of biological amines, disulphide compounds and thiols. *Int. J. Radiat. Biol.* **5:** 543–57.

CHAPTER 8

PROTECTION BY THIOLS AGAINST POISONING BY RADIOMIMETIC AGENTS

Z. M. Bacq

Liège, Belgium

8.1. INTRODUCTION

The analogy between the effects of some alkylating agents and those of ionizing radiation has often been stressed (see for instance Bacq and Alexander, 1961) and, not surprisingly, a number of experimental studies have attempted to detect a protective effect of thiols against these agents.

Cysteamine (MEA), cysteine, aminoethylisothiourea (AET), glutathione, thiourea, dimercaprol (BAL), and other less well known —SH protective agents (and even thiols which are inactive against ionizing radiation) may protect mammals and *in vitro* living systems against radiomimetic alkylating agents used in cancer chemotherapy (nitrogen mustards (HN2), sarcolysine, busulfan, etc.*) (Brandt and Griffin, 1951; Weisberger *et al.,* 1952; Peczenik, 1953; Deysson and Truhaut, 1953a, b, 1956; Truhaut and Deysson, 1954; Dunjic *et al.,* 1955; Desaive, 1955; Truhaut *et al.,* 1956; Cima and Pozza, 1960a; Hastrup, 1961; Maisin and Dunjic, 1962; Connors and Elson, 1962; Herrádi *et al.,* 1962; Asano *et al.,* 1962, 1963; Brimcker, 1964; Bacq, 1965). Connors (1966) has devoted an intelligent review to this question; there is no reason why one should not accept the logic of his presentation.

*   HN2   : $H_3C-N\begin{cases} CH_2-CH_2Cl \\ CH_2-CH_2Cl \end{cases}$

Sarcolysine (Merophan®) : $CH_2-\overset{\overset{\displaystyle NH_2}{|}}{CH}-COOH$, $N\begin{cases} CH_2-CH_2Cl \\ CH_2-CH_2Cl \end{cases}$

Busulfan (Myleran®) : $H_3C-SO_2-O-(CH_2)_4-O-SO_2-CH_3$

This effect of certain thiols is again strictly "protective", i.e. the substance must be administered before exposure to the radiomimetic agent. Kirrmann (1966) stresses this point in his *in vitro* studies with the intestine of the chick embryo in organotypic culture. Cysteamine protects against HN2 only if applied at non-toxic concentrations (12 mM) which do not inhibit the oxygen consumption of the organ. A concentration of 64 mM does protect against radiation but not against nitrogen mustards.*

The protection by thiols against alkylating agents seems to be a universal phenomenon. It has been observed not only in mammals, but with plant cells (Deysson and Truhaut, 1953a, b, 1954, 1956), bacteria (Hernádi *et al.*, 1962), isolated mammalian cells (Therkelsen, 1961), and model systems as discussed below. This universality of action is also an important feature of the protection against ionizing radiation by the sulfur-containing substances (Bacq, 1965).

Therkelsen (1961) observed good protection of mouse fibroblasts against HN2 in tissue culture by both MEA and cystamine although with the same material he failed to see any protection against X-ray irradiation. He believes that the destruction of some vital —SH groups in the cell plays a central part in the effect of the nitrogen mustard on cells.

As pointed out by Therkelsen, the technique followed by Deysson and Truhaut (1953, 1954) demonstrates that MEA (not cystamine) reacts *in vitro* with the nitromine (HN2 oxidized on the N) and not that the cells of *Pisum sativum* are protected. The French authors exposed the cells to a mixed solution of MEA and the agent in Knop's medium.

8.2. IS THERE A CORRELATION BETWEEN THE PROTECTIVE POWER OF VARIOUS THIOLS AGAINST RADIOMIMETIC AGENTS AND IONIZING RADIATION?

The answer is clearly no, as shown by the data of Table 1 collected by Connors (1966). Large doses of cysteine which give about the same protection (to mice or rats) against X-ray irradiation as 5 to 6 times less MEA or AET protect more efficiently against sarcolysine and still better against HN2. Aminoethylisothiourea is a better protective agent against sarcolysine than MEA. Using mice Goldenthal *et al.* (1959) have also

---

*Kirrmann (1966) does not accept Connors' (1966) general interpretation (direct chemical reaction) because when he applies MEA and HN2 simultaneously to his test, he does not observe any protection.

TABLE 1. COMPARATIVE PROTECTION GIVEN TO RATS OR MICE BY THREE THIOLS AGAINST
X-RAYS AND TWO ALKYLATING AGENTS (COMPUTED BY CONNORS, 1966) EXPRESSED AS
DOSE REDUCTION FACTORS.[a] MTD = MAXIMAL TOLERATED DOSE

Thiol	MTD (mg/kg)	X-rays	HN2	Merophan
MEA	150	1.8–2.0	2.0	1.3
AET	200	1.8–2.0	2.0	2.0
Cysteine	1000	1.8	7.0	4.2

[a] There is a variation in the DRF found for different strains of animals. These figures are the highest recorded in the literature. The dose DRF is obtained from the ratio LD_{50} animals pretreated with the thiol/LD_{50} (or LD_{99}) of irradiated animals or animals given the alkylating agent only. The thiol is given at the previously determined optimum time to give the greatest protection, usually 5–30 min before the alkylating agent or irradiation. In most cases thiol pretreatment does not alter the slope of the dose–mortality curve, so that the DRF obtained applies to all doses of X-rays or alkylating agents.

found that cysteine gives better protection than MEA against HN2; these two substances do not protect against tretamine (triethylenemelamine), probably because their chemical reaction with this carcinostatic agent is too slow.

Thus it appears that the mechanisms of protection against radiomimetic agents are different from those which have been carefully analyzed and discussed as far as ionizing radiations are concerned (see Bacq, 1965; Bacq and Goutier, 1967).

8.3. THE HYPOTHESIS OF COMPETITIVE REMOVAL
(Connors, 1966)

Immediate chemical reaction of mustards (and other war poisons) with thiols is a well-known phenomenon (Bacq, 1942, 1946a, b; Bacq *et al.*, 1947; Goldenthal *et al.*, 1959; Contractor, 1963); detoxication in the body by reaction with the —SH of cysteine is also clearly demonstrated for busulfan (Roberts and Warwick, 1958, 1961), a bifunctional antileukaemic agent, the toxicity of which is also decreased by previous administration of MEA (Dunjic, 1966). Thus the hypothesis of a competition between thiol functions and other sites (more important for the cytostatic effects) for the alkylating agent seemed logical and has been carefully studied.*

* Salerno and Friedell (1954) (who observed protection of mice by cysteine or MEA) have proposed a mechanism which involves the "chemical" inactivation of the nitrogen mustard by the —SH group of the thiols. Therkelsen (1958) rejects this possibility which at that time was little substantiated by adequate experiments and was not expressed as it should be in the terms of competition.

Alkylation is the substitution of a hydrogen atom of a molecule by an alkyl (RCH_3-) group

$$R.CH_2X + HR' \longrightarrow R.CH_2R' + XH$$

The reactions of the agent with a tertiary amine (to form a quaternary ammonium compound) or with an ionized acid (to form an ester) are also alkylations. In the case of the halogenated mustards, a highly reactive transient carbonium ion is formed in the presence of water. This intermediate combines rapidly with the nucleophilic centers (negatively charged atoms or atoms of high electron density) of many molecules. Such sites are, for instance, the thiol, amino, carboxyl groups of proteins. But it is the reaction with DNA at the level of guanine which is thought to be the mechanism responsible for cytotoxicity.

Since ionized thiols are extremely reactive toward alkylating agents, it may be expected that if added in sufficient concentration they may compete successfully, remove a significant proportion of the toxic molecules before they reach the DNA, and in this way decrease DNA alkylation.

This hypothesis postulates several corollaries.

8.4.   TOXICITY OF THE PROTECTOR AND COMPETITION FACTOR

The best protective thiols would have (a) little toxicity in order to be present at higher concentration when the alkylating agent is administered, (b) a high competition factor. This factor has been measured for sulfur mustard (Ogston, 1948), which may be considered as representative of this class of alkylating agents, in conditions approaching that which occur in the body. Table 2 (from Connors, 1966) shows that the thiols (cysteine and thiosulfate), at approximately equal doses, with a higher competition factor protect more effectively against HN2 than the poorly competitive thiourea.

Connors and Elson (1962) studied the ability of various thiols to protect rats against lethal doses of sarcolysine and other alkylating agents. Cysteine, thiourea, AET, and a thiazolidine reduce the toxicity of sarcolysine and more chemically reactive agents but not the less reactive ones (bisulfan and dimethylmyleran, for instance). Cysteamine and penicillamine have little protective effect.

TABLE 2. PROTECTION OF RATS OR MICE AGAINST THE ACUTE TOXICITY OF HN2
(NITROGEN MUSTARD) BY VARIOUS CHEMICALS (Connors, 1966)

Chemical	Maximal tolerated dose (mg/kg)	Competition factor	Dose reduction
L-Cysteine	1000	1.2×10^3	7.0
Thiosulfate	2000	2.7×10^4	5.0
Thiourea	1200	1.5×10^2	2.0
Diethyldithiocarbamate	350	3.4×10^4	2.0
Dimercaptopropanol	100	7.8×10^2	1.0

Diethyldithiocarbamate has a good competition factor but is much more toxic and cannot be injected in large quantities. Dimercaprol (BAL) which combines the two defects—high toxicity and poor competition—does not protect significantly.

One might wonder why thiosulfate which has a higher competition factor and smaller toxicity than cysteine is not at least as good a protector as the amino acid. As shown by Connors (1966), thiosulfate protects as well as cysteine against HN2, but is nearly ineffective against sarcolysine although cysteine is about equally active against sarcolysine as against HN2. The reason might be that thiosulfate does not easily cross the cell membranes and accordingly remains in the plasma and interstitial fluid; it is known to protect extracellular structures (fibers and polysaccharides of connective tissue for instance) against ionizing radiations but does not decrease the lethal properties of irradiation in mammals which are due mainly to intracellular lesions. The fact that thiosulfate does protect well against mustards means that a large fraction of the injected mustard is "neutralized" in the extracellular space. There are other facts which, in connection with the inability of thiosulfate to penetrate into cells, might explain why this thiol does not protect well against sarcolysine. The mechanism of alkylation by HN2 is very complex (see Ross, 1962), and not the same as that by sarcolysine. Sarcolysine acts mainly by formation of an intermediate carbonium ion, and thiosulfate cannot compete with this very reactive ion appearing inside the cell. On the contrary, alkylation by HN2 starts by the formation of a transition complex between the agent and nucleophilic centers. Dissociation then takes place to give the alkylated product. With this mechanism, the rate of alkylation is markedly influenced by the concentration of nucleophilic centers. HN2 injected in an animal treated with thiosulfate will meet more reactive centers in the plasma and interstitial fluid before entering the cell; more HN2 will react extracellularly; less HN2 will be available for alkylation of the nucleic acids.

For a given good protective agent, the protective effect is proportional to the dose. The LD_{50} of sarcolysine in rats is not increased by cysteine 125 mg/kg; the dose reduction factor (DRF)* rises to 1.8 for 250 mg and reaches 4.2 for 1000 mg/kg.

In order to react with an alkylating agent in the body, the thiol must be available in its free form. Since it is known that many thiols when injected in the body are rapidly "fixed" to proteins to give mixed disulfides (see Chapter 8.5), one would expect the time-course of protection to correspond rather closely to that of the concentration of the free thiol in the tissues. This has been found to be true for cysteine against sarcolysine (Calcutt *et al.*, 1963). The DRF is high when sarcolysine is injected 15 or 30 min after cysteine. It is slightly lower at 60 min when free cysteine in the tissues has significantly decreased; it is still much lower, 2 hr after the injection. Unfortunately it is difficult to interpret the results obtained at 15 min or before 15 min because some injected cysteine is still present in the peritoneal cavity when sarcolysine is injected by the same route. This phenomenon differentiates protection against alkylating agents from that against X-rays irradiation. In the latter case there is no time correlation between the intensity of protection and the concentration of the *free* thiol (see Bacq, 1965; Bacq and Goutier, 1967). It has been most regularly observed that protection (by MEA or cystamine) is higher 10 min after injection than at 30 min, although the concentration of the *free* thiol in the tissues is higher at 30 min (see also Chapter 5).

The competitive removal theory also postulates that for a given thiol the DRF should be greater with highly reactive than with less reactive alkylating agents. If one takes as a measure of general reactivity the approximate half life of the agent in water, this corollary is found to be true (Connors, 1966). In Table 5 it is stated that cysteine does not protect against busulfan, a slow-reacting alkylating agent (see also Kelly *et al.*, 1960; Asano *et al.*, 1963, about AET), but according to Dunjic (1966)

---

* Dose reduction factor is the factor by which the radiation dose has to be multiplied after administration of a radioprotective agent in order to obtain the same death rate as with controls. For instance, a DRF of 2 means that a LD_{50} (30 days) of 500 is increased to 1000.

By extension, the protection by chemicals against radiomimetic substances is expressed in the same way. The DRF is the factor by which one must multiply the dose of a cytostatic in order to obtain the same mortality in animals treated with a protective thiol as in controls.

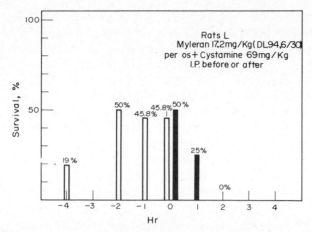

FIG. 1. Survival of rats given a 95% lethal dose of busulfan per os plus i.p. injections of MEA at various moments before or after the busulfan (Maisin, personal communication, 1963).

MEA and cystamine protect rats against busulfan. Figure 1 shows that MEA is equally effective in reducing mortality when injected a very short time *after* busulfan; this fact is explainable by the lowered reactivity of busulfan. The dose reduction factor of these two amines injected intraperitoneally (i.p.) (60 mg/kg) 1 hr after the oral ingestion of lethal doses of busulfan) is 1.35. If ten times more cystamine is given orally 1 hr before the lethal dose of busulfan (also by oral route) the DRF rises to 3.43, but in this case, direct chemical inactivation may occur in the intestinal tract before absorption of busulfan (Dunjic, 1966).

8.5. INCREASED EXCRETION OF DETOXICATION PRODUCTS

If the injected protective thiol competes with the natural nucleophilic centers within the body, it should be possible to detect an increased urinary output of metabolites of the alkylating agent. After administration of ^{14}C-labeled HN2, rats excrete 15% of the radioactivity in 24 hr; if pretreated with a protective amount of cysteine, the percentage excreted increases to 43% (Goldenthal *et al.*, 1959). Control mice excrete 64% of the label in 24 hr; in MEA-pretreated mice (DRF=2) 95% of the radioactivity is recovered in the same time (Contractor, 1963). These observations are interpreted very differently by these authors. Goldenthal *et al.* are in favor of a competition, of a direct reaction between the protective agent and HN2; they show that the excess of radioactive material in the urine of protected rats is a reaction product of cysteine and HN2. Contractor believes that MEA inhibits the reaction of HN2 with the sensitive sites by mixed disulfide formation. This opinion does not seem logical if one recalls (a) that MEA reacts with S—S groups of proteins (to form mixed disulfides) and that the disulfide bridges are not preferential sites for reaction with HN2; if Contractor's interpretation were correct, only cystamine which blocks —SH functions should protect against alkylating agents; (b) the time course of protection does not follow the curve of the concentration of bound protective agent in the tissues; one should expect, according to Contractor's hypothesis, a much higher protection 5 min after injection of MEA than after 30 min; it is indeed a correlation of the concentration of the *free* form with protection against alkylating agent which has been observed; (c) MEA does not react with DNA, i.e. with the guanine site which is believed to be most important for the cytostatic and lethal effect, and according to Contractor should be unable to protect DNA.

There is no increase in urinary excretion of tritium by ^{3}H-labeled melphalan treated rats after protective treatment with cysteine (Ball and Connors, 1967); but the binding of melphalan to proteins is unaltered by cysteine and only 6% of the radioactivity is excreted in 4 days. This observation as explained by Ball and Connors is not a serious objection to the competitive removal hypothesis.

8.6.   PROTECTION OF NUCLEIC ACIDS

Ball and Connors (1967) have shown both *in vitro* and *in vivo* that the protection by thiols can be wholly explained by a decreased alkylation of DNA and RNA. They separated the nucleic acids, nucleoproteins, and cytoplasmic proteins from homogenates of Yoshida sarcoma cells treated with ^{3}H-labeled melphalan* in the presence or absence of thiol protective agent. The specific activity of the isolated fractions was measured according to the classical techniques. Free cysteine reaches a maximal concentration of 6.5 mcmol/g wet weight in the tumor 30 min after i.p. injection of 1 g/kg of cysteine, but the concentration is still high (5 mM)

---

*Melphalan (Alkcran®) is a phenylalanine mustard derivative: 4-*N,N*-di(2-dichlor-ethyl)-amino-L-phenylalanine; it was ^{3}H-labeled in position 2.

TABLE 3. REACTION OF ^{3}H-MELPHALAN WITH CELL FRACTIONS OF THE YOSHIDA SARCOMA *in vivo*. MELPHALAN IS INJECTED 30 MIN AFTER CYSTEINE; RATS ARE KILLED 1 HR AFTER MELPHALAN INJECTION (Ball and Cannors, 1967)

Cell fraction	Control, specific activity (counts/min/mg) after H^3-melphalan at dose stated (Mean ± S.E.)		Cysteine pretreated, specific activity (counts/min/mg) with cysteine treatment before H^3-melphalan (Mean ± S.E.)		Hydrolyzed melphalan activity
	4 mg/kg	8 mg/kg	4 mg/kg	8 mg/kg	4 mg/kg
DNA	102 ± 4	241 ± 17	25 ± 3	40 ± 4	< 5
RNA	174 ± 9	366 ± 19	40 ± 4	70 ± 3	< 5
Nuclear protein	165 ± 22	312 ± 1	62 ± 12	64 ± 5	19 ± 4
Cytoplasmic protein	283 ± 24	550 ± 30	281 ± 27	298 ± 19	334 ± 25

90 min after the injection; the approximate half life of the alkylating agent is 90 min. The results are given in Table 3. The labeling of DNA, RNA, and nucleoproteins is drastically reduced; that of cytoplasmic proteins is unchanged when 4 mg/kg of melphalan are used. Hydrolyzed, inactivated melphalan does not bind to nucleic acids but still reacts with cytoplasmic proteins.

TABLE 4. EFFECT OF VARIOUS THIOLS IN REDUCING ALKYLATION OF DNA BY ^{3}H-MELPHALAN *in vitro* (Ball and Connors, 1967)

Compound	Concentration (mM)	Specific activity of DNA (% control)
Sodium thiosulfate	0.0005	99.8
	0.005	88.9
	0.05	4.3
	0.5	0.6
L-Cysteine	0.05	98.5
	0.5	57.5
	5.0	21.0
	50.0	9.8
Glutathione	0.5	71.0
Dihydrolipoic acid	0.5	45.0
DL-Homocysteine	0.5	78.5
2,3-Dimercapto-propanol	0.5	41.5
AET	0.5	70.0
Thiourea	0.5	72.0
MEA	0.5	76.0
Sodium chloride[a]	0.5	100.0
	5.0	80.0
	50.0	21.0

[a] Effect of sodium chloride concentration—as per cent of 0.5 mM control.

Model *in vitro* research shows that isolated tumor DNA is protected from alkylation by concentrations of protective agent which are titrated in the tumor after i.p. injection. The better protective agents (cysteine, thiosulfate) are those thiols which at equivalent concentration decrease more efficiently the labeling of the DNA (Table 4). Protection by thiosulfate against HN2 adds to that of cysteine (to reach the remarkable DRF of 9.6), but the same thiosulfate decreases the protection afforded by cysteine against sarcolysine; Connors *et al.* (1964) suggest that this last fact might be due to thiosulfate preventing cysteine from entering cells.

8.7. PROTECTION OF HEMATOPOIETIC TISSUES

The reactions of the hematopoietic system have been particularly studied because the damage to this system constitutes a limiting factor in the use of alkylating agents for cancer chemotherapy.

Protection of the bone-marrow is proved by observations on the bone-marrow or spleen as well as on the peripheral blood. In mice, Therkelsen (1956) described protection of the spleen and bone-marrow against HN2 by MEA; better and earlier regeneration in the protected animals was obvious.

Cysteine markedly decreased the effect of sarcolysine on blood lymphocytes and neutrophils in the rat. In this animal, sarcolysine induces lymphopenia (maximal at 2 days) and granulopenia (maximal at about 4 days) followed by recovery and overshoot (very important as far as neutrophils are concerned). Both phases are similarly "damped" by cysteine (1 g/kg) pretreatment (Connors, 1966). The DRF is again about 4 (Connors *et al.*, 1965a). Brandt and Griffin (1951) fail to find significant protection by cysteine against the decrease in white blood count induced by HN2 in mice; this contrasts with the good protection observed against the lethal effect.

Intravenous injection of 600 mg/kg L-cysteine in the rabbit just before i.v. injection of 3 mg/kg HN2 allows recovery of the bactericidal properties of the blood in 6 days, instead of 20 days as in controls (Donaldson and Miller, 1959).

A good quantitative test of the toxicity of alkylating agents for bone-marrow are the DNA and RNA contents of this tissue (Connors *et al.*, 1965a, Table 5). If one calculates the dose of sarcolysine needed to cut by half the DNA content of the bone-marrow of rats, one obtains a dose

TABLE 5. REDUCTION OF TOXICITY OF SARCOLYSINE BY CYSTEINE IN RATS
(Connors *et al.*, 1965a)

Pretreatment	LD_{50} (mg/kg)	DRF	50% fall in bone-marrow DNA[a] (mg/kg)	Bone-marrow DRF	Bone-marrow SH 30 min after cysteine (mcg/g wet wt)
None	3.67		1.7		121 ($\pm$34.5)
Cysteine (250 mg/kg i.p.)	6.50	1.8			142 ($\pm$21.5)
Cysteine (500 mg/kg i.p.)	11.02	3.0	5.0	2.9	178 ($\pm$27.0)
Cysteine (1000 mg/kg i.p.)	15.24	4.2	7.4	4.4	261 ($\pm$38.5)

[a] The dose of sarcolysine to give 50% in fall in the bone-marrow DNA concentration.

reduction factor of 4.4 for 1 g/kg of cysteine, a DRF identical to that given by studies of the lethal effect.

8.8.   PROTECTION OF TUMORS

A logical consequence of the facts analyzed in the preceding paragraphs is that thiols must protect tumor cells as well as normal cells against alkylating agents. Peczenik's (1953) observation that MEA may increase the effect of HN2 on tumors has never been confirmed; but several authors (see Rutman *et al.*, 1961; Therkelsen, 1958) observed some increase of the therapeutic index in experimental tumors. Cysteine inhibits the cytostatic effect of melphalan on the Yoshida sarcoma *in vivo*; the dose reduction factor is about 2, i.e. about the same as for the lethal or cytostatic action on normal blood cells. This is very unfortunate

TABLE 6. EFFECT OF CYSTEINE PRETREATMENT ON THE THERAPEUTIC INDEX OF SARCOLYSINE
(Connors, 1966)

Tumor	Treatment	LD_{90} (mg/kg)	LD_{50} (mg/kg)	Therapeutic index[a]
ADJ/PC5	Sarcolysine alone	2.3	4.2	1.9
Plasma cell tumor	Sarcolysine + cysteine	8.5	10.6	1.3
Walker carcinoma	Sarcolysine alone	0.24	3.4	14.2
	Sarcolysine + cysteine	1.6	19.0	11.9
Yoshida sarcoma	Sarcolysine alone	0.2	3.4	17.0
	Sarcolysine + cysteine	2.2	16.0	7.3

[a] The therapeutic index is the ratio LD_{50}/LD_{90} (the dose to give 90% tumor inhibition), and is a measure of the selectivity of the drug.

because it prevents improvement of the therapeutic index, i.e. the selectivity of cytostatic drugs in cancer chemotherapy. Table 6 (from Connors, 1966) shows that cysteine pretreatment reduces the therapeutic index of sarcolysine in the treatment of three experimental tumors. Administration of AET (which concentrates less in certain tumors than in normal tissues, see Chapter 5) increases the therapeutic index of sarcolysine against a mouse plasma cell tumor (Connors *et al.*, 1965b; Back and Ambrus, 1959).

There has been much discussion about the correlation between resistance of tumors to alkylating agents (and to ionizing radiation) and content of free or protein-bound —SH (see, for instance, Connors, 1966).

One should not forget in discussions about the reactions of —SH groups with alkylating agents that three main natural intracellular small molecules may be concerned. The greatest bulk of free non-protein —SH is *glutathione* maintained in free reduced (SH) form by the action of glutathione reductase; but as pointed out by Connors (1966) when discussing the question of reaction and sensitivity to mustards, glutathione has little importance since it is not particularly reactive to these agents and since injection of large amounts of this polypeptide fails to confer any increased resistance.* *Lipoic acid* is not devoid of protective effect (see Table 4) when put in competition *in vitro* for DHA alkylation by melphalan, but its intracellular concentration is probably kept constant within strict limits. After administration of an alkylating agent to an animal, nobody has observed any deficiency in biochemical reactions in which this thiol acts as coenzyme. Similarly no deficiency in *coenzyme A* is mentioned in the literature after alkylation although the final —SH group of the MEA moiety of this molecule must be highly reactive. To our knowledge, no systematic search has been carried out. Failure of inactivation of CoA may be due to the fact that the final S of the coenzyme is constantly "covered" (and consequently protected) by one of the numerous radicals (acetyl, etc.) which it activates.

8.9. PROTECTION OF THE ADRENAL CORTEX

David (1968) claims that pretreatment with AET favorably influences the secretion and synthesis of adrenal hormones in rats poisoned with nitrogen mustard.

---

*As far as ionizing radiations are concerned, glutathione is a moderately good protective agent.

8.10. NITROSOALKYLAMINES, CARBON TETRACHLORIDE, FUNGISTATICS

The inhibitory effects of carcinogenic *N*-nitrosoalkylamines on incorporation of amino acids in rat liver is prevented by MEA (Emmelot *et al.*, 1962). Conversely, the *N*-nitrosodialkylamines inhibit the hepatic glycogenolysis which is so characteristic an effect of MEA and cysteine.

Cysteamine has no protecting effect against rat liver necrosis induced by CCl_4, but prevents the decrease in NADP and NADPH seen in the control necrotic livers (Slater *et al.*, 1966).

The fungistatic effect of many substances (some of them halogenated and being really alkylating agents) is reduced by cysteine and thioglycolate by virtue of their reaction with the $-SH$ group of the protective agents (Zsolnai, 1962).

8.11. CONCLUSIONS

Connors (1966) summarizes the facts analyzed in his review in the following way: "Although thiols may protect against both X-irradiation and alkylating agent induced toxicity, there is evidence that the protective mechanism is not the same in both cases. All compounds that have so far been shown to give good protection against alkylating agents attain a high concentration in free form in the animal and are very reactive towards alkylating agents. It is likely that they will react directly *in vivo* with administered alkylating agents and such a reaction would restrict their alkylation of DNA and could thus account entirely for the protective effect. The application of thiol protection to cancer chemotherapy is of doubtful value since even if protective amounts of thiol could be administered protection to the host would be likely to be paralleled by protection to the tumor with no gain in selectivity of action of the alkylating agent."

REFERENCES

ASANO, M. M., McDONALD, T. P. and ODELL, T. T. JR. (1962) Effects of nitrogen mustard on mouse tissue and modification by AET. *Int. J. Rad. Biol.* **4:** 591–600.

ASANO, M., ODELL, T., McDONALD, T. and UPTON, A. (1963) Radiomimetic agents and X-rays in mice and AET protectiveness. *Arch. Path.* **75:** 250–63.

BACK, N. and AMBRUS, J. L. (1959) The use of *S*-(2-aminoethylisothiouronium bromide hydrobromide (AET) to localize the effect of alkylating agents and to extend their therapeutic index in the treatment of neoplastic ascites. *Cancer* **12:** 1003–8.

BACQ, Z. M. (1942) Inactivation des vésicants et des lacrymogènes par réaction avec des composés sulfhydrylés: essai thérapeutique. *Bull. Acad. Roy. Méd. Belg.* **7**: 500–27.
BACQ, Z. M. (1946a) Réaction des toxiques de guerre avec les groupes thiols des protéines, du glutathion et de la cystéine. *Bull. Acad. Roy. Méd. Belg.* VIth series **11**: 137–64.
BACQ, Z. M. (1946b) Substances thioloprives. *Experientia* **2**: 349–54 and 385–90.
BACQ, Z. M. (1965) *Chemical Protection against Ionizing Radiation.* American Lecture Series no. 599, Ch. C. Thomas, Springfield, U.S., p. 328.
BACQ, Z. M. and ALEXANDER, P. (1961) *Fundamentals of Radiobiology,* 2nd ed. Pergamon Press, Oxford, 555 p.
BACQ, Z. M. and GOUTIER, R. (1967) Mechanisms of action of sulphur containing radioprotectors, pp. 241–62. In: *Brookhaven Symposia No. 20, Recovery and Repair Mechanisms in Radiobiology.*
BACQ, Z. M., DESREUX, V. and GOFFART, M. (1947) Action of mustard gas (ββ'-dichlorethylsulfide) on thiol groups of proteins. *Nature* **159**: 478.
BALL, C. R. and CONNORS, T. A. (1967) Reduction of the toxicity of "radiomimetic" alkylating agents by thiol pretreatment. VI. The mechanism of protection by cysteine. *Biochem. Pharmacol.* **16**: 509–19.
BRANDT, E. L. and GRIFFIN, A. C. (1951) Reduction of toxicity of nitrogen mustards by cysteine. *Cancer* **4**: 1030–5.
BRIMCKER, H. (1964) Protection of C_3H mice against toxic effects of endoxan by means of cysteine hydrochloride. *Acta Path. Microbiol. Scand.* **61**: 321–2.
CALCUTT, G., CONNORS, T. A., ELSON, L. A. and ROSS, W. C. J. (1963) Reduction of the toxicity of "radiomimetic" alkylating agents in rats by thiols. II. Mechanism of protection. *Biochem. Pharmacol.* **12**: 833–7.
CIMA, L. and POZZA, F. (1960a) Influenza del dietilditiocarbammato sulla tossicita della mecloretamina. *Bol. Soc. Italiana Biol. Speriment.* **36**: 1123–6.
CIMA, L. and POZZA, F. (1960b) Influenza di radioprotettori sulla tossicita della mecloretamina. *Ricerca Scientifica* **5**: 680–5.
CIMA, L. and POZZA, F. (1960c) Dietilditiocarbammato sodico e coefficiente terapeutico della mecloretamina. *Ricerca Scientifica* Suppl. **12**: 2387–90.
CONNORS, T. A. (1966) Protection against the toxicity of alkylating agents by thiols: The mechanism of protection and its relevance to cancer chemotherapy. *Europ. J. Cancer* **2**: 293–305.
CONNORS, T. A. and ELSON, L. A. (1962) Reduction of the toxicity of "radiomimetic" alkylating agents in rats by thiol pretreatment. *Biochem. Pharmacol.* **11**: 1221–32.
CONNORS, T. A., JENEY, A. and JONES, M. (1964) Reduction of the toxicity of "radiomimetic" alkylating agents in rats by thiol pretreatment. III. The mechanism of the protective action of thiosulphate. *Biochem. Pharmacol.* **13**: 1545–50.
CONNORS, T. A., DOUBLE, J. A., ELSON, L. A. and JENEY, A. JR. (1965a) Reduction of the toxicity of "radiomimetic" alkylating agents in rats by thiol pretreatment. IV. Protection against bone-marrow damage. *Biochem. Pharmacol.* **14**: 569–77.
CONNORS, T. A., JENEY, A. JR. and WHISSON, M. E. (1965b) Reduction of the toxicity of radiomimetic alkylating agents in rats by thiol pretreatment. V. The effect of thiol pretreatment on the anti-tumor action of Merophan. *Biochem. Pharmacol.* **14**: 1681–3.
CONTRACTOR, S. F. (1963) Protection against nitrogen mustard by cysteine and related substances, investigated using (^{3}H) methyl-di-(2-chloroethyl)amine. *Biochem. Pharmacol.* **12**: 821–32.
DAVID, G. (1968) Zur radiomimetischen Wirkung des Stickstofflostes. II. Funktionsveränderungen der Nebenniere bei experimenteller Strahlenkrankheit und bei Stickstofflost-Vergiftung. Die bei Gave von AET auftretenden Änderungen. *Radiobiol. Radiother.* (*East Berlin*) **9**: 61–5.

DESAIVE, P. (1955) Influence des doses élevées de méthyl-bis(2-chloroéthyl) amine sur l'ovaire de la lapine adulte, avec ou sans préparation par la bétamercaptoéthylamine. In: *Radiobiology Symposium, Liège* 1954. BACQ, Z. M. and ALEXANDER, P. (eds.). Butterworths, London, pp. 340–57.

DEYSSON, G. and TRUHAUT, R. (1953a) Recherches sur l'action cytotoxique des composés dits radiomimétiques. Protection exercée par la β-mercaptoéthylamine vis-à-vis des effets toxiques sur les cellules végétales de la β, β′, β″-trichoéthylamine. *Bull. Soc. Chim. Biol.* **35**: 1019–26.

DEYSSON, G. and TRUHAUT, R. (1953b) Action protectrice de la β-mercaptoéthylamine vis-à-vis des effets toxiques sur les cellules d'*Allium cepa* d'un composé du groupe des radiomimétiques: la β, β′, β″-trichloréthylamine. *C. R. Acad. Sc.* **236**: 2329–32.

DEYSSON, G. and TRUHAUT, R. (1954) Action protectrice de la β-mercaptoéthylamine vis-à-vis des effets toxiques sur les cellules végétales d'une "moutarde azotée" oxydée à l'azote: le chlorhydrate de méthyl-bis(β-chloréthyl)amine *N*-oxyde. *C.R. Acad. Sc.* **238**: 1725–7.

DEYSSON, G. and TRUHAUT, R. (1956) Nouvelles recherches sur l'action protectrice exercée par divers composés sulfhydrylés vis-à-vis de la toxicité des "moutardes azotées" et de la triéthylène-mélanine pour les cellules végétales. *C.R. Soc. Biol.* **150**: 1171–3.

DONALDSON, M. D. and MILLER, M. L. (1959) Depression of normal serum bactericidal activity by nitrogen mustard. *J. Immunol.* **82**: 69–74.

DUNJIC, A. (1966) Au sujet de l'action protectrice de la cystéamine et de la cystamine chez le rat ayant reçu des doses létales de Myleran. *Pathologie Biologie* **14**: 554–8.

DUNJIC, A., MAISIN, H. and MAISIN, J. (1955) De la protection par la mercaptoéthylamine de rats injectés d'ypérite. *C.R. Soc. Biol.* **149**: 1684–97.

EMMELOT, P., MIZRAHI, I. J. and KRIEK, E. (1962) Prevention by cysteamine on the inhibitory effect of carcinogenic *N*-nitrosoalkylamines on incorporation of amino acids in rat liver. *Nature* **193**: 1158–61.

GOLDENTHAL, E. J., NADKARNI, M. V. and SMITH, P. K. (1959) A study of comparative protection against lethality of triethylenemelanine, nitrogen mustard, and X-irradiation in mice. *Radiation Res.* **10**: 571–83.

HASTRUP, J. VON (1961) Die kombinierte Behandlung homologer Maüse-Tumoren mit Cysteamin und Endoxan. *Arzneimittel Forsch.* **11**: 177–9.

HERNÁDI, F., VÁLYI-NAGY, T., NAGY, ZS. and JENEY, A. (1962) Protection against the toxic effects of X-ray and nitrogen mustard on *E. coli* O 111 by radioprotectors. *Radiation Res.* **16**: 464–70.

KELLY, M. G., RALL, D. P., TRIVERS, G. E., O'GARA, R. W. and ZUBROD, C. G. (1960) Actions of *S*,2-aminoethylisothiouronium Br, HBr (AET). Toxicity and protective effect against nitrogen mustard toxicity. *J. Pharmacol.* **129**: 218–30.

KIRRMANN, J. M. (1966) Sur l'action protectrice exercée par la cystéamine contre les effects d'une substance radiomimétique, l'ypérite azotée, appliquée à un organe embryonnaire cultivé *in vitro*. *C.R. Acad. Sc.* (*Paris*), Série D **222**: 1296–8.

MAISIN, J. (1963) Personal communication.

MAISIN, J. and DUNJIC, A. (1962) Personal communication.

OGSTON, A. G. (1948) The replacement reactions of β-β′dichlorodiethyl sulphide and of some analogues in aqueous solution: the isolation of β-chloro-β-hydroxy diethyl sulphide. Part I. The kinetics of hydrolysis and replacement reactions of β-β′-dichlorodiethyl sulphide. *Trans. Faraday Soc.* **44**: 45–56.

PECZENIK, O. (1953) Influence of cysteinamine, methylamine and cortisone on the toxicity and activity of nitrogen mustard. *Nature* **172**: 454–5.

ROBERTS, J. J. and WARWICK, G. P. (1958, 1961) Studies on the mode of action of alkylating agents. *Biochem. Pharmacol.* **1**: 60–75; **6**: 205–16; **6**: 217–27.

ROSS, W. C. J. (1962) *Biological Alkylating Agents*. Butterworths, London, p. 148.

RUTMAN, R. J., LEWIS, F. S. and PRICE, C. (1961) An effect of 1-mercapto-2-aminobutane (MAB) on the antitumor activity of nitrogen mustards. *Biochem. Pharmacol.* **8:** 72.

SALERNO, P. R. and FRIEDELL, H. L. (1954) Studies on the nature of the protective action of β-mercaptoethylamine and cysteine against X-rays and a nitrogen mustard. *Radiation Res.* **1:** 228.

SLATER, T. F., SAWYER, B. C. and STRAULI, U. D. (1966) Liver NADP and NADPH₂ in liver necrosis induced by carbon tetrachloride: the modifying action of protective agents. *Biochem. Pharmacol.* **15:** 1273–8.

THERKELSEN, A. J. (1956) Protective effect of cysteamine on mice injected with nitrogen, pp. 260–6. In: *Progress in Radiobiology, Proc. 4th Int. Conf. Radiobiology,* Cambridge, 1955, MITCHELL, J. S., HOLMES, B. E. and SMITH, C. L. (eds.). Oliver & Boyd. Edinburgh.

THERKELSEN, A. J. (1958) Studies on the mechanism of the protective action of sulphydryl compounds and amines against nitrogen mustard (HN2) and roentgen irradiation in mice. *Biochem. Pharmacol.* **1:** 258–66.

THERKELSEN, A. J. (1961) Protection of cells in tissue cultures by means of cysteamine and cystamine against the action of nitrogen mustard and X-rays. *Biochem. Pharmacol.* **8:** 269–79.

TRUHAUT, R. (1954) Sur l'action protectrice de la β-mercaptoéthylamine vis-à-vis des effets toxiques des composés de la série des moutardes. *Acta contra Cancrum* **10:** 182–7.

TRUHAUT, R. and DEYSSON, G. (1954) Etude des effets, sur les mitoses des cellules végétales, du 1,4-diméthylsulfoxybutane. Essais de protection par la β-mercaptoéthylamine. *C.R. Acad. Sc.* **238:** 1833–5.

TRUHAUT, R., PAOLETTI, C., BOIRON, M. and TUBIANA, M. (1956) Sur l'action protectrice de la β-mercaptoéthylamine vis-à-vis de la méthyl-bis(choroéthyl)amine chez le rat. *C.R. Soc. Biol.* **150:** 1363–8.

WEISBERGER, A. S., HEINLE, R. W. and LEVINE, B. (1952) The effect of L-cysteine on nitrogen mustard therapy. *Amer J. Med. Sc.* **224:** 201–11.

ZSOLNAI, T. (1962) Versuche zur Entdeckung neuer Fungistatica. V. *Biochem. Pharmacol.* **11:** 515–33.

CHAPTER 9

IMPORTANCE OF PHARMACOLOGICAL EFFECTS FOR RADIOPROTECTIVE ACTION

Z. M. Bacq

Liège, Belgium

IN A preliminary paper (Bacq and Alexander, 1964) and a monograph (Bacq, 1965) a series of arguments is given in favor of the so-called "biochemical shock" theory to explain radiation protection by some sulfur-containing substances.

At the macromolecular level, in radiation chemistry of phages, the mechanism of protection by thiols may be considered to be quite well understood at the present time. At the cellular level, although much more information is available, many difficulties persist. But as far as the whole mammal is concerned one feels the need of a drastic revision since all the hypotheses available are unsatisfactory.

The following concept—expressed in general terms because it is not possible to give more precision—seems, in the author's opinion, to outline a logical frame for future research and to agree with the present experimental evidence.

When a mammalian organism is suddenly flooded with a large dose of a thiol or disulfide protective agent, a series of events takes place: (a) in a few minutes, most of the substance is bound to protein; the intracellular equilibrium between free and bound —SH together with the regulation of the redox potential is deeply disturbed; (b) the binding of the radioprotective substance to proteins (and maybe to other compounds) of intracellular structures causes the discharge of substances (enzymes, glutathione, etc.); (c) during the following hour(s), the cells slowly recover and regain their normal state.

In step (a), the mixed disulfide formation is important; it is a necessary preliminary reaction for step (b); non-radioprotective thiols or disulfides

319

do not seem capable of inducing step (b).

Protein binding by itself at the molecular level has little or no importance in radioprotective action; it is important for the general physiology of the cell, which is modified in the direction of a greater radioresistance. Steps (b) and (c) contribute to radioprotection in a manner which so far cannot be traced with precision.

The main arguments in favor of these ideas are: (1) that there does not seem to be a close correlation between protection and tissue levels of either the bound or the free form of the protective agent; (2) that a certain delay—about 10 min—is needed for full development of protection against ionizing radiation. This observation on mice has been confirmed with isolated cells (Sato *et al.*, 1970).

The detailed study by different technical approaches of the cellular reactions to radioprotective concentrations of thiols and disulfides becomes the most promising avenue for research in this field. The discovery of some natural intracellular substance which might play an important role in chemical protection is not excluded, when it has been displaced or activated by a sufficient concentration of a radioprotective agent. Modig and his associates (1971) have worked along this line.

Straightforward extrapolation to the whole mammal of mechanisms which are clearly identified with phages and isolated cells is dangerous although there is no objection to the assumption that these mechanisms (instantaneous repair, free radical scavenging, energy transfer) do operate in the whole mammal. When phages or yeast cells are irradiated it is not difficult to know exactly what the physical and chemical condi-

TABLE 1. COEFFICIENTS OF DECREASED SENSITIVITY (DOSE REDUCTION FACTORS) TO GAMMA-IRRADIATION OF *E. coli* 15 TAU-ʙᴀʀ ACCORDING TO GROWTH CONDITIONS AND VARIOUS CONTACTS WITH β-MERCAPTOETHYLAMINE (Ginsberg, 1966)

Growth phase	Logarithmic	Early stationary
No MEA	1	±2
MEA 0.044 M present during irradiation; no previous incubation	±4	±8
MEA absent during irradiation but having been in contact with culture for 2 hr before irradiation	±2	±2
MEA present during irradiation and during 2 hr before irradiation	±8	±8

tions are. Irradiation of a mammal after injection of cysteamine (MEA) or aminoethyliosothiourea (AET) involves a most heterogeneous system: various types of cells respond differently to ionizing radiation and also concentrate the protective agent and react to it in various ways. It is not surprising that the details of this complicated mosaic and the relative importance of its different patterns are not fully understood even after 20 years of relentless research.

The importance of metabolic changes in protection against ionizing radiation by MEA is clearly indicated by the observations of Ginsberg (1966) on *E. coli*. This microorganism was irradiated with adequate controls in various conditions with respect to the growth phase and time of exposure to MEA.

The results of Ginsberg may be summarized in Table 1 and interpreted in the following way:

(a) When the microorganism is in a stationary phase, i.e. in a resting metabolic condition, MEA protects only if it is present during irradiation; this may be interpreted as the expression of a physico-chemical mechanism of protection (free radical scavenging probably).

(b) It is well known that growing cells are more sensitive to ionizing radiation than non-growing ones; but, after treatment for 2 hr with MEA, whether the amine is present or not during irradiation, the radio-sensitivity of growing and non-growing cells is the same. Indeed, after a certain time of action of MEA, the logarithmically growing culture acquires the properties of a stationary culture. The synthesis of proteins stops and DNA synthesis is progressively inhibited. Mitosis is blocked.

(c) If one considers the reactions of the growing cells three stages of increasing protection may be seen: (1) Cysteamine acting for 2 hr, but removed during irradiation, (2) MEA acting only during irradiation, and (3) MEA being present before and during irradiation.*

(d) The only logical interpretation of these data assumes that two independent mechanisms are acting synergistically: (1) a physico-chemical one which operates on stationary cells, (2) a biochemical one which operates only on actively metabolizing cells.

It has taken about 20 years to understand that *as far as mammals are concerned,* the physico-chemical mechanism is of very little importance because the concentration of the protective agent (whether free or bound) reached inside the cell is always too small to be significant. Smaller (1963)

---

* The technical conditions of the experiments are such that MEA is never present after irradiation, because the medium in which the cells are suspended is diluted for plating as soon as irradiation ceases.

has shown that, in order to inhibit by 20% the EPR (electron paramagnetic resonance)* signal produced by irradiation on yeast cells, one must have 0.1% MEA (by weight) in the system. The highest concentration ever reached in the cells of mammals never exceeded 0.01%. Latarjet and his associates (1963) using aqueous solutions of thymine have shown that five to ten molecules of cystamine are needed for each thymine molecule in the solution in order to protect the base against peroxidation by irradiation. Such a ratio (one to five) of the sensitive substrate to the protective agent is unobtainable in mammals because of the toxicity of these sulfur-containing radioprotective compounds. The physico-chemical mechanisms of protection have been frequently investigated on model systems and are very interesting for the radiochemist but cannot be extrapolated to the mammalian organism without the greatest precautions (Adams, 1967; Davies *et al.*, 1968; Sanner and Pihl, 1968; Lenherr and Ormerod, 1970; Loman *et al.*, 1970; Vos *et al.*, 1970).

It is the biochemical mechanism which is of greatest importance in mammals. At present, it is difficult to spot which of the numerous actions of these substances are the really important steps for radioprotective agents. Is it the mitotic delay as proposed by Bacq and Goutier (1967)? A new mechanism of chemical protection involving cyclic AMP has been proposed by Langendorff and Langendorff (1972); so far, it has not been discussed by competent radiobiologists. Already several hypotheses may be built on the existing data which represent an important contribution both to pharmacology and radiobiology.

REFERENCES

ADAMS, G. E. (1967) The general application of pulse radiolysis to current problems in radiobiology. *Curr. Topics in Radiat. Res.* **3:** 35–94.

BACQ, Z. M. (1965) *Chemical Protection against Ionizing Radiation.* Ch. C. Thomas, Springfield, Ill., U.S.A., p. 344.

BACQ, Z. M. and ALEXANDER, P. (1964) Importance for radioprotection of the reaction of cells to sulphydryl and disulphide compounds. *Nature* **203:** 62–4.

BACQ, Z. M. and GOUTIER, R. (1967) Mechanisms of action of sulfur-containing radio-protectors, pp. 241–62. In: *Recovery and Repair Mechanisms in Radiobiology,* no. 20, Brookhaven Symposia in Biology.

DAVIES, J. V., EBERT, M. and SHALEK, R. J. (1968) The radiolysis of dilute solutions of lysozyme. II. Pulse radiolysis studies with cysteine and oxygen. *Intern. J. Radiat. Biol.* **14:** 19–27.

GINSBERG, D. M. (1966) Effects of β-mercaptoethylamine on growth and radiation sensitivity of *Escherichia coli* strain 15 tau-bar. *Radiation Res.* **28:** 708–16.

---

* Some authors prefer the term ESR (electron spin resonance).

LANGENDORFF, H. and LANGENDORFF, M. (1972) Adenosin-Nukleotide und Strahlenempfindlichkeit. *Strahlenther.* **144:** 451–6.

LATARJET, R., EKERT, B. and DEMERSEMAN, P. (1963) Peroxidation of nucleic acids by radiation. *Radiation Res.* suppl. **3:** 247–56.

LENHERR, A. D. and ORMEROD, M. G. (1970) Electron reactions in γ-irradiated thymidine and cystamine. *Nature (London)* **225:** 546–7.

LOMAN, H., VOOGT, S. and BLOK, J. (1970) Indirect radioprotection by sulfhydryl compounds: a model chemical system. *Radiation Res.* **42:** 437–45.

MODIG, H. G., EDGREN, M. and RÉVÈSZ, L. (1971) Release of thiols from cellular mixed disulfides and its possible role in radiation protection. *Intern. J. Radiat. Biol.* **22:** 257–68.

SANNER, T. and PIHL, A. (1968) Sulfhydryl groups in radiation damage. *Scand. J. Clin. Labor. Invest.* **22:** Suppl. **106:** 53–63.

SATO, F., SHIKITA, M., TERASINA, T. and AKABOSHI, S. (1970) Gradual development of radioprotection in HeLa S₃ cells during treatment with β-mercaptoethylguanidine. *Radiation Res.* **44:** 660–9.

SMALLER, B. (1963) Detection of radiation products. *Radiation Res.* suppl. **3:** 153–70.

VOS, O., GRANT, G. A. and BUDKE, L. (1970) Protection against X-irradiation employing cysteamine derivatives in tissue cultures and in mice. *Intern. J. Radiat. Biol.* **18:** 111–26.

AUTHOR INDEX

Page references in *italic figures* indicate pages on which reference lists appear

Abe, M. 2
Ackermann, D. 63, *74*
Adams, G. E. *322*
Aebi, H. 172, 173, 190, 193, *200, 202, 268, 270*
Akaboshi, S. 18, 23, *36*, 289, *300*, 320, *323*
Åkerfeldt, S. 18, 22, *32*
Albano, V. 21, *32*
Alexander, P. 1, 8, *11, 12, 126*, 215, *270, 303, 316*, 319, *322*
Allen, J. M. 99, 100, *103*
Ambrus, J. L. 314, *315*
Amoore, J. 156, *158*
Anderson, A. A. 266, *271*
Andrews, J. R. 53, *57*, 134, *135*
Arbusow, S. J. 16, *32*, 107, 108, *126*, 171, 172, 193, *200*
Arient, M. 95, *102*
Asano, M. M. 303, 308, *315*
Auerbach, C. 5, *12*
Auerswald, W. 66, *74*

Back, N. 84, *88*, 314. *315*
Bacq, Z. M. 1, 2, 4, 5, 6, 7, 8, 9, 11, *12, 13*, 15, 17, 18, 19, 21, 23, 25, 26, 27, 28, *32, 33, 36*, 41, 42, 43, 44, 45, 46, 47, 48, 49, 51, 53, *56, 57*, 60, 61, 62, 63, 64, 66, *74, 75, 76*, 77, 78, 79, 81, 84, 85, 86, 87, *88, 89*, 90, 91, 93, 94, 96, 97, 99, 100, *101, 102, 103*, 108, 109, 118, 119, 120, 121, 122, *126, 127*, 132, 134, *135*, 138, 140, *141, 142*, 143, *158*, 161, 166, 167, 169, 170, 171, 188, 189, 191, 192, 194, 195, 196, *200*, 209, 213, 214, 215, 221, 223, 227, 234, 243, 260, 264, 269, *270, 271, 272, 273*, 277, 279, 283, 295, *299*, 303, 305, 308, *316*, 319, *322*
Baddiley, J. 2, *12*
Ball, C. R. 180, 181, *200*, 310, 311, *316*

Barac, G. 51, *56*, 91, 94, *101*
Barakina, N. F. 216, 217, 219, *274*
Barnes, J. H. 84, *88*
Barnett, M. 23, *34*
Baron, C. 120, *127*
Bartley, W. 156, *158*
Basanow, V. A. 16, *32*, 171, 172, 193, *200*
Bassleer, R. 286, 290, *299*
Baugnet-Mahieu, L. 291, 292, 295, 296, *299, 300*
Baur, H. 63, *75*
Bautista, S. C. 84, *88*
Beaumariage, M. L. 18, *33, 36*, 41, 42, 45, 47, 48, 49, *56, 57*, 59, 61, 62, 63, 64, *74*, 77, 78, 84, 85, 86, 87, *88, 89*, 92, 93, 95, 96, 97, *101, 102*, 105, 109, 119, 122, *126, 127*, 132, *135*, 137, 138, 140, *141, 142*, 213, 260, 264, *271, 279*
Beccari, E. 19, *33*
van Bekkum, D. W. 1, *12*, 196, *200*, 214, 218, 220, *271, 281*
Belokonskii, I. S. 212, *271*
Benabid, Y. 244, *271*
Benedetti, L. 214, *273*
Benigno, P. 107, 108, *126*
Benson, R. E. 19, 22, 29, *33*, 60, *74*, 105, *126*
Berg, T. L. 292, *300*
van de Berg, F. 21, *36*
van de Berg, L. 21, *36*, 47, 48, ·*57*, 58, 119, *128*
Bernard, J. 96, *101*
Bernheim, F. 266, 267, *271, 281*
Betz, E. H. 210, 211, 212, 213, 214, 216, 219, 223, 228, 229, 231, 239, 240, 243, 246, 247, 249, *271, 277, 280*
Bianchi, C. 19, *33*
Bicheikina, N. I. 242, 264, *271*
Bieri, J. G. 266, *271*

Billen. D.   289, *301*
Bing, R. J.   223, *274*
Blackburn, E. W.   22, *33*
Blavier, J.   5, *12*, 19, 21, *33*
Bleiman, C.   223, 224, 227, *273*
Bloch, R. J.   27, *34*
Blok, J.   322, *323*
Boeri, E.   269, *271*
Bohrenstayn, C.   59, 68, 69, 70, *75*
Boiron, M.   303, *318*
Bombardieri, G.   *75*
Bonnichsen, R. K.   269, *271*
Booth, J.   269, *271*
Boquet, P. L.   188, *200*
Borgers, M.   145, 153, 157, *159*, 214, *275*
Børesen, H. C.   165, *201*
Bourdon, V.   94, *103*
Boyland, E.   269, *271*
Bradford, R. H.   175, 196, *200*, 295, 296, *299*
Brandt, E. L.   303, 312, *316*
Braun, H.   86, *89*, 147, *158*
Bremer, J.   156, *159*, 165, 166, *201, 203*, 222, 229, 242, 244, 245, 246, 247, 248, 249, 250, 251, *273, 280*, 295, *299*
van den Brenk, H. A. S.   226, *275*
Brimcker, H.   303, *316*
Brodie, B. B.   269, *271*
Brois, S. J.   2, 19, 20, *34*
Bronzetti, P.   93, *101*
Brousolle, B.   48, 52, 54, *57*, 106, 107, 108, 112, 119, 120, 121, 122, 125, *127*, 131, *135*
Brown, P. E.   294, 295, *299*
Brues, A.   1, *12*
Bucher, T.   223, *271, 275*
Budke, M.   284, 285, *301*, 322, *323*
Bulat, M.   64, *74*
Bulbring, E.   109, *126*
Bunge, R. P.   148, 149, 155, 157, *159*, 187, *202*
Burdon, K. L.   68, 70, *76*
Burnett, W. T. Jr.   16, 17, 18, 19, 20, 22, *33, 36*, 109, *126, 201*
de Busk, B. G.   248, *279*

Caffarati, E.   21, *33*
Calcutt, G.   180, *200*, 308, *316*
Callebaut, M.   26, *35*
van Caneghem, P.   28, *33, 36*, 41, 42, 47, 48, 49, *56*, 61, 62, 63, 64, *74*, 77, 78, 79, 80, 81, 82, 83, 84, 86, *88, 90*, 98, *103*, 119,

126, 132, *135*, 137, 138, 139, 140, *141, 142*, *271*
Cannizzaro, G.   65, *76*
Caputto, R.   266, *273*
Carey, M. M.   94, *101*
Carpentier, M. P.   266, *273*
Casier, H.   199, *202*
Cater, D. B.   216, 217, *271*
van Cauwenberge, H.   60, 68, 69, 70, 71, 72, *75, 76*, 93, 94, 95, 96, *103*, 138, *142*
Cavallini, D.   63, 65, *74*, 175, 181, 182, 183, 189, *201, 202*, 241, *272*
Cession-Fossion, A.   43, 44, 46, 51, *56, 57*, 60, 61, 62, 64, 66, *76*, 77, 78, *89*, 91, 93, *101, 103*, 108, 120, *127*, 132, *135*, 138, 140, *142*
Chance, B.   221, 226, 251, 260, *272*
Chang, C. Y.   144, *158*
Chapman, W. H.   *33*
Charlier, R.   51, *57*, 68, 72, *74, 272*
Chasseaud. L. F.   269, *271*
Chefurka, W.   238, *272*
Chenau, U. A.   266, *273*
Chèvremont, M.   143, 144, *158*, 260, *272*, 286, *299*
Chèvremont-Comhaire, S.   260, *272*, 286, 290, *299*
Chevron, F.   2
Christophersen, B. O.   265, 266, 267, *272*, *280*
Ciccarone, P.   *201*, 214, 230, 231, 242, 243, *271, 272*
Cima, L.   303, 316
Cirstea, M.   66, *74*
Cohen, G.   268, *272*
Cohen, P.   226, *272*
Colclough, N. V.   18, 19, 22, 23, *34*
Coletta, M.   *75*
Colinet-Lagneaux, D.   79, *89*
Condit, P. F.   53, *57*, 134, *135*
Congdon, C. C.   1, *13*, 144, *159*
Connors, T. A.   180, 181, *200, 201*, 303, 304, 305, 306, 307, 308, 310, 311, 312, 313, 314, 315, *316*
Contractor, S. F.   305, 309, *316*
Cooper, D. Y.   269, *273*
Cooperstein, S. J.   222, *272*
Corwin, L. M.   266, *272*
Coulon, R.   68, 72, *74*
Cousens, S.   1, *12*
Couvreur, P.   19, 23, *35*
Cronkite, E. P.   22, *33*
Crough, B. G.   22, *33*

de la Cruz, B.   84, *88*
Csagoly, E.   *300*
Cuminge, D.   155, *159*
Curzon, G.   32, *33*
Cuypers, Y.   215, 221, *271*

Dacquisto, M. P.   22, *33*
Daft, F. S.   27, *36*
Dale, W. M.   3, *12*
Dallner, G.   269, 270, *278*
Dalos, B.   *300*
Damjanovich, S.   124, *127*
Dasler, W.   27, *33*
David, G.   95, *102*, 314, *316*
Davidović, J.   93, *102*, 120, *126*
Davies, G. E.   65, 68, 72, *74*
Davies, J. V.   *322*
Davies, R.   264, *273*
Davis, E. M.   290, *301*
Davison, Cl.   94, 95, *102*, 193, *203*
Deakin, G.   295, *299*
Deanović, Z.   64, *74*
Debijadji, R.   93, *102*, 120, *126*, *128*
Dechamps, G.   5, *12*, 19, 21, *33*
Deknudt, G. H.   24, *35*
Della Bella, B.   41, *57*, 110, 111, 112, 115,
   118, 119, *126*, *127*, 269, *273*
Delrez, M.   284, 285, *299*
Deltour, G.   71, *74*, 93, 96, *101*, *103*
Demaree, G. L.   62, *75*, 76
Demerseman, P.   322, *323*
Denstedt, O. F.   268, *274*
Desaive, P.   303, *317*
Desreux, V.   305, *315*
Deysson, G.   288, *299*, 303, 304, *317*, *318*
Dickens, E. A.   *201*
Diemer, K.   221, *273*
Dienstbier, Z.   52, 53, *58*, 95, *102*
Distefano, V.   15, *33*, 42, 49, 50, 54, *57*,
   106, 107, 109, 112, 117, 119, 121, 122,
   125, *126*, 130, 132, 133, *135*
Dobrovolskii, N. M.   226, *273*
Doherty, D.   1, *12*, *13*, 16, 17, 18, 19, 20,
   22, 31, *33*, *35*, *36*, 49, *57*, 106, 107, 109,
   112, 117, 119, 121, 122, 125, *126*, *135*,
   144, *159*, 175, 196, *200*, *201*, *202*, 295,
   296, *299*
Doleschel, W.   66, *74*
Domenjoz, R.   68, 69, *76*, 93, 96, *103*
Donaldson, D. M.   71, *76*, 312, *317*
Double, J. A.   312, 313, *316*
Doudney, C. O.   16, *34*

Doull, J.   2, 19, 20, 31, *34*, *36*
Downs, W. L.   19, 22, 29, *33*, 60, *74*, 105,
   126
DuBois, K. P.   27, 31, *34*, *36*, 37, 99, *104*,
   234, 253, 254, 255, 256, 257, 258, *273*, *281*
Duchesne, P. Y.   96, 97, *102*, 122, *127*
Duncan, I. W.   268, *280*
Dunjic, A.   19, 23, *35*, 138, *142*, 303, 305,
   308, 309, *317*
Duyckaerts, C.   223, 224, 225, 227, *273*
Dyer, H. M.   15, *34*

Ebert, M.   *322*
Edgren, M.   *301*, 320, *323*
Edlbacher, S.   63, *75*
Edman, K. A. P.   66, *75*
Eker, P.   144, *158*, 286, 290, 297, *299*
Ekert, B.   322, *323*
Ekstrand, V.   268, *280*
Elčić, S.   93, *102*, 120, *126*, *128*
Eldjarn, L.   1, 2, *12*, *13*, *36*, 99, *102*, *103*,
   163, 164, 165, 166, 167, 170, 171, 172,
   188, 190, 192, 194, 199, *201*, *202*, *203*,
   214, 222, 229, 230, 233, 242, 244, 245,
   246, 247, 248, 249, 250, 251, *273*, *278*,
   280, 295, *299*, *300*
El-Khatib, S.   266, *273*
Elson, L. A.   303, 306, 308, 312, 313, *316*
Elvin, P. A.   264, *273*
Ely, J. O.   228, *279*
Emmelot, P.   214, 270, *273*, *278*, 315, *317*
Ephrati, E.   3, *13*
Erdos, E. G.   66, *75*
Ernster, L.   266, 269, 270, *275*, *278*
Ershoff, B. H.   29, *36*
Estabrook, R. W.   269, *273*
Evrard, E.   215, 221, *271*

Faredi, L.   95, *102*
Fausto, N.   296, *300*
Fedoseev, V. M.   178, *204*
Fehér, O.   124, *127*
Felder, E.   19, *33*
Fernandez, J. P.   2
Ferrone, S.   85, *89*
Filippovich, I.   88, *89*, 293, 298, *300*, *301*
Firket, H.   147, 157, *158*, 173, *201*, 214,
   273, *277*, 284, 285, *299*
Fischer, P.   5, *12*, 19, 21, *33*, 45, *57*, 93, 96,
   99, *101*, *102*, *103*, 166, 191, 196, *200*,
   201, 227, 228, *271*, *273*

Fitzpatrick, T.   137, *142*
Flemming, K.   94, *102*
Flohé, L.   268, *279*
Fluharty, A.   166, *201*
Fong, C. T. O.   263, *280*
Foris, G.   *300*
Foster, W. C.   99, *102*
Fox, M.   1, *12*
Foye, W. D.   18, *34*
Franchimont, P.   61, *75*, 93, *101*, 138, *142*
Francoeur, M.   268, *274*
Frederic, J.   260, *274*
Fredericq, H.   119, *127*
Freeman, G. L.   66, *76*
Frenk, E.   137, *142*
Fridman-Manduzio, A.   15, 30, 31, *35*, 143, 144, 153, *159*
Friedell, H. L.   215, 221, 243, *279*, 305, *318*
Froede, H. C.   232, *274*
Fromageot, P.   188, *200*
Fukuda, M.   2
Fumigalli, P.   228, *274*
Furstenberg, H.   84, *89*

Galeotti, T.   226, *274*
Ganty-Mandell, L.   86, *89*
Gantz, J. A.   31, *34*
Garbus, J.   156, *159*
Gebicki, J. M.   263, 264, 265, *274*, *275*
Geierhaas, B.   94, *102*
de Gennes, J. L.   71, *74*
Gensicke, F.   171, 189, *201*
Gerasi, G.   232, *274*
Gerzki, K.   84, *90*, 98, *103*, 227, *280*
Gilles, A.   288, *300*
Gilles, R.   227, *273*
Gillette, J. R.   269, *271*
Ginsberg, D. M.   288, 289, 296, *300*, 320, 321, *322*
Goblet, J.   68, 71, *75*
Goffart, M.   49, 54, *57*, 91, *102*, 109, 110, 111, 112, 115, 116, 117, 118, *127*, 129, 130, 131, 132, 133, 134, *135*, 139, *142*, 305, *316*
Goldenthal, E. J.   304, 305, 309, 310, *317*
Goldzieher, M. A.   94, *102*
Goldzieher, Y. W.   94, *102*
Goutier, R.   6, *12*, 15, *32*, 144, *158*, 283, 286, 287, 291, 292, 295, 296, *299*, *300*, *301*, 305, 308, *316*, *322*
Graevsky, E. Y.   298, *300*
Graham, W. D.   239, *274*

Granger, R.   2
Grant, G. A.   285, 322, *323*
Gray, L. H.   3, *12*, 215, 220, *274*
Grayevsky, E. Y.   216, 217, 219, *274*
Green, D. E.   156, *158*, 259, *280*
Gregoire, S.   167, 189, 192, 194, 195, *204*
Grenan, M.   42, *58*
Gresham, P. A.   23, *34*
Grévisse, J.   120, *127*, 129, 130, 131, 132, 133, 134, *135*
Griffin, A. C.   303, 312, *316*
Griffith, W. H.   15, *34*
Grover, P. L.   269, *274*
Gudbjarnason, S.   223, *274*
Gunsalus, I. C.   *279*
Gunter, S. E.   220, *276*

Hahn, J.   269, *279*
Hajdukovic, S.   64, 65, *76*, 96, 97, *102*, 119, 122, *127*, *128*, 269, *281*
Halász, P.   124, *127*
Hallmann, M.   259, *274*
Hanna, C.   18, 19, 22, 23, *34*
Hansell, J.   144, *158*
Harman, D.   28, *34*
Harrer, C. J.   269, *280*
Hartree, E. F.   235, 269, *275*
Harvengt, C.   84, *89*
Hasegawa, A. T.   23, 31, *34*, *35*, 46, *58*
Hassinen, I.   258, 259, *274*
von Hastrup, J.   303, *317*
Heckmann, U.   96, *102*
Heiffer, M. H.   31, *35*, 43, 50, 51, *57*, *58*, 59, 61, 62, *75*, *76*, 78, 84, 88, *89*, 92, 93, 96, 98, *102*, *103*, 105, *127*, 133, 134, *135*, 166, 190, 191, 192, *201*, *202*, 221, *274*
Heiniger, J. P.   268, *270*
Heinle, R. W.   303, *318*
Hellstrom, M.   18, 22, *32*
Hemker, H. C.   250, *274*
Henriques, O. B.   66, *76*
Henrotte, J. G.   79, 81, *89*, *90*
Heppel, L. A.   269, *274*
Herbert, F.   187, *203*
Herberts, G.   66, *75*
Hernádi, F.   289, 296, *301*, 303, 304, *317*
Hertzberg, O.   27, *35*
Herve, A.   1, 4, 5, 6, *12*, *13*, 19, 21, *33*, 143, *158*, 196, *200*
Heusghem, C.   18, *33*, *36*, 84, 85, 86, *89*, 93, *103*, 264, *279*
Hewitt, R. R.   188, *201*

Hietbrink, B. E. 31, *34*, *37*, 227, 256, 257, *273*, *275*
Highman, D. 144, *158*
Hilgertova, J. 238, *280*
Hilmoe, R. J. 269, *274*
Hoag, W. 46, *58*
Hochstein, P. 266, 268, *272*, *275*
Hodge, H. C. 19, 22, 29, *33*, 60, *74*, 105, *126*
Hodges, C. 5, *13*
Hoffsten, P. E. 264, 265, *275*
Hofmann, F. G. 94, 95, *102*
Hohorst, H. J. 223, *275*
Hollaender, A. 1, *13*, 16, *34*, 220, *275*
Holsti, L. R. 95, *102*
Honjo, I. 289, *300*
Horgan, V. J. 266, *275*
Hornberger, C. S. Jr. 248, *279*
Horvath, F. 288, *300*
Hosek, B. 208, *278*
Howland, J. W. 19, 22, 29, *33*, 60, *74*, 105, *126*
Hubener, H. J. *275*
Huber, R. 2, 17, *34*
Huff, J. W. 266, *281*
Hugon, J. 23, *35*, 143, 145, 153, 157, *159*, 178, 179, 184, 185, 186, *202*, 214, *275*, 290, *301*
Hulse, E. V. 15, 23, *34*, 127
Hulsmann, W. C. 250, *280*
Hunter, F. E. Jr. 263, 264, 265, *274*, *275*

Innes, J. R. 95, *102*
Irwin, R. L. 287, *300*
Ishizaka, K. 67, *75*
Ishizaka, T. 67, *75*
Ivanov, I. I. 21, *34*

Jackson, F. L. 222, *281*
Jackson, J. F. 290, *300*
Jackson, R. W. 27, *34*
Jacobus, D. P. 76
Jaenicke, L. 248, *275*
Jager, A. 95, *103*
Jakovlev, V. G. 21, *34*
Jamieson, D. 226, *272*, *275*
Janoff, A. 84, *89*
Jean, G. 85, *89*
Jeanjean, M. 84, *89*
Jellum, E. 293, 294, 295, *300*
Jeney, A. J. 180, *201*, 303, 304, 312, 313, 314, *316*, *317*

Jobsis, F. 226, *272*
Johnston, C. D. 198, *202*, 239, *275*
Jokay, I. 66, 68, 70, 74, *75*
Jones, M. 312, *316*
Jauany, J. M. 48, 52, 54, *57*, 99, *102*, 106, 107, 108, 112, 119, 120, 121, 122, 125, *127*, 131, *135*
Jucker, P. 63, *75*
Juliani, G. 21, *34*
Jurtshuk, P. 259, *280*

Kalkwarf, D. 1, *13*
Kari, G. 289, 296, *301*
Karpova, E. V. 67, *75*
Kaslander, J. 199, *202*
Kassay, L. 66, 68, 70, 74, *75*
Katayama, E. 287, *300*
Katzen, H. M. 269, *275*
Kawamura, F. 287, *300*
Keilin, D. 235, 269, *275*
Kelly, M. G. 308, *317*
Kessler, M. 221, *275*
Khym, J. X. 196, *202*
King, C. G. 269, *280*
Kirrman, J. M. 147, 155, *159*, 289, *300*, 304, *317*
Kiselev, P. N. 67, *75*
Kiss, A. 66, 68, 70, 74, *75*
Kitajima, T. 287, *300*
Klahn, J. 42, 50, *57*, 109, 121, *126*, 130, *135*
Klavins, J. V. 29, *34*
Kleivert, H. 96, *102*
Klemm, D. 17, *34*
Klingenberg, M. 222, 223, 251, *271*, *275*
Kneebone, G. 52, *58*
Knott, D. H. 22, *35*, 52, *57*, 105, *127*, 133, 134, *135*
Kobayashi, J. 287, *300*
Koch, G. 167, 170, *203*
Koch, R. 1, *13*, 17, 18, 19, *34*, 86, 89, 147, *158*, 233, *276*
Kochtcheenko, N. N. 88, *89*, 293, 298, *301*
Kohn, H. T. 220, *276*
Kolar, V. 21, *34*
Kolesnikov, E. E. 298, *300*
Kollmann, G. 23, *35*, 173, 174, 175, 176, 177, 194, 195, *202*, *203*, 294, *300*
Konopolanikov, A. G. 226, *276*
Konstantinova, M. H. 216, 217, 219, *274*, *281*, 298, *300*
Korn, P. S. 50, 54, *57*, 112, 117, 121, *126*, 133, 135

Kotatko, J.   52, 53, *58*
Kourilek, K.   95, *102*
Kovács, P.   289, 296, *301*
Krasnykh, I. G.   31, *37*
Krebs, H. A.   225, *281*
Kreutz, F. H.   223, *275*
Kriek, E.   315, *317*
Krstić, M.   64, *76*
Kudryashov, Y. B.   226, *276*, *280*
Kuhn, R.   99, *102*
ter Kuile, C. A.   42, 43, 45, *58*, 108, *127*
Kuna, P.   48, *57*
Kunkel, H. A.   96, *102*
Kushakovskii, M. S.   212, *276*
Kuznets, E. I.   31, *37*
Kuznetsov, V. I.   212, 245, *276*

Labeyrie, F.   233, *276*
Laborit, H.   48, 52, 54, *57*, 106, 107, 108, 112, 119, 120, 121, 122, 125, *127*, 131, *135*
La Du, B. N.   269, *271*
Lajtha, L. C.   286, *301*
Lambiet, M.   30, *35*, 143, 144, *158*, *159*, 286, 287, 292, *300*
van Lancker, J. L.   296, *300*
Landahl, H. D.   23, *34*, *35*
Lange, R.   233, *276*, *279*
Langendorff, H.   1, *13*, *142*, 166, 233, *276*, 322, *323*
Langendorff, M.   *142*, 322, *323*
Lansagen, L.   84, *88*
Lardy, Ha.   249, *276*
Laroche, Cl.   71, *74*
Latarjet, R.   3, *13*, 322, 323
Lauber, K.   172, 173, 190, 193, *200*, *202*, 268, *270*
Lazar, J.   1, *12*
Leary, D. E.   42, 49, 50, 54, *57*, 106, 107, 109, 112, 117, 119, 121, 122, *126*, 130, 132, 133, *135*
Lebihan, H.   5, *12*, 19, 21, *33*
Lecomte, J.   4, 5, *12*, 19, 21, *33*, 39, 41, 43, 44, 45, 46, 47, 48, 49, 50, 51, 53, *56*, *57*, 59, 60, 61, 62, 63, 64, 66, 68, 69, 70, 71, 72, *75*, *76*, 77, 78, *89*, 91, 93, 96, *101*, *102*, *103*, 108, 119, 120, 121, *128*, 129, 130, 132, 134, *135*, 138, 140, *142*, 220, *276*
Leddy, J. P.   66, *76*
Leffingwell, T. P.   16, 19, *35*
Legallais, V.   226, *272*
Lehninger, A. L.   88, *89*, 230, 250, 259,

260, 261, 262, 263, *276*, *278*, *279*
Leifheit, H. C.   *202*
Lelièvre, P.   147, 157, *158*, 161, 167, 168, 173, 182, *201*, *202*, 205, 210, 211, 212, 213, 214, 216, 219, 223, 228, 229, 230, 231, 232, 233, 239, 240, 241, 243, 245, 246, 247, 248, 249, *271*, *273*, *276*, 277
Lenherr, A. D.   322, *323*
Léonard, A.   23, 24, 26, 31, *35*, 144, 145, 157, *158*, *159*, 174, 178, 179, 184, 185, 186, *202*, 214, *277*, 286, 287, 290, 292, *300*, *301*
Levine, B.   303, *318*
Levy, A. H.   53, *57*, 134, *135*
Lewis, F. S.   313, *318*
Libon, J. Cl.   43, 44, *57*, 60, 61, 62, 64, 66, *76*, 77, 78, *89*, 93, *103*, 108, 120, *127*, 132, *135*, 138, 140, *142*
Liébecq, C.   205, 209, 222, 223, 224, 225, 227, 269, 270, *271*, *273*, *275*, *277*, 283, *299*
Liébecq-Hutter, S.   77, *89*, 109, *126*, 209, 213, 260, *271*
Lieberman, I.   296, *301*
Lindahl-Kiessling, K.   290, *300*
Lipmann, F.   2, *12*, 249, *278*
Little, C.   266, 267, *277*, *278*
Little, K. D.   50, *57*, 117, *126*, 132, *135*
Litwins, J.   95, *103*
Locker, A.   109, *127*, 208, 213, *277*
Loman, H.   322, *323*
Lomonos, P. I.   99, *103*
Long, D. A.   68, 70, *76*
Lorber, A.   86, *89*
Lowe, J. S.   65, 68, 72, *74*
Lowman, D. M. R.   84, *88*
Lubbers, D. W.   221, *275*, *277*, *280*
Lumper, L.   266, *277*
Lund, P.   225, *281*
Luz, A.   66, *76*
Lynen, F.   2, *12*, 248, *275*

Maisin, H.   303, *317*
Maisin, J. R.   1, *13*, 15, 19, 23, 24, 26, 27, 30, 31, *35*, 143, 144, 145, 153, 157, *158*, *159*, 161, 174, 178, 179, 184, 185, 186, 194, *202*, 214, *275*, 286, 287, 290, 291, 292, *300*, *301*, 303, 309, *317*
Makinodan, T.   1, *13*
Malamed, S.   156, *159*
Malaspina, A.   228, *274*
Maley, G. F.   249, *276*
Manson, B.   72, *76*

Mansour, T. E. 232, *274*
de Marco, C. 63, 65, *74, 75,* 175, 181, 182, 183, 189, *201, 202,* 241, *272*
Marcus, D. 71, *76*
Martin, D. 173, *203,* 290, *300*
Martini, O. 269, *279*
Maruyama, Y. 100, *103*
Masurovsky, E. B. 148, 149, 155, 157, *159,* 187, *202*
Mattelin, G. 15, 26, 30, 31, *35,* 143, 144, 153, *159*
Maxwell, G. 52, *58*
Mayer, D. 226, *274*
Maynard, E. A. 19, 22, 29, *33,* 60, *74,* 105, *126*
McDonald, T. P. 303, 308, *315*
McIlwain, H. 230, *277*
McKee, R. W. 228, *277*
Mechler, F. 124, *127*
van der Meer, C. 42, 43, 45, *58,* 108, *127,* 141, *147,* 214, 216, 217, 218, 219, *281*
Mehlman, B. 43, 51, *57, 58,* 59, 61, *76,* 78, 84, 88, *89,* 92, 93, 96, 98, *102, 103,* 166, 190, 191, 192, *201,* 221, *274*
Mekhtieva, S. M. 226, *276*
Melching, H. 1, *13*
Meldrum, N. U. 268, *277*
Melville, G. S. Jr. 16, 19, *35*
Meredith, W. J. 3, *12,* 86, *89*
Meriwether, B. P. 249, *278*
Merlevelde, E. 199, *202*
Mewissen, D. J. *271*
Meyerhof, O. 266, *277*
Meyers, W. M. 68, 70, *76*
Michaelson, S. M. 19, 22, 29, *33,* 60, *74,* 105, *126*
Michailov, M. Ch. 46, *58*
Migone, L. 84, *89*
Milani, R. 214, 230, 231, 242, *272*
Miller, M. L. 312, *317*
Mills, G. C. 268, *277, 278*
Milvy, P. 295, *301*
Misuskova, J. 208, *278*
Mitchell, H. H. 27, *35*
Mitchell, P. 252, *278*
Mitznegg, P. *142*
Mizrahi, I. J. 214, 270, *273, 278,* 315, *317*
Modig, H. G. 295, 298, *301,* 320, *323*
Mole, R. 5, *13*
Mondovi, B. 63, 65, *74,* 175, 181, 182, 183, 189, *201, 202,* 241, *272*
Mongar, J. L. 66, *75*

Moreau, R. 1, *13*
Morgan, W. 26, *35*
Morsdorf, K. 68, 69, *76,* 93, 96, *103*
Mudd, S. H. 249, *278*
Mundy, R. L. 31, *35,* 43, 50, 51, *57, 58,* 59, 61, 62, *75, 76,* 78, 84, 88, *89,* 92, 93, 96, 98, *102, 103,* 105, *127,* 133, 134, *135,* 166, 190, 191, 192, *201, 202,* 221, *274*

Naccarato, R. 214, *273*
Nadkarni, M. V. 304, 305, 309, 310, *317*
Nagy, Z. S. 289, 296, *301,* 303, 304, *317*
Nakken, K. F. 166, *201, 202*
Nekatschalowa, I. J. 16, *32,* 171, 172, 193, *200*
Nelson, A. 18, 22, 27, *32, 35,* 173, *202*
Nesbakken, R. 164, *202,* 214, 230, 242, *278*
Neubert, D. 88, *89,* 250, 261, 262, *276, 278*
Newsome, J. R. 22, *35,* 105, *127*
Neyhoff, J. A. 42, 43, 45, *58,* 108, *127*
Niaussat, P. 48, 52, 54, *57,* 106, 107, 108, 112, 119, 120, 121, 122, 125, *127,* 131, *135*
Nicholls, P. 269, *275*
Nickerson, M. 95, *102*
Nizhnik, G. V. 174, *202*
Noble, J. F. 19, *34*
Norum, K. 248, *278*
Novak, L. 205, 206, 207, 208, 209, 213, 214, *278, 279*
Novelli, G. D. 144, *159*
Novoselova, G. S. 19, 23, *36*
Nuzhdin, N. I. 174, *202*
Nygaard, O. 99, *102, 103,* 171, 172, 194, *201,* 235, 239, *278*

O'Brien, P. J. 266, 267, *277, 278*
Odell, T. T. Jr. 303, 308, *315*
O'Gara, R. W. 308, *317*
Ogston, A. G. 306, *317*
Okada, S. 297, *301*
Oliva, L. 21, *32*
Oliveira, M. C. 66, *76*
Onkelinx, C 25, *35*
Onoyama, Y. 2
Opitz, E. 221, *278*
Ord, M. G. 295, *299*
Ormerod, M. G. 322, *323*
Orrenius, S. 269, 270, *278*
Orso, G. P. 21, *34*
Ottolenghi, A. 266, *278*
Ovakimov, V. G. 178, *204*

Overman, R. R.   22, *33, 35,* 52, *57,* 105, *127,* 133, 134, *135*
Owen, J.   84, *89*

Palazzoadriano, M.   65, *76,* 107, 108, *126*
Palyga, G. F.   178, *204*
Pany, J. E.   63, *76,* 109, *127,* 208, 213, *277*
Paoletti, C.   303, *318*
Paribok, V. P.   2
Park, C. R.   249, *278*
Park, J. H.   249, *278*
van der Parren, J.   15, 30, 31, *35,* 143, 144, 153, *159*
Patalowa, W. N.   16, *32,* 171, 172, 193, *200*
Pathak, M.   137, *142*
Paton, D. W.   115, 116, 117, *127,* 132, *135*
Patt, H.   1, 4, 5, 6, *12, 13,* 21, 22, *36,* 143, *159,* 213, *279*
Pearson, G.   86, *89*
Peczenik, O.   27, *36,* 303, 313, *317*
Perry, W. L. M.   124, *127*
Pesesse, M. P.   138, *142*
Petelina, W. W.   16, *32,* 171, 172, 193, *200*
Peters, K.   144, *159*
Peters, R. A.   214, *279*
Petkovic, M. Z.   67, *76*
Pfaff, E.   251, *275*
Philpot, J. St. L.   5, *13,* 266, *275*
Picarelli, Z. P.   66, *76*
Pihl, A.   1, *36,* 144, *158,* 163, 164, 165, 166, 167, 170, 171, *203,* 233, *273, 276, 279,* 286, 290, 297, *299, 301,* 322, *323*
Piret, J.   109, *127,* 139, *142*
Pirie, A.   268, *279,* 286, *301*
Pirotte, M.   21, *33,* 93, *101,* 166, 191, *201*
Pivanova, P. S.   99, *103*
Pizzagalli, G.   93, *101*
Pliess, J.   187, *203*
Plock, H. J.   266, *277*
Plomteux, G.   18, *33, 36,* 84, 85, 86, 87, *89,* 264, *279*
Plzak, V.   2, 19, 20, 31, *34, 36*
Polikarpova, L. I.   93, *103*
Ponlot, R.   27, *33*
Porter, B. W.   266, *275*
Pospíšil, J.   52, 53, *58,* 95, *102,* 205, *279*
Pozza, F.   303, *316*
Praga, C.   85, *89*
Preston, R. L.   29, *36*
Price, C.   313, *318*
Pullman, I.   195, *301*
Purdue, J.   156, *158*

Quadbeck, G.   99, *102*

Raaflaub, J.   260, *279*
Racker, E.   269, *279*
Radivojević, D. V.   62, *74*
Rall, D. P.   308, *317*
Rall, J. E.   99, 100, *104*
Rall, T. W.   230, *279*
Ramioul, H.   96, *101*
Randall, H. P.   268, *278*
Randon, M.   2
Rasmussen, H.   263, *280*
Rausa, L.   65, *76*
Rawls, W. R.   94, *102*
Rayet, P.   5, *12,* 19, 21, *33,* 167, 169, 170, 171, 189, 192, 194, 195, *204*
Raymund, A. B.   27, 31, *34, 37,* 99, *104,* 227, 234, 253, 254, 255, 256, 257, 258, *273, 275, 281*
Razorenova, V. A.   21, *36*
Reed, L. J.   248, *279*
Rein, H.   275
Remmelts, M.   216, 219, *281*
Renson, J.   94, *103*
Repplinger, T. E.   99, *102*
Révész, L.   295, 298, *301,* 320, *323*
Reynier, M.   48, 52, 54, *57,* 106, 107, 108, 112, 120, 121, 122, 125, *127,* 131, *135*
Reyss-Brion, M.   26, *36*
Richert, D. A.   235, *279*
Riley, M. V.   263, *279*
Rinaldi, R.   244, *271*
Rixon, R. H.   95, *103*
Robaye, B.   94, *103*
Robbe, Y.   2
Robbers, H.   41, 47, 48, 49, 50, 54, *58,* 61, *76,* 77, 78, *89,* 106, 107, 108, *127,* 130, 131, *135*
Roberts, J. J.   305, *317*
Robson, J.   5, *12*
Rocha e Silva, M.   71, *76*
Romantsev, E. F.   88, *89,* 209, 242, 243, 264, 266, 267, *271, 279,* 293, 298, *300, 301*
Ronnback, C.   18, 22, 27, *32, 35*
Roodyn, D. B.   266, *275*
Root, M.   31, *36*
Rosenthal, O.   269, *273*
Rosenthal, R. L.   95, *103*
Roskam, J.   93, *103*
Ross, M. H.   228, *279*
Ross, W. C. J.   307, 308, *316, 317*
van Rossum, G.   226, *274*

Rothe, W.   42, *58*
Rotkovska, D.   208, *278*
Rousanov, A. M.   19, 23, *36*, 175, *203*
Rudinger, J.   263, *280*
Rutman, R. J.   313, *318*
Ryan, B. A.   227, *275*
Rytoemaa, T.   95, *102*

Sablayrolles, C.   2
Salerno, P. R.   215, 221, 243, *279*, 305, *318*
la Salle, M.   289, *301*
Salvador, R. A.   193, *203*
Sanadi, D. R.   166, *201*
Sanner, T.   297, *301*, 322, *323*
Sarcione, E.   84, *90*, 98, *103*, 227, *280*
Sato, F.   18, 23, *36*, 320, *323*
Savitch, A. V.   209, 243, *279*
Sawada, S.   297, *301*
Sawyer, B. C.   315, *318*
Scaife, J. F.   255, *279*
Scandurra, R.   198, *201*
Schamowa, E. K.   16, *32*, 171, 172, 193, *200*
Schauer, R.   269, *279*
Schild, H. O.   66, *75*
Schindler, F.   226, *272*
Schliep, H. J.   46, *58*
Schmidli, B.   193, *200*
Schmidt, U.   86, *89*
Schneider, A.   264, 265, *275*
Schneider, F.   268, 269, *279*
Schneider, M.   221, 260, 261, *276*, *278*
Schneider, R.   23, *34*
Schnieden, H.   32, *33*
Schoener, B.   226, *272*
Schoessler, M. A.   263, *280*
Schultze, M. O.   269, *280*
Schwartz, I. L.   263, *280*
Schwarz, E. E.   23, *35*, 174, 175, 176, 177, 194, 195, *202*, *203*
Schwarze, W.   17, 18, 19, *34*
Scott, A.   264, 265, *275*
Scott, C. A.   215, *274*
Scott, E. M.   268, *280*
Scott, J. K.   19, 22, 29, *33*, 60, *74*, 105, *126*
Scott, O.   1, *13*
van Scott, E. J.   53, *57*, 134, *135*
Sebrell, W. H.   27, *36*
Seidel, D. M.   31, *37*, 99, *104*
Seiter, I.   17, *34*
Sekusu, I.   259, *280*
Selye, H.   72, *76*, 95, *103*

Semal, M.   292, 295, 296, *299*
Semenov, L. F.   217, 219, *281*
Shalek, R. J.   *322*
Shapira, R.   17, 18, 19, 20, *33*, *36*, 175, 196, *200*, *202*, 295, 296, *299*
Shapiro, B.   23, *35*, 173, 174, 175, 176, 177, 194, 195, *201*, *202*, *203*, 290, *300*
Shapiro, I. M.   217, 219, *274*
Shapiro, O. W.   266, *281*
Shashkov, V. S.   31, *37*
Sheffield, H.   156, *159*
Sherbova, E. N.   21, *36*
Sheremetyevskaya, T. N.   298, *300*
Shigetoshi, A.   178, *203*
Shikita, M.   18, 23, *36*, 320, *323*
Shinoda, M.   18, 23, *36*
Shoemaker, W.   85, *90*
Silver, L.   263, *280*
Simić, M. M.   67, *76*
Simon, E.   144, *158*
Simons, H. A. B.   290, *301*
Sims, P.   269, *271*, *274*
Sinha, H. K.   *127*
Skrede, S.   156, *159*, 222, 246, 247, 248, 249, 250, 251, 252, 265, 266, *280*
Slater, E. C.   *280*
Slater, T. F.   250, 270, *280*, 315, *318*
Slijivić, V. S.   67, *76*
Small, D. L.   99, 100, *103*
Smaller, B.   321, *323*
Smirnova, I. B.   216, 217, *274*
Smith, D. E.   4, 5, 6, *13*, 21, 22, *36*, 143, *159*, 213, *279*
Smith, J. C.   124, *127*
Smith, P. K.   193, *203*, 304, 305, 309, 310, *317*
Smoliar, V.   173, *201*, 210, 211, 212, 213, 214, 216, 219, 223, *271*, *277*, *280*
Sochorova, M.   238, *280*
Soetens, R.   215, 221, *271*
Sokal, J.   84, *90*, 98, *103*, 227, *280*
Sonka, J.   238, *280*
Sørbo, B.   295, *301*
Spector, W. G.   93, *104*
Spence, D. L.   94, *101*
Spode, E.   2, 17, *34*, 171, 189, *201*
Stapleton, G.   1, *13*, 220, *275*
Starlinger, H.   221, *280*
Staudinger, H.   266, *277*
Steger, R.   84, *88*
Stein, F.   80, 81, 82, 86, *90*, 138, *142*
Stenger, E. G.   68, 69, *76*, 93, 96, *103*
Stepanović, S.   64, 65, *76*, 119, *128*, 269, *281*

Stetten, D. Jr. 269, *275*
Stocken, L. A. 259, *280*, 295, *299*
Stotz, E. 269, *280*
Straube, R. 1, 4, 5, 6, *13*, 21, 22, *36*, 143, *159*, 213, *279*
Strauli, U. D. 315, *318*
Strömme, J. H. 197, 198, 199, *203*, 235, 236, 237, 238, *280*
Sudduth, H. C. 259, *276*
Sugahara, T. 67, *75*
Sumarukov, G. V. 226, *280*
Sumegi, J. 297, *301*
Sümner, J. B. 235, 239, *278*
Supek, Z. 64, *74*
Suvorov, N. N. 31, *37*
Szabo, G. 137, *142*
Sztanyik, L. *300*

Takagi, Y. 18, 23, *36*
Takamori, Y. 289, *300*
Tanaka, Y. 95, *103*
Tank, L. I. 245, *276*
Tanka, D. 95, *102*
Tappell, A. L. 266, *280*
Tarasenko, A. G. 178, *204*, 298, *300*
Tarr, H. L. A. 268, *277*
Tchoe, Y.-T. 289, *300*
Tentori, L. 175, 181, 182, 183, 189, *201*, *202*
Terasina, T. 18, *36*, 320, *323*
Theismann, H. 21, *36*
Theobald, W. 68, 69, *76*, 93, 96, *103*
Therkelsen, A. J. 17, 19, 27, 31, *36*, 144, *159*, 286, *301*, 304, 306, 312, 313, *318*
Thiele, E. H. 266, *281*
Thomas, L. 84, *89*
Thomou, A. 269, *277*
Thompson, R. H. S. 259, *280*
Thors, M. B. 222, *281*
Tietze, F. 269, *275*
Tiunov, L. A. 2
Todd, R. H. 66, *76*
Trivers, G. E. 308, *317*
Troquet, J. 79, *89*
Trucco, R. E. 266, *273*
Truhaut, R. 288, *299*, 303, 304, *317*, *318*
Tsukada, K. 296, *301*
Tubiana, M. 303, *318*
Tyree, E. 4, 5, 6, *13*, 21, 22, *36*, 143, *159*, 213, *279*

Ueno, Y. 146, *159*

Ullberg, S. 173, *202*
Upton, A. 1, *13*, 303, 308, *315*
Urbach, F. 196, *203*
Urbain, M. F. 167, 169, 170, 171, 189, 192, 194, 195, *204*
Uyeki, E. 215, *279*

Vacek, A. 205, 208, 209, *278*
Valdsteyn, E. A. 2
Válentin, M. 2
Valkenburg, P. W. 42, 43, 45, *58*, 108, *127*, 216, 219, *281*
Valyi-Nagy, T. 289, *301*, 303, 304, *319*
Vandeberg, A. 245, *281*
Vandergoten, R. 292, 295, 296, *301*
Vanderlinde, R. 235, *279*
Vandermeulen, R. 46, *56*, 93, *101*
Vandersmissen, L. 68, 72, *74*
Varagić, V. 64, 65, *76*, 93, *102*, 119, 120, *126*, *128*, 269, *281*
Vasilyev, G. A. 2
Vaughan Smith, S. 23, *34*
Velick, S. F. 233, *281*
Venker, P. 171, 189, *201*
Vergroesen, A. J. 214, *281*, 284, 285, 286, *301*
Verly, W. G. 167, 169, 170, 171, 188, 189, 192, 194, 195, *203*, *204*, 213, *281*
Vittorio, P. V. 99, 100, *103*
Viviani, C. 93, *101*
Vladimirov, V. G. 183, *204*
Vliers, M. 68, 71, *75*
Vokrouhlicky, L. 48, *57*
Vollmer, E. P. 94, *101*
Voogt, S. 322, *323*
Vos, O. 214, *281*, 284, 285, *301*, 322, *323*

Waaler, P. E. 286, 290, 297, *299*
Wajda, I. 109, *126*
Wald, N. 95, *103*
Wang, R. I. H. 31, *34*, 46, *58*
Warwick, G. P. 305, *317*
Wase, A. W. 99, *102*
Wasmuth, W. 63, *74*
Weber, B. 48, 52, 54, *57*, 99, *102*, 106, 107, 108, 119, 120, 121, 122, 125, *127*, 131, *135*
Weinbach, E. 156, *159*
Weinstein, J. 264, 265, *275*
Weisberger, A. S. 303, *318*
Weiskopf, R. D. 124, *127*

Weissmann, G. 84, *89*
Wellers, G. 27, *36*
Wells, A. 29, *36*
Wels, P. 138, *142*
Westerfeld, W. W. 235, *279*
Whisson, M. E. 180, *201*, 314, *316*
White, D. 144, *158*
Wiese, J. B. 259, *276*
Wilbur, K. M. 266, *281*
Wilhelm, D. L. 72, *76*
Wilkens, H. 84, *88*
Wilkinson, A. E. 266, *281*
Williams, G. R. *272*
Williams, K. 251, 269, *271*
Williamson, D. H. 225, *281*
Williamson, J. R. 226, *272*
Willoughby, D. A. 93, *104*
Wills, E. D. 266, *281*
Wilson, S. 42, *58*
Winand-Devigne, J. 223, 224, 227, *273*
Wohler, J. R. 66, *75*

Wolff, J. 99, 100, *104*

Yam, K. M. 31, *36, 37*
Yamano, K. 146, *159*
Yarmonenko, S. P. 31, *37*, 178, *204*

Zaalberg, O. 1, *12*, 214, 220, *271, 281*
Zaim, R. H. 18, *34*
Zalkin, H. 266, *280*
Zeitounian, K. A. 217, 219, *281*
Zherebchenko, P. G. 31, *37*
Zhulanova, Z. I. 266, 267, *279*
Zins, G. R. 31, *37*, 99, *104*, 234, 253, 254, 255, 256, *281*
Zsolnai, T. 315, *318*
Zubrod, C. G. 308, *317*
Zuppinger, A. 172, 173, 190, 193, *200, 202*
Zweifach, B. 84, *89*
Zwemer, R. L. 94, *101*

SUBJECT INDEX

48/80   61, 62, 69

ABMT   3
    effects on nervous system   112, 113, 117
Abscess induction   72
ABT   50
    effects on nervous system   112, 113,
        117, 123
N-Acetoacetylcysteamine   9
Acetyl choline   7, 112, 115, 117
    nicotinic effects   115
    parasympathetic system   118
    receptors   119, 124
    synthesis   124
N-Acetylcysteamine   9
N-Acetylmethylcysteamine   9
Acid phosphatase test   153, 155
Acidosis   214
Aconitase, fluorocitrate inhibition   214
ACTH   60, 67, 68, 69, 71, 93, 95
Adenosine triphosphatase   250
Adrenal cortex   93, 314
Adrenal medulla
    action of MEG   46
    catecholamines in   43, 51, 91, 93
    effect of MEA   91, 99, 117
Adrenolytics, action of   46
AEMMT   3, 9
    cardiovascular effects   42
    effects on nervous system,   112, 113, 117,
        123
AEMT   3, 9
    effects on nervous system   112, 113, 117
AET   2, 6, 8, 9, 303
    cardiovascular effects   42, 45, 48, 49,
        51, 53
    cellular effects   143
    distribution   173, 174, 183, 184, 185
    ECG disturbances due to   52
    effect on coagulation   85

effect on corticosteroids   95
effects on nervous system   105, 106, 109,
    112, 113, 117, 119, 120, 121, 123,
    124
effects on respiration   208, 216
effects on smooth muscle   129, 130,
    131, 132, 133, 134
excretion   194
metabolic effects   234, 238, 253
metabolism   194
mode of action   54
toxicity   15, 285, 287
    LD_{50} 18, 19
transguanylation   11
Agglutination, amine release with   66
Albumin/globulin ratio   81
Alcoholic detoxication   235
Aletheine   9
Alkylating agents
    half-life   311
    toxicity   312
Allergic reaction   48, 70
Allium cepa   288
Alloxan diabetes   234
2-Aminobutylisothiuronium bromide hy-
    drobromide   see under ABMT
Aminoethane sulfinic acid   189
2,2-bis(2-Aminoethyl)-1,1′-ethylenebisisothi-
    uronium bromide dihydrobromide
    see under EbAET
S-2, Aminoethylisothiourea   see under AET
2-Aminoethyl-N′-methylisothiuronium bro-
    mide hydrobromide   see   under
    AEMT
2-Aminoethyl-N′,N″-methylisothiuronium
    bromide hydrobromide   see under
    AEMMT
2-Aminoethylthiol   see under MEA
S-2, Aminoethylthiosulfuric acid   9
p-Aminophenol   226
p-Aminopropiophenone   see under PAPP

337

3-Aminopropyl-*N*,*N*′-dimethylisothiuro-
    nium bromide hydrobromide *see
    under* APMMT
2,2-bis(3-Aminopropyl)1,1′-ethylenebisiso-
    thiuronium bromide hydrobromide
    see under EbAPT
S-2, Aminopropylisothiourea *see under*
    APT
3-Aminopropyl-*N*′-methyl-*N*″-(2-hydroxy-
    ethyl) isothiuronium bromide hydro-
    bromide *see under* APMHET
o-Aminothiophenol 10
Ammonium dithiocarbamate 10
AMPT, cardiovascular effects 42, 50
Anaphylaxis 66, 70, 73
    shock 70
Anesthesia 105, 122
    barbiturate effect of MEA 269
    effect of toxicity 31
    local 109, 122, 139
Antabuse *see under* Disulfiram
Antigen–antibody reaction 66
Antihistamines 48, 49, 51, 59, 60, 138
    anti-inflammatory action 68, 71
    used with MEG 46
Anti-inflammatory agents 67
Antioxidants 265
APMHET 3
    effects on nervous system 114, 117
APMMT 3
    effects on nervous system 114, 117
Aprotinin 48, 61
APT 2
    cardiovascular effects 42, 50
    effects on nervous system 112, 114, 117,
        121, 124
    LD$_{50}$ 20
Arthritis, kaolin-induced 72
Atropine 41, 48, 49, 50, 106, 132
Azide 6

Bacteria 7, 8, 16, 288, 289
    endotoxins 66
Bacteriophage 3
Barbiturate action 106, 107, 108, 122
Becaptan *see under* MEA
S-Benzylcysteamine 9
Bezold–Jarisch reflex 125, 126
Biochemical shock theory 8, 319
Blood 166, 167, 169, 185, 186, 190, 191,
        192, 229, 235, 236, 237, 244
    coagulation 85

composition
    cations 79
    effect of sulfur-containing radioprotec-
        tive agents 79
    enzymic 84
    hemoconcentration 79, 86
    plasma proteins 81
    pressure 72
BOL 148 64
Bone 167, 174, 177, 185, 216, 217, 218,
        219, 287, 290, 312
Bradycardia 45, 48, 51, 52, 119, 121
Bradykinin 73
    formation 65
    modification of pharmacological effects
        65
Brain 166, 169, 235, 240
British antilewisite (BAL) *see under*
        Dimercaprol
Bronchospasm 64
Busulfan 303, 305, 308, 309

Cadaverine 293
Carbohydrate metabolism (*see also under*
        Krebs cycle)
    effects of sulfur-containing radioprotec-
        tive agents 213
    gluconeogenesis 228
    glycogenolysis 227
    glycolysis 227
    pentose phosphate shunt 238, 242, 245
    regulation of 98
Carbon tetrachloride 315
Carotid occlusion 126
Cat 48, 91, 106, 110, 111, 115, 116, 117,
        118, 120, 121, 124, 125, 132
Catalase 262, 268, 269
Catecholaminemia 51
Catecholamines 7, 130, 131
    adrenergic system 119
    hypertension due to 44
    organ contents 120
    receptors 119
    release 88, 91, 93, 98, 100, 118, 132, 225
    stores 42, 43, 51
Cell cultures 283, 320
    bone-marrow 289
    Chang 286, 290
    Chinese hamster fibroblast 284, 285
    fibroblast 304
    human kidney 284, 285
    human leucocyte 290

Cell cultures—*cont.*
  L-cell cultures 286
  lymphatic 289
  survival of cells 284
Cerebral cortex 108
Chelation 10
Chemo-receptors 121
Chicken 41, 55, 62, 125, 143, 153, 260
Chlorazol blue 60, 69
Chloroform 69
Chlorpromazine 226
  effects on toxicity 31
Cocaine 116
Connective tissue, permeability 71
Corticoids, synthesis 94
Corticotropin *see under* ACTH
Croton oil 69, 73
Cyanide 6, 214
Cystamine 53, 60, 61, 294
  anti-inflammatory effect 73
  cardiovascular effects 41, 42, 43, 47, 48
  diacetyl 252
  distribution 167, 182
  effects on nervous system 105, 106, 107, 109, 117
  effects on respiration 208, 211, 212, 213, 219, 220, 239, 246
  effects on skin 137
  excretion 188
  metabolic effects 227, 246, 247, 250, 290
  metabolism 163, 164, 166, 188
  shock effects 77, 88, 141
  site of action 53
  sulfoxide 233
  tetramethyl 252
Cysteamine *see under* MEA
Cysteamine-*N*-acetic acid 9
Cysteine 3, 4, 5, 6, 7, 8, 9, 21, 28, 65, 66, 94, 124, 243, 303
  anti-inflammatory properties 68
  distribution 161, 180
  effects on nervous system 117
  effects on respiration 207, 216, 219
  excretion 161, 187
  metabolism 161, 166, 181, 187
    decarboxylation 187, 188
  toxicity 285, 289
Cystine 3, 9
Cytochrome *c* 198, 234, 235, 256, 269
Cytochrome oxidase 222, 266, 269
  affinity for oxygen 221
  inhibition by AET 254
  inhibition by GED 255

Cytochrome *P*-450 269, 270
Cytostatic drugs 313, 314

DCI 225
Decamethonium 111, 112, 123
DEDTC 3, 10, 31, 307
  effects on respiration 211
  excretion 196
  metabolic effects 234, 256
  metabolism 196
Demethylation of drugs 269, 270
Dense bodies 157
Diabetes 99
N,S-Diacetylcysteamine 9
Diamine oxidase 166, 189, 241
Diammonium-amidophosphorothioate 22
  DRF 18
Diarrhea 105
Dichloroisoproterenol *see under* DCI
Di (ethylaminoethyl) sulfide 9
N,N-Diethylcysteamine 9, 32
Diethyldithiocarbamate *see under* DEDTC
Dihydroergotamine 98
Dimercaprol 303, 307
Dimethylammonium - dimethyldithiocarbamate 31
N-Dimethylcysteamine 9
4,6-Dimethyl-2-mercaptopyrimidine 10
Dimethyl sulfoxide, cellular effects of 144
Dinitrophenol 250
Diphenhydramine 98
Disulfide 162, 233, 247, 298
  DEDTC 196
  Detoxication 192
  effects on mitochondria 261, 262
  formation 163, 167, 220, 295, 299, 308, 310, 319
  reduction 163
  5-thiopenthylamine 183
Disulfiram 196, 234, 239
  excretion 197, 198, 199
  metabolic effects 258, 259
  metabolism 197, 198, 199
Dithiopentaerythrit 10
2,3-Dithiopropanol 5, 10
Dithiothreitol 298
Dog 9, 17, 19, 21, 22, 23, 50, 54, 55, 59, 61, 84, 91, 92, 93, 105, 125, 133, 166, 170, 191
Dose reduction factor *see under* DRF
DRF 3, 7, 308
Dysplasia 137

Ear 47
E-avitaminosis 266
EbAET 3
  cardiovascular effects 42
  effects on nervous system 112, 113, 117, 123
EbAPT 3
Eczema 71
Edema
  atopic 71
  following scalding 72, 73
Edrophonium 112
EDTA, effects on respiration 212
EEG 107
Eosinopenia 95, 96
Eosinophilia 95
Ergotamine 99, 234
Ergothioneine 10
Erythrocytes *see under* Blood
Escherichia coli 288, 289, 294, 296, 321
Ethanolamine 111
Ether, effect of toxicity 31
N-Ethyl maleimide 95
Evans blue 59, 60
Eye 110, 122, 139, 134, 182, 286

933F 133
Fibroblast 143
Fluoracetate 209
Fluorescein 71
Fluoroacetylation 246
Fluorocitrate, accumulation in kidney 246
Formate 3
Formol 69
Frog 4, 41, 109, 110, 115, 119, 129
Fungistatics 315

Gallamine 112
Ganglion
  blockade 124
  dorsal root 148, 149
  parasympathetic 125
  superior cervical 115
GED 2, 23, 164, 174, 294
Glucagon 99
Glucose-6-phosphate dehydrogenase 238, 268
Glutathione 3, 4, 7, 8, 9, 22, 30, 31, 65, 66, 94, 111, 117, 124, 235, 294, 303, 314
  cellular effects 145, 233, 247, 260, 264
  distribution 161, 181

  effects on respiration 211
  excretion 161
  metabolism 161, 163, 164, 181, 268
  peroxidase 262, 268
  reduction 164, 166, 220, 229, 230, 237, 268, 314
Glutathione-homocystine transhydrogenase 269
Glycemia 84
Glyceraldehyde dehydrogenase 232, 239
Goitrogen 100
Golgi complex 149
GSH *see under* Glutathione
CSSG *see under* Glutathione
Guanethidine 125
Guanidoethyl disulfide *see under* GED
Guanylthiourea 9
Guinea-pig 47, 63, 64, 65, 66, 70, 72, 94, 107, 109, 119, 120, 125, 130, 137, 188, 266, 287

Hamster 249
Heart 41
Hematopoietic tissues 312
Hemolysin, formation 67
Hexamethonium 115, 116, 120, 131
Hexobarbital, oxidation of 269
Hexokinase 229, 234
Histamine 7
  action 214
  catabolism 63
  effects on respiration 212
  modification of pharmacodynamic properties 63
  release 69, 72, 123, 140
    after MEA administration 61, 69, 138
    after MEG administration 63
Histone *see under* Nucleoproteins
Hodgkin's disease 5
Homocysteine 10
  thiolactone 9
Hydroxylation of drugs 269, 270
5-Hydroxytryptamine *see under* Serotonin
Hyperglycemia 93, 94, 224, 227
Hypoglycemia 234
Hypoproteinemia 81
Hypotension 41, 42, 43, 45, 47, 48, 51, 53, 54, 132
Hypothalamus 91, 96

Idiosyncrasy 70
Inflammation 59, 61

Inflammatory agents 59, 70
Inosine 245
Insulin 234, 262
Intestine 45, 62, 63, 66, 95, 129, 130, 131, 132, 133, 153, 169, 171, 174, 193
  crypt cells 143, 145, 146, 150, 151, 152, 154, 184, 287, 290, 291
  villus-absorbing cells 145, 153
Iodoacetate 4
Ischemia 223
Isocysteine 147

Kallidin 65, 73
Kallikrein 65, 73
Kidney 24, 25, 31, 166, 169, 170, 172, 184, 240, 253, 256
  pyruvate dehydrogenase in 27
Kinins (*see also under* Bradykinin; Kallikrein) 65
Krebs cycle 166, 228, 247, 249, 255

Labaz 1935 62, 63, 69
Lambratene *see under* MEA
Leucocytes 74
Leukemia 96
  myeloid 195
  strain L5178Y 297
Lewis triad, production by MEA 59
Lewisite-induced lesions 5
Lipemia 84
ᴸ yldehydrogenase 248
Liver 31, 166, 169, 170, 172, 174, 182, 183, 217, 219, 240, 243, 253, 256, 286
  glycogen 96, 98, 227
Lundsgaard effect 4
Lungs 27, 62, 66, 130
Lymphoid tissue, tumors of 5
Lymphopenia 312
Lysosome 26, 153, 155, 157, 158
  effects of thiols on 88

Magnesium sulfate, effect on toxicity 31
Malate dehydrogenase 254
Mammary gland 216
Man 17, 21, 52, 59, 70, 71, 100, 134, 166, 212
MEA 2, 5, 6, 8, 9, 10, 11, 21, 53, 59, 62, 65, 94, 98, 303, 320
  administration 28
  cardiovascular effects 41, 42, 43, 44, 47, 48, 49, 51, 53

cellular effects 143
distribution 167
DRF 7, 320
effects on nervous system 105, 107, 108, 110, 117, 119, 120
effects on respiration 208, 209, 211, 212, 213, 219, 239, 247
effects on skin 137
effects on smooth muscle 129, 130, 131, 132, 133, 134
excretion 188
in inflammatory reactions 66, 73, 93
local anesthetic power 109
metabolic effects 227
metabolism 166, 188
mode of action 54
nicotinic action 91, 100, 132
shock effects 77, 86, 191
storage 16
toxicity 15, 285, 288, 297
  cellular 17
  LD_{50} 18, 19
MEG 2, 8, 23, 93, 121, 247, 255, 295
  cardiovascular effects 45
  distribution 174, 196
  effects on respiration 211, 212, 213, 219
  metabolism 196
  oxidation of 11
  toxicity 18
  vasomotor effects 46
Megakaryocyte 185, 186
Melphalan 310, 311, 313, 314
Mercaptamine *see under* MEA
1-Mercapto-7-aminoheptane 10
1-Mercapto-5-diethylaminopentane 10
Mercaptoethanol 17, 86, 162
β-Mercaptoethylamine *see under* MEA
Mercaptoethyldithiocarbamate 257
Mercaptoethylguanidine *see under* MEG
5-Mercaptomethylpyridine 147
Mercaptopropylamine *see under* MPA
3-Mercaptopropylguanidine *see under* MPG
4-Mercaptopyridoxine 17, 86, 147
5-Mercaptopyridoxine 17, 86, 147
Mercaptosuccinic acid 10
2-Mercaptothiazoline 10
Merkamine *see under* MEA
Methemoglobin 198, 237
Methionine 9
Methylamine 6
S-Methylcysteamine 9
α-Methylcystenine 10

Methylene blue 229
N-Methylphenylcysteamine 9
Methysergide 60, 61, 138
Mitochondria 145, 146, 147, 149, 153, 156, 158, 166, 221
  effects of thiols on 88
  enzymes 245
  lipid peroxidation 264
    detoxication 268
    role of thiols 266
  oxidation by 248, 249
  permeability 246, 250, 260
  protoplasts 264
  swelling 260
    effects of disulfides 262
    effects of thiols 260
Mitosis 143, 144
  activity 286
  effects of sulfur-containing radioprotective agents 283
  index 285, 286, 287
  metaphase 287
  prophase 285
Monkey 9, 22
Monoamine oxidase 65
N-Monomethylcysteamine 9
S-2 (1-Morpholyl) ethylisothiourea bromide hydrobromide 9
Motor end-plate 110, 112
Motor nerve 110, 123
Mouse 4, 5, 9, 10, 19, 20, 21, 22, 23, 27, 28, 30, 32, 42, 54, 55, 60, 62, 64, 69, 70, 93, 108, 121, 129, 137, 144, 146, 150, 151, 152, 154, 168, 169, 171, 172, 173, 180, 184, 185, 195, 205, 206, 207, 208, 213, 216, 286, 287, 290, 291
MPA 2, 10
  effects on respiration 242
  LD_{50} 19
MPG 3, 10
Mucopolysaccharides 7
Muscle
  skeletal 110
  smooth, action of sulfur-containing radioprotective agents on 129
  striped 115
Mustards 5, 162, 307, 314
  chemical reactions 305
  detoxication 305
  halogenated 306
  nitrogen (HN2) 303, 304, 306, 308, 309, 312, 314

Mydriasis 106, 129, 134

NADPH oxidase 269
Narcotics *see under* Anesthesia; Barbiturate action
Nausea 105
Nervous system
  autonomic 115, 124
  central 105, 121, 171
Neuromuscular blockade 110
Neuromuscular junction 110, 112, 123
Neurosecretion 96, 100
Nictitating membrane 106, 115, 116, 117, 132
Nitriles 6
Nitritoid crisis 53
Nitroglycerol reductase 269
Nitrosoalkylamines 315
Norepinephrine *see under* Catecholamines
Nucleic acid
  alkylation 308
  protective action 310
  structure, effects of sulfur-containing radioprotective agents on 293
  synthesis 321
    effects of sulfur-containing radioprotective agents on 289
    inhibition 298
Nucleolus 153, 158
Nucleoproteins 293, 294
  electron spin resonance studies 295

Oriza sativa 288
Ovalbumin 70
Oxidative phosphorylation 249
  chemi-osmotic theory 252
  effects of cystamine on 250
  effects of MEG 255
  effects of sulfur-containing radioprotective agents 213, 214
  uncoupling 249, 251, 259
2-Oxoglutarate dehydrogenase 247
Oxytocin 262

Pain 122
Pancreas 98, 179
Pantetheine 9
PAPP 3
Penicillamine 307
Pentachlorophenol 156

Pentamethonium 131
Pentobarbital (*see also under* Barbiturate action) 23, 31
Peristalsis 130, 131, 133
Peritoneal cavity 166
  cells 62
Peroxides 4
Phages 319
Phenothiazine 46
Phentolamine 133
N-Phenylcysteamine 9
Phosphofructokinase 231
Phrenic nerve 112
Phyto-hemagglutination 290
N-Piperidylcysteamine 9
Pisum sativum 288, 304
Pituitary
  anterior 91
  posterior 96
Polymyxine B 62
Pressor-receptors 121
Procaine 110
Promethazine (*see also under* Antihistamines) 67, 68
Prostigmine 111
Protein synthesis, effects of sulfur-containing radioprotective agents 296
Pyridoxal-5-phosphate 166
Pyruvate
  dehydrogenase 258
  metabolism 241
  utilization 254, 258

Rabbit 19, 23, 47, 60, 63, 70, 71, 81, 107, 110, 120, 125, 138, 139, 166, 174, 191, 286
Radiomimetic agents
  competitive removal hypothesis 305
  effects 293
  protection against poisoning by 303
Rat 9, 10, 19, 20, 21, 22, 24, 25, 26, 29, 43, 54, 55, 60, 61, 64, 65, 66, 69, 78, 79, 80, 82, 83, 84, 85, 86, 87, 93, 94, 98, 100, 107, 112, 120, 130, 147, 148, 166, 167, 168, 172, 180, 192, 209, 210, 211, 212, 216, 224, 228, 232, 253, 256, 286, 287, 291, 292, 309, 312, 314
Redox potential *see under* Respiration
Respiration 105, 106, 107, 122
  anoxia 3, 7, 8, 39, 51, 105, 214, 215, 216, 220, 223, 226

carbon dioxide production 207, 209
  cellular 239
  cytochromes 222
  deoxygenation 215
  effects of sulfur-containing radioprotective agents 205, 223
  hypoxia 8, 122, 212, 214, 219, 220, 228, 267
  oxygen consumption 207, 209, 211, 213
  oxygen effect 212
  oxygen tension 215, 222
    extracellular 219
    heterogeneity of 221
    measurement 226
  redox potential 221
    cellular 222
    cytoplasmic 223
    mitochondrial 225
    of bound nucleotides 226
    respiratory quotient 209
Reticular formation 122
RNA polymerase 292, 296
Rough endoplasmic reticulum 145, 153

Saccharomyces fragilis 264
Sarcolysine 303, 304, 306, 312
  therapeutic index 313
  toxicity 313
    LD$_{50}$ 308
Sciatic nerve 110
Serotonin 3, 7, 61, 138
  alterations in pharmacodynamic properties 64
  catabolism 65
  cellular effects 144
  content 140
  depressor effects 44, 46, 47
  effects on respiration 212
  release 64, 73, 123
  toxicity 29
Shock 77, 87
  cardiovascular collapse 77
  enzyme liberation produced by 84
Shwartzman phenomenon 70, 73
Sialic acid 81
Skin 61, 71, 95, 190, 193
  blood vessels 138
  dehydrogenase 138
  effects of cystamine on 137
  effects of MEA on 137
  irritants 69, 138
  oxygen tension 141

Skin—*cont.*
  pigmentation 137
  pilous system 140
    hair growth 137
  temperature 139
  tuberculin, reaction to 70
Sodium mercaptoethane sulfonate 86
Sodium tellurite 138
Spermatogenesis
  effect of phenylalanine on 28
  effect of sulfur-containing radioprotective
    agents 30, 31
Spermatogonia 145
Spermatozoa 174
Splanchnic nerve stimulation 118
Spleen 27, 133, 147, 167, 172, 174, 177,
  180, 182, 183, 184, 216, 217, 218, 219,
  291
Starling's heart–lung preparation 50
Streptomycin 71, 166
Succinate dehydrogenase
  inhibition by AET 254
  inhibition by GED 254
Sulfanilamide, acetylation of 245
Sulfhydryl compounds, toxicity 17
Sulfur 3
Sulfur-containing radioprotective agents
  analysis
    autoradiography 173, 178, 183
    biochemical techniques 167
    chemical techniques 175, 181
  cardiovascular effects 39, 41
  cellular effects
    electron microscope studies 143, 145
    optical microscope studies 144
  effects on embryos 25
  excretion of detoxication products 309
  history 3
  metabolism 6
  nomenclature 1
  pharmacology 39
  toxicity 8, 15
  of mixtures 30, 32
Supraoptic nucleus 97
Sympathetic nervous system 93
Sympathomimetic amines *see under* Catecholamines

Tachyphylaxis 61, 62, 116
Taurine, excretion 188
Teeth 187
Temperature regulation 109
  hypothermia 213, 224

Tenesmus 106
Testis 167, 179, 182
Tetraethylammonium 115
N,N'-Tetramethylcystamine 9, 230
Tetrathionate 10, 233
Thioacetamide 10
Thiobarbituric acid test 164
Thioctic acid 166
Thiocyanate 10
Thioglycollic acid 3, 10, 162
1(−)-2-Thiolhistidine 10
Thiols 8, 308
  alkylation of 162
  detoxication of 162
  energy transfer agents 167
  oxidation of 162, 285
  protective action 165
  reactivity 162
  toxicity of 284
Thiourea 3, 5, 10, 99, 303
Thrombocytes, agglutination 66
Thymidine-cytosine deoxyribosyl trans-
  ferase 298
Thymidine kinase 292, 296, 298
Thymus 95, 287, 291, 297
Thyreostimulin 100
Thyroid 99, 171
Thyroxine 260, 261
α-Tocopherol 264, 265, 266
Tolazoline 133
Tortoise 41, 118, 125
Trasylol 138
Tretamine 305
Trihydroxyethylrutosid 138
Trypan blue 60
Tryptophan 3
d-Tubocurarine 110, 112, 115, 123
Tumors (*see also under* Leukemia) 181, 315
  ascites 287, 295
  DNA 312
  Ehrlich ascites 173, 298
  mammary 195
  plasma cell 180, 313
  Walker carcinoma 313
  Yoshida hepatoma ascite 230, 242
  Yoshida sarcoma 180, 310, 313

Ubiquinone factor 259
Urine 170, 190, 191, 194
Uterus 130, 131, 133

Vacuoles, autophagic 155

Vagotomy 45, 50, 52
Vascular permeability 59, 73
  tests for changes in 69
Vasopressin 262
  receptor combination 263

X-rays
  peroxidation effects 266
  protection from 3, 211, 315, 319
    with cysteine 4
    with MEA 5, 25, 28, 155, 290